Perspectives in Medical Geography

I0883938

Medical geography is a fascinating area of rapidly evolving study that aims to analyse and improve worldwide health issues based on the geographical factors which have an impact on them. *Perspectives in Medical Geography* will appeal to both novice and seasoned researchers looking to be informed on the latest theories and applications in the field. Chapters represent a wide range of industries, ranging from private/public universities to private companies to non-profit foundations. Contributors describe ways in which map and geography librarians can engage in public health research – creating data standards, archiving map collections and providing mapping/GIS services. In addition to compiling current theories and practices related to medical geography, this volume also features commentaries from two pre-eminent geography librarians, sharing their perspectives on this emerging field and how map and geographic information librarians can engage in health-related research through their profession.

This book was originally published as two special issues of the *Journal of Map & Geography Libraries*.

Amy J. Blatt earned her Bachelor of Science degree in Biological Sciences from Stanford University, USA; Master of Science degree in Biology from the University of Houston, USA; and Ph.D. degree in Geography from the University of Cincinnati, USA. She is certified by the GIS Certification Institute as a Geographic Information Systems Professional (GISP).

Perspectives in Medical Geography

Theory and Applications for Librarians

Edited by
Amy J. Blatt

Routledge
Taylor & Francis Group
LONDON AND NEW YORK

First published 2012
by Routledge

2 Park Square, Milton Park, Abingdon, Oxfordshire OX14 4RN
711 Third Avenue, New York, NY 10017

Routledge is an imprint of the Taylor & Francis Group, an informa business

First issued in paperback 2017

This book is a reproduction of the *Journal of Map & Geography Libraries*, volume 7, issues 1 and 3. The Publisher requests to those authors who may be citing this book to state, also, the bibliographical details of the special issue on which the book was based.

British Library Cataloguing in Publication Data
A catalogue record for this book is available from the British Library

ISBN 13: 978-0-415-69782-8 (hbk)
ISBN 13: 978-1-138-06141-5 (pbk)

Typeset in Baskerville
by Taylor & Francis Books

Publisher's Note
The publisher would like to make readers aware that the chapters in this book may be referred to as articles as they are identical to the articles published in the special issue. The publisher accepts responsibility for any inconsistencies that may have arisen in the course of preparing this volume for print.

Contents

Notes on Contributors

Paige G. Andrew is the Maps Cataloging Librarian and a member of the Maps Cataloging Team, Cataloging and Metadata Services Department, at Pennsylvania State University, USA. He received a Bachelor of Arts degree in Geography from the Western Washington University, USA, and a Master of Library Science degree from the University of Washington, USA. Mr. Andrew received the 2009 Nancy B. Olson Honors Award for outstanding service to the Online Audiovisual Catalogers and the Librarianship profession.

Andrew Bazemore is the Medical Director for Policy Research at the Robert Graham Center for Policy Studies in Family Medicine and Primary Care in Washington, DC, USA. He received his Bachelor of Arts degree from Davidson College, USA; his medical degree from the University of North Carolina, USA; and his Masters of Public Health degree from Harvard University, USA. He also completed residency training and a faculty development fellowship at the University of Cincinnati, USA.

Amy J. Blatt earned her Bachelor of Science degree in Biological Sciences from Stanford University, USA; Master of Science degree in Biology from the University of Houston, USA; and Ph.D. degree in Geography from the University of Cincinnati, USA. She is certified by the GIS Certification Institute as a Geographic Information Systems Professional (GISP).

Jeff Blossom earned a Bachelor of Science degree in Environmental Science from Willamette University, USA; and a Master of Arts degree in Geography from the University of Denver, USA. He is currently employed as a Senior GIS Specialist at the Center for Geographic Analysis, Harvard University, USA. Jeff also teaches the class "Geographic Communication Today" at the Harvard Extension School.

James Boxall is the Director of the GISciences Centre at Dalhousie University in Halifax, Nova Scotia, Canada. He is Adjunct Professor and Lecturer in the Faculties of Architecture and Planning; Management; and Science at Dalhousie. He is a Fellow of the Royal Geographical Society and has been elected to the College of Fellows for the Royal Canadian Geographical Society.

Bonnie Burns has worked at Harvard University, USA, for 11 years, and is currently the Librarian for Geographic Information Services. Prior to Harvard, Bonnie was a GIS Specialist for the National Parks Service (USA), and attended the University of Massachusetts at Amherst, Massachusetts, USA.

Sarah Cordivano earned her Bachelor of Arts degree in Geography and Urban Studies from Temple University, USA and her Masters degree in Urban Spatial Analytics from the University of Pennsylvania, USA. She is a GIS analyst and researcher in Philadelphia, Pennsylvania, USA.

Ellen K. Cromley earned her Bachelor of Arts degree in Urban and Environmental Studies from Case Western Reserve University, USA; Master of Arts degree in Geography from The Ohio State University, USA; and Ph.D. degree in Geography from the University of Kentucky, USA. She co-authored with Sara McLafferty *GIS and Public Health*, now in its second edition.

Julia L. Finkelstein received her Bachelor of Science degree from McGill University, Canada; Masters of Public Health degree from Brown University, USA; and Master of Science and Doctor of Science degrees in Nutrition and Epidemiology from the Harvard School of Public Health, USA. Julia is co-PI of IndiaMap and contributes to the AfricaMap and WorldMap projects at the Center for Geographic Analysis, Harvard University. Julia is currently a faculty member in the Division of Nutritional Sciences, College of Human Ecology, at Cornell University, and a Fellow at the Center for Geographic Analysis at Harvard University.

Jane Garb is an Epidemiologist at Baystate Health and Research Assistant Professor at Tufts University School of Medicine, USA. She holds a Masters of Public Health degree in Epidemiology, a Certificate in Geographic Information Systems, and is a certified Geographic Information Systems Professional (GISP). She has published over 100 papers, book chapters, and a book entitled *Understanding Medical Research: A Clinician's Guide.*

Weihe Wendy Guan is the Director of GIS Research Services at the Center for Geographic Analysis, Harvard University, USA, since the Center's establishment in 2006. Wendy has a Ph.D. in Ecology and GIS; a Master of Arts degree and a Master of Science degree in Geography and Resource Management, and a Bachelor of Science degree in Biology. She taught GIS in various universities, including the Harvard Extension School.

Seiji Hayashi is the Chief Medical Officer for the Bureau of Primary Health Care at the Health Resources and Services Administration, USA. Dr. Hayashi received his Bachelor of Arts degree in Studio Art from Vassar College, USA, and his medical degree from the Albert Einstein College of Medicine, USA. He completed the Family and Community Medicine Residency Program at the University of California, San Francisco, USA, and received his Masters of Public Health degree from the Harvard School of Public Health (USA) as a Fellow with the Commonwealth Fund/Harvard University Fellowship in Minority Health Policy.

Ezekiel Kalipeni is a Professor in the Department of Geography at the University of Illinois at Urbana Champaign, USA. His research interests focus on demographic, health, environmental, and resource issues in sub-Saharan Africa. He has authored or co-edited 11 books, among them *HIV/AIDS in Africa: Beyond Epidemiology* (Blackwell Publishing, 2004) and *Strong Women, Dangerous Times: Gender and HIV/AIDS in Africa* (Nova Science Publishers, 2009).

Shaun Langley received his Bachelor of Science degree in Wildlife Ecology from the University of Wisconsin–Madison, USA; Master of Science degree in Entomology from Michigan State University, USA. He is working towards his Ph.D. in Geography at Michigan State University, USA, with a focus on Volunteered GIS.

Jessica McIntyre is an Assistant Clinical Professor in the Department of Family Medicine at Loyola Stritch School of Medicine and serves as faculty for the Loyola-Cook County-Provident Family Medicine Residency program in Chicago, Illinois, USA. Dr. McIntyre received her Bachelor of Arts degree in Anthropology from the University of Notre Dame, USA, and her medical degree from Loyola University Chicago-Stritch School of Medicine, USA. She completed her family medicine residency through Georgetown University-Provident Hospital in Washington, DC, USA, and a Fellowship in Faculty development through Cook County, Illinois, USA.

Joseph P. Messina is an Associate Professor of Geography with the Department of Geography, the Center for Global Change and Earth Observations, and AgBioResearch at Michigan State University, USA. He received his Ph.D. in Geography from the University of North Carolina at Chapel Hill, USA.

Thomas J. Miyoshi is an analyst at the Arkansas Center for Health Improvement in Little Rock, Arkansas, USA. He has been on the faculties at Denver University (USA), the University of Colorado Health Sciences Center (USA), the University of Rochester (USA) and New York University (USA). He is certified by the GIS Certification Institute as a Geographic Information Systems Professional (GISP).

Imelda Moise is a Ph.D. candidate in the Department of Geography at the University of Illinois at Urbana-Champaign, USA. She received her Master of Science degree in Geography (Health Geography concentration) from the same institution and her Bachelor of Arts degree in Environmental Studies and Geography (double major) from the University of Oregon, USA.

John Olson earned a Bachelor of Science degree in Geography from Lock Haven University of Pennsylvania, USA; a Bachelor of Arts degree in Geology from Mercyhurst College, USA; and an MILS degree in Information and Library Studies from the University of Michigan, USA. He is currently the Maps/GIS, Geography, Earth Sciences and Government Documents Librarian at Syracuse University, USA.

Robert L. Phillips is Director of the Robert Graham Center in Washington, DC, USA. He earned a Bachelor of Science degree in Biological Sciences from the Missouri University for Science and Technology, USA; a medical degree from the University of Florida, USA; and a Masters of Science in Public Health from the University of Missouri, USA. He is a member of the National Academy of Sciences' Institute of Medicine.

Grace Ting serves as Health Services Director, Clinical Health Policy at WellPoint, Inc., overseeing the corporate agenda to address health disparities and increase the organization's capacity to offer culturally and linguistically appropriate services to members. She is responsible for developing pilot initiatives and training programs for providers, communities-at-large, and WellPoint associates. Grace received her Bachelor of Science degree in Biology from the University of California, Los Angeles, USA; and her Master of Health Administration degree from the University of Southern California, USA.

Zachary Vernon currently serves as a Senior Health Information Consultant in Wellpoint's Health Equity, Cultural and Linguistics Program Office. His primary role is to provide analytic support for WellPoint's work to address health disparities. Zachary received his Bachelor of Arts degree in Economics from the University of the South, USA.

Richard Wait is currently Chief of Surgery at Baystate Medical Center in Springfield, and Professor of Surgery at Tuft's University School of Medicine in Boston. A strong advocate for new technologies in medical education, Dr. Wait helped establish the GIS program at Baystate. A member of numerous medical and scientific societies, he has authored more than 70 articles in scientific journals, and serves as editorial reviewer for several.

Katherine H. Weimer is Associate Professor, Curator of Maps at the Texas A&M University Libraries, College Station, Texas, USA. In addition to being a recipient of the 2008 Distinguished Achievement Award for Librarianship from Texas A&M University, USA, she is past chair of the American Library Association's Map and Geography Round Table, and curator/project lead on the digital version of the *Geologic Atlas of the United States*. She holds a Bachelor of Science degree from Texas A&M University, USA, and a Master of Library and Information Science degree from Louisiana State University, USA.

Leo C. Zulu is an Assistant Professor in the Department of Geography at Michigan State University. He obtained his Bachelor of Science degree in Ecological Sciences at the University of Edinburgh, Scotland; Master of Arts degree in GIS and International Development at Clark University, Massachusetts, USA; and Ph.D. degree in Human Geography at the University of Illinois at Urbana-Champaign, Illinois, USA. He conducts research on geospatial applications in medical geography, land use and land cover change, and nature-society interactions, focusing on environmental governance and development in Africa.

Editor's Acknowledgements

I would like to gratefully acknowledge the many people who have supported me throughout the development of this book. I would like to thank Paige Andrew (Pennsylvania State University) and Kathy Weimer (Texas A&M University) for their continued support and mentorship during this entire process. I have been very fortunate to work with two of the most interesting and collegial geography librarians on earth. I am also grateful to Mary Larsgaard (University of California, Santa Barbara), whose enthusiastic support helped launch this project in the beginning.

I would like to express my sincerest gratitude to the wonderful, patient, and cheerful editorial staff at Taylor & Francis/Routledge. Emily Ross has been a godsend in helping make this book possible. Stacy Stanislaw, Beth Schad, and John Nosal have also been invaluable in the publication of the *Journal of Map & Geography Libraries*, on many levels. In addition, I would like to thank the editorial board members of the *Journal of Map & Geography Libraries* for their diligent and thoughtful review of the manuscripts that comprise this special collection.

I would like to thank the geographers who contributed to this volume. Their professional biographies can be found within these pages, but more interestingly, their high-quality research and development of the field of medical geography are showcased here. As this volume first took form three years ago, I have been very impressed and humbled by the breadth and depth of the public health and medical geographic research which have informed health care policies and practitioners alike. I am proud to have worked with this select group of researchers, from the academic, business, and non-profit arenas.

I am indebted to Dr. Susanna Tong, who has been, and continues to be, a role model to me in many different ways.

Finally, my family has been the bedrock and foundation of my academic and intellectual pursuits. My husband Gary – an accountant by training and a geographer at heart – is a true reflection of everything I love about this world. My parents, Shiow-Ling Yeh Liu and Henry Kun-Ling Liu, established the solid foundation and support of my love of learning during my formidable years. Lastly, my brother, Jerry, continues to provide the "comic relief" that is so necessary in all of life's endeavors.

Chapter Acknowledgements

Chapter 2: *The Role of the Map and Geographic Information Library in Medical Geographic Research* (Ellen K. Cromley)

Patrick McGlamery, Michael Howser, Bill Miller, and Jeffrey Dunn of the Map and Geographic Information Center, Homer Babbidge Library, and University of Connecticut are acknowledged for their assistance in accessing resources in the collection.

Chapter 3: *Enabling Geographic Research Across Disciplines: Building an Institutional Infrastructure for Geographic Analysis at Harvard University* (Weihe Wendy Guan, Bonnie Burns, Julia L. Finkelstein and Jeffrey C. Blossom)

The authors wish to thank HMC and CGA colleagues for their input and support to the work represented in this manuscript, especially those from Professor Peter Bol, the Charles H. Carswell Professor of East Asian Languages and Civilizations and director of the CGA.

Chapter 4: *Transforming Community Health and Primary Care Education Using Clinical and Administrative Data and Geographic Information Systems* (Arthur Seiji Hayashi, Andrew Bazemore and Jessica McIntyre)

The authors would like to thank the following people for their contributions to the original research activity: Eleina Preston, Ranit Mishori, Ernest Brown, Jeff Weinfeld, and Guy White.

Chapter 5: *Harnessing Geographic Information Systems (GIS) to Enable Community-Oriented Primary Care* (Andrew Bazemore, Robert L. Phillips and Thomas Miyoshi)

This article is being reprinted with permission from the *Journal of the American Board of Family Medicine*. It is available at http://www.jabfm.org/cgi/content/full/23/1/22. This article was externally peer reviewed.

Chapter 6: *Embracing the Open-Source Movement for Managing Spatial Data: A Case Study of African Trypanosomiasis in Kenya* (Shaun A. Langley and Joseph P. Messina)

This research was supported by The National Institutes of Health, Office of the Director, Roadmap Initiative, and NIGMS: Award RGM084704A.

Foreword

It is with great zeal that we introduce *Perspectives in Medical Geography*. This collection had its beginnings in 2008, when first considered as a possible theme issue of the *Journal of Map & Geography Libraries*. The topic was a brainchild of current and former JMGL co-editors Paige Andrew and Mary Larsgaard, and guest editor, Amy Blatt. In response to the increasing national interest about health care and medical research, the editors sought to bring awareness about the subject's emerging sub-specialty that integrates geographic information systems (GIS), and decided to devote both issues 7(1) and 7(3) of JMGL to the topic. Dr. Blatt proceeded to gather an excellent panel of authors with wide-ranging backgrounds and interests to share their experiences and thoughts on this considerable topic.

The use of GIS for health care and medical research is a relatively young specialty; however, as the sub-specialty has expanded, and continues to further expand, the spatial data needs of the researchers will become more demanding. Librarians and information professionals should be cognizant of these researchers' data requirements and their role in spatial data management, and be prepared to respond. A joint workshop held during February 2011 between the U.S. National Institutes of Health and the Association of American Geographers, and a related initiative called the "AAG Initiative for an NIH-Wide GIS Infrastructure," speaks to the large-scale attempts at building geospatial infrastructures for the medical research community.

What is presented in this volume is a wide-ranging collection that speaks broadly to the importance of geographic information in health and medical research by providing specific research applications using GIS, as well as the role of the librarian or information professional in the management and delivery of the spatial data. Taken as a whole, the content between the covers of this book are diverse yet interrelated, important, and especially meaningful. We fully expect that others will use the outcomes and challenges provided within to further expand the areas of medical, public health, health care delivery, and even software applications research to the greater benefit of individuals worldwide.

In the concluding remarks to her introductory chapter, Dr. Blatt asks: "Can geography libraries act as enablers in the distribution of resources to the nontraditional and nonacademic audiences of health care practitioners and service providers?" We think the answer is obvious, and, thanks to her engaging leadership, inquisitive mind, and many months of hard work and dedication to this project, we feel confident that you will agree that the theme of *Perspectives in Medical Geography* has been met with success in these pages.

Paige Andrew and Katherine H. Weimer
Co-Editors, *Journal of Map & Geography Libraries*

Maps, Geography Libraries, and Health Outcomes: Gazing into the Future of Medical Geography

AMY J. BLATT
Quest Diagnostics, West Norriton, Pennsyslvania, USA

This article introduces issues and concepts related to current opportunities in medical geography. The opportunities described herein pertain to not only the academic geographer, but also to the nonacademic researcher wishing to utilize geographic insights. These opportunities lend themselves to map and geography reference librarians who oversee the databases and archives that support these research endeavors. As these special theme issues on "Geographic Opportunities in Medicine" will reveal, map and geography libraries can act as "enablers" to distribute geographic databases and resources to a wider, nontraditional and nonacademic audience of health care delivery and service providers.

INTRODUCTION

According to Meade and Earickson (2000), "the development of medical geography has been part of a response to inadequate theory, methodology, and understanding of health and disease in our society." Although the perspective of medical geography can be traced back to Hippocrates (ca. 400 BC) in his treatise "On Airs, Waters, and Places," this article focuses on its renewal as a specialization of the discipline of geography. Modern medical geography has an illustrious and distinguished history, both among medical practitioners (such as Dr. John Snow, a founding father of epidemiology, and Dr. Jacques May, father of modern medical geography) and social scientists. However, the goal here is not to review the history of medical geography—others have provided excellent reviews and compilations (May 1950; Banks 1959; Armstrong 1965; Paul 1985; Meade and Earickson 2000; Gessler 2003)—but to highlight a series of issues that have extended the access and reach of medical geography to the nonacademic geographer. It also serves as an introduction to this special theme volume in the *Journal of Map and Geography Libraries* on "Geographic Opportunities in Medicine."

"Geographic Opportunities in Medicine" describes the content of this special theme volume well because its articles highlight ways in which both the academic and nonacademic geographer can utilize geographic insights to improve the quality of health care services and delivery to patients. It is our collective belief that the exciting future of medical geography will most likely be populated with health care providers and social scientists using geographic data and tools to enhance direct patient care.

Following this introduction will be a review of two major research questions of medical geography (adapted from Amedeo and Golledge 1975) and how geography libraries can respond to them. In addition, I will discuss how academic map and geography libraries can act as "enablers" to distribute geographic databases and resources to a wider, nontraditional and nonacademic audience of health care delivery and service providers. As map and geography library resources become more widely adopted and accessible, they will play a more important role in enabling a broader array of health care providers to use geographic data and tools to improve the quality of care and services available to patients. Hence, the articles in this theme volume point more to current trends and opportunities for involvement of the medical geographic community and less to the librarian performing actual medical geography.

A REVIEW OF TWO MAJOR RESEARCH QUESTIONS IN MEDICAL GEOGRAPHY

In 1975, Amedeo and Golledge formulated six major research questions for the discipline of geography.

1. Why is a phenomenon distributed in a particular way?
2. Why are facilities and businesses located where they are?
3. Why do people move in certain directions for certain distances?
4. Why do innovations spread as they do?
5. Why do people vary in their perception of the environment?
6. How do objects, ideas, processes, and living beings interact to characterize and constitute places?

Although these six questions were originally used to describe the discipline of geography, they can also be applied to research in medical geography (Meade and Earickson 2000), where they may be stated as:

1. Why does the prevalence or incidence of a disease or medical condition vary throughout the world?
2. Why are health care facilities located where they are?
3. Why do people move in certain directions for certain distances to obtain health care services?
4. Why do medical innovations (such as new medical devices and diagnostic tests) spread as they do?
5. Why do some people vary in their perception of the effects of a certain disease or medical condition?
6. How will regional and community-based health care facilities meet the needs of a more diverse population in the future?

Of these, the first two questions are the most often addressed in medical geographic research by nonacademic geographers and geography librarians (as will be demonstrated by the contributors in this volume). For this reason, I will explore the implications of these two questions and also describe how geography librarians can respond to them.

In terms of medical geography, the first question can be further divided into two subquestions: How are diseases and medical conditions distributed throughout the world? and Why is there such great variation in the incidence and prevalence of a disease or medical condition from place to place? To address the first subquestion, we need only look at the myriad of atlas and map compilations that have been produced concerning the distribution and incidence of disease (Brewer 2006; Brewer and Pickle 2002). Examples include Cliff and Haggett's (1988) *Atlas of Disease Distributions*; Shannon and Pyle's (1993) medical atlas of the 20th century; and the *Dartmouth Atlas of Health Care* (Wennberg et al. 2008). The answers to the first subquestion naturally lend themselves to the second subquestion concerning the spatial variations in the incidence of disease. Researchers from both academia and industry have long used multivariate statistical analyses, along with geodemographic and socioeconomic data, to derive models to explain distributions.

For instance, at Quest Diagnostics, a series of HealthTrends reports have been developed to identify and track disease trends and wellness benchmarks. These reports use the nation's largest databases of laboratory test results to help educate patients, health professionals, and policy-makers about the current status of the nation's health and to help them make decisions using this multidimensional data source (Quest Diagnostics 2010). In the area of cardiovascular health, for example, Quest Diagnostics conducted a retrospective study of nearly 80 million low-density lipoprotein (LDL) cholesterol tests performed by its laboratories across the United States from 2001 through 2004. These tests had been ordered on behalf of U.S. adults 20 years of age and older under a physician's care. The study found a significant and steady decline in average LDL cholesterol levels of approximately 10 percent

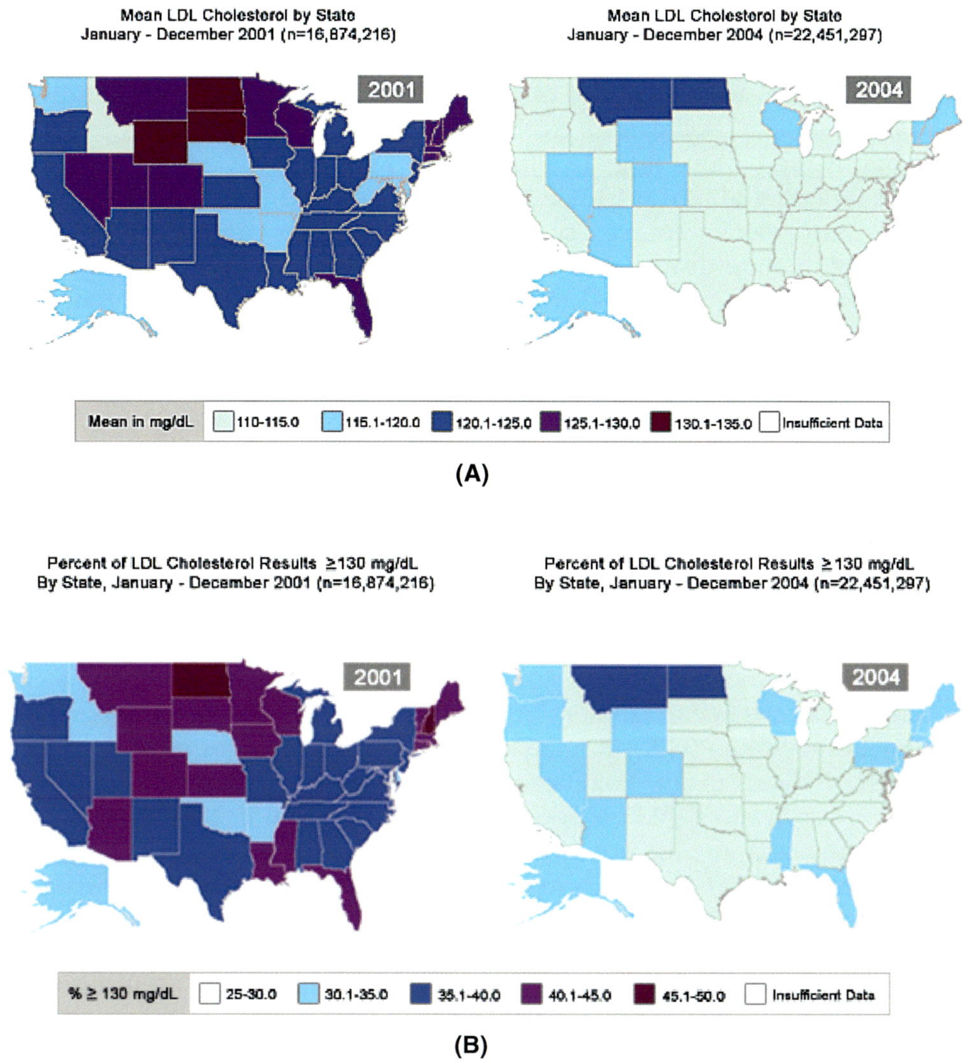

FIGURE 1A AND 1B Results from a Quest Diagnostics HealthTrends report, which indicates a steady decline in low-density lipoprotein (LDL) cholesterol levels throughout the United States. (Source of Figure 1A: http://www.questdiagnostics.com/brand/business/healthtrends/hearthealth/bystate.html, accessed September 22, 2010; Source of Figure 1B: http://www.questdiagnostics.com/brand/business/healthtrends/hearthealth/percentabove130.html, accessed September 22, 2010).

over the four-year period throughout most of the United States (Figures 1A and 1B). There is speculation that this decline is due to the proliferation of cholesterol-lowering medications in the U.S. marketplace.

In "Geographic Opportunities in Medicine," both Vernon and Ting (2011) and Garb and Wait (2011) use advanced statistical analyses to address the issues of spatial variation in the medical population. Some questions concerning spatial variation are best answered using interviews and field surveys to make connections between cultural and demographic patterns and disease prevalence (Senior et al. 1993). Other health patterns and disease transmission rates can be explained by examining vegetation patterns, topography, and climatology (Kalkstein and Davis 1989; Cutter and Solecki 1989; Kalipeni et al. 2011; Langley and Messina 2011). Map and geography libraries are obvious sources of information for these types of questions because of the interdisciplinary nature of the investigations. Geography reference librarians can respond to this question by facilitating collaborative exchanges of material between the social sciences collections, physical sciences collections, and computer sciences collections, as well as any others needing to be consulted. As mapping software systems proliferate across college campuses, it becomes imperative for the map librarian to conduct significant and meaningful outreach seminars to educate people on their resources, archives, and repositories of geospatial data. Place and space have become important factors in research outside the discipline, and geography reference libraries that welcome interdisciplinary collaborations will see their investments multiply.

The second question, Why are health care facilities located where they are? transforms medical geography from a purely academic discipline to an applied social science. Bazemore et al. (2011) explore the use of geographic information systems (GIS) in analyzing the service areas of a primary care network of clinics in the Baltimore, Maryland, area. In Philadelphia, Pennsylvania, Cordivano (2011) reports that approximately 23,000 women give birth in the city annually; however, thirteen labor and delivery-care units in the city have ceased operation in the past decade. She uses GIS to analyze the impact of these closures, and makes recommendations for the opening of new facilities in the area.

Health care facilities need to be located in areas that optimize their operational efficiencies and revenues (Cromley and Albertsen 1993; Albert and Gessler 1997; Peters and Hall 1999). Albert and Gessler address the health care policy implications of multiple locations of medical practice. They conclude that future research on physician access and availability must consider a physician's work time at secondary and other locations in the measurement of physician-to-population ratios and that the mere location of physicians within an area is an insufficient indicator of access. This study made extensive use of maps and geographical insight. Locations of health and medical facilities should be a staple in libraries that are concerned with local and community health issues. Although the data themselves may not be physically stored in the reference library, the reference librarian should be able to assist the community researcher or planner in obtaining the necessary data. For this reason, reference librarians must foster relationships with local health and medical organizations so that public-access information is easily available for medical geographical research.

MAP AND GEOGRAPHY LIBRARIES AS ENABLERS

Map and geography libraries have traditionally been the source of information for geographic research (University of South Maine: Theunissen 2007; Saint Anselm College: Walsh 2004; Library of Congress: Mangan 2007). With the advent of the Internet, most data and information storage occurs electronically (Croner 2004; Olson 2004b). Geography libraries are well-poised to be guardians of electronic geospatial information and data storage. Some current examples include the New York State Public Library (Strasser 1998), Washington State university libraries (Suh and Lee 1999), Syracuse University (Olson 2004a), and Harvard University (Guan et al. 2011). Can geography libraries act as enablers in the distribution of resources to the nontraditional and nonacademic audience of health care delivery and service providers? A number of issues concerning the distribution of geographic data need to be addressed before this question can be fully answered.

As map curator James Boxall (2004) eloquently stated, the map and geography library "must be about participation and empowerment. Libraries . . . will be at the forefront of community use and individual exploration of information and ideas." His use of the term "geolibrary" is especially appropriate in the context of medical geographic research because of the digital revolution in which geography librarians are immersed. As the director and curator of the GIS Centre and Map Collection at Dalhousie University in Nova Scotia, Boxall heads the initiatives in medical geography at the library, which comprise half of the research that the GIS Centre undertakes.

Providing access and services associated with digital geospatial information is also an integral aspect of Harvard University's Center for Geographic Analysis (Guan et al 2011; Blossom et al. 2011), which is similar to the organization and structure of Boxall's GIS Centre at Dalhousie. The Center for Geographic Analysis and the Harvard Map Collection together play a leadership role in providing an infrastructure and the technical expertise needed to provide geographic analysis, bringing these various groups together to advance GIS research in health, medicine, and other disciplines across the campus. This includes data acquisition; development and sharing; software license management; lab and equipment management; credit courses and noncredit training; help-desk services; spatial-analytic services; consultation for projects and grant proposals; managing outsourced contracts; developing and hosting spatial database and Web services; monitoring and evaluating new technologies; authoring and publishing guidelines, procedures, and best practices; and organizing seminars, workshops, and colloquia.

As the Harvard case study illustrates, a useful and functional geographic reference service must possess the infrastructure and personnel to support the spatial data infrastructure (SDI) that cutting-edge research demands. Although geolibraries and SDIs exist in different flavors and forms throughout the globe, the lesson learned from most of them is that more needs to be known about how user needs develop and are met through the services of a digital library system (Smith 2003). Because medical geography is a relatively young—yet rapidly evolving—discipline, a stakeholder's analysis of a reference library's users must be performed annually to assess whether the needs of the research community are being met. In addition, as more nontraditional geographers are using geographic insights in their research, geographic information literacy must remain at the helm of educating the public on the proper use and dissemination of geographic materials (Jablonski 2004).

CONTRIBUTIONS TO "GEOGRAPHIC OPPORTUNITIES IN MEDICINE"

Map and geography libraries play a prominent role in the development of medical geography because of the depth and breadth of their resources that are made available to the wider research community. As Dr. Ellen K. Cromley of the University of Connecticut School of Medicine explains first in this theme issue, map and geography libraries play a crucial role in her medical geographic research, both in the U.S. and in other countries (Cromley 2011). As GIS databases become more widely shared resources, medical researchers are beginning to use map archives and geographic databases to improve health outcomes for patients. In two articles, one in each theme issue, Dr. Weihe Guan of Harvard University describes the research teams she collaborates with in supporting geospatial analysis in medical research. More and more nontraditional geographers and physicians are utilizing geographic insights to enhance health care delivery and service. In the second issue (Vol. 7, No. 3) in this theme, a group of physicians and epidemiologists from Baystate Health in Massachusetts will discuss their use of GIS in a number of applications ranging from research to direct patient care to disaster preparedness. As this series of articles demonstrates, the contributors to this special theme volume on "Geographic Opportunities in Medicine" were chosen for their broad experience in medical geography and their contributions to the database design and applications that play a vital role in developing the geographic and cartographic offerings within map and geography libraries.

This volume begins with several articles that describe the different roles map libraries can play in medical geographic research, both within the U.S. and internationally. One of these articles focuses specifically on unique and novel database-design issues about which map libraries should be concerned (Langley and Messina 2011). These researchers propose formal ontological and data structures for a data repository that promotes the efficient organization and management of data, facilitating importation, storage, modeling, and retrieval. Using a Kenya-based African trypanosomiasis project, they propose an innovative framework for the management and storage of multidimensional data. In addition, Hiyashi et al. (2011) present a novel way of satisfying the residency review committee requirements for graduate medical education in family medicine. By using administrative patient information and census data, these researchers were able to design a residency curriculum that used GIS to help residents in family medicine analyze community health data to enhance patient care and outcomes. This presents a perfect opportunity for engaging medical librarians to compile the necessary geographic databases for the curriculum and expand their geographical collections.

The forthcoming second theme issue presents applications in medical geography that deal with spatial data issues from the continental (Kalipeni et al. 2011) to the local scale (Garb and Wait 2011). Employing sophisticated spatial interpolation techniques, Kalipeni et al. produced statistically and visually meaningful maps for areas in Africa where little or no data on HIV/AIDS prevalence exists. The role of map and geography libraries in investigating infectious diseases in Africa is also described in an article from Harvard University researchers (Blossom et al. 2011), as well as other case studies that utilize their map archives and databases in medical geographic research. Health care disparities in the United States and direct patient care are the focus of the two articles by Vernon and Ting (2011) and Garb and Wait (2011). Vernon and Ting's research involves the development of a GIS-based, race-prediction model (used by WellPoint, Inc.) to determine areas where interventions can best facilitate the reduction of health disparities. With a prediction accuracy rate of 86.2 percent for all members, this model derives indirect race and ethnicity information for members for whom this information is lacking. Furthermore, in their article "Spatial Analysis in Healthcare," Garb and Wait describe some of the ways in which Baystate Health has used GIS to address problems in health care. Baystate is the parent corporation of an integrated health care system that has been recognized for its innovative and wide-ranging use of GIS in health.

CONCLUDING REMARKS

Can geography libraries act as enablers in the distribution of resources to the nontraditional and nonacademic audience of health care practitioners and service providers? As this volume on "Geographic Opportunities in Medicine" illustrates, the answer is a resounding "yes!" A number of suggestions and challenges have surfaced in our gaze into the future of medical geography. Map and geography librarians must foster and promote interdisciplinary investigations within their organizations. They must form relationships with local health and medical organizations, so that public-access data and information can be disseminated without difficulty. The appropriate infrastructure and personnel must be in place to support the digital archival process. A stakeholders' analysis must be performed annually, to ensure that the needs of the research community are being met. Geographic information literacy must be a top priority in geography libraries, because only the appropriate use of information can result in meaningful research. It is my hope that the contents of this volume will inspire current and future geography libraries to take a more diverse and active role in supporting medical geographic research in academia, industry, and nonprofit organizations.

REFERENCES

Albert, D. P., and W. M. Gesler. 1997. Multiple locations of practice in North Carolina: Findings and health care policy implications. *Carolina Health Services and Policy Review* 4: 55–75.

Amedeo, D., and R. G. Golledge. 1975. *An introduction to scientific reasoning in geography*. New York: Wiley.

Armstrong, R. W. 1965. Medical geography: An emerging specialty? *International Pathology* 6: 61–63.

Banks, A. L. 1959. The study of the geography of disease. *Geographical Journal* 125: 199–216.

Bazemore, A., R. L. Phillips, and T. Miyoshi. 2011. Harnessing geographic information systems (GIS) to enable community-oriented primary care. *Journal of Map and Geography Libraries* 7(1): 71–86.

Blossom, J., J. L. Finkelstein, B. Burns, and W. W. Guan. 2011. Applying GIS methods to public health research. *Journal of Map and Geography Libraries* 7(3): Forthcoming.

Boxall, J. 2004. Advances and trends in geospatial information accessibility—part I: Geolibraries. *Journal of Map and Geography Libraries* 1(1): 7–40.

Brewer, C. A. 2006. Basic mapping principles for visualizing cancer data using geographic information systems (GIS). *American Journal of Preventive Medicine* 30(2S): S25–S36.

Brewer, C. A., and L. Pickle. 2002. Evaluation of methods for classifying epidemiological data on choropleth maps in series. *Annals of the Association of American Geographers* 92(4): 662–681

Cliff, A., and P. Haggett. 1988. *Atlas of disease distributions: Analytical approaches to epidemiological data*. Oxford: Blackwell.

Cordivano, S. 2011. Maternity ward closures in Philadelphia: Using GIS methods to measure disruptions in essential health services. *Journal of Map and Geography Libraries* 7(3): Forthcoming.

Cromley, E. K. 2011. The role of the map and geographic information library in medical geographic research. *Journal of Map and Geography Libraries* 7(1): 13–35.

Cromley, E. K., and P. C. Albertsen. 1993. Multiple-site physician practices and their effect on service distribution. *Health Services Research* 28(4): 503–522.

Croner, C. M. 2004. Public health GIS and the Internet. *Journal of Map and Geography Libraries* 1(1): 105–135.

Cutter, S. L. and W. D. Solecki. 1989. The national pattern of airborne toxic releases. *Professional Geographer* 41(2): 149–161.

Garb, J. L., and R. Wait. 2011. Spatial analysis in healthcare. *Journal of Map and Geography Libraries* 7(3): Forthcoming.

Gessler, W. 2003. Medical geography. In *Geography in America at the dawn of the 21st Century*, ed. C. G. Willmott and G. Gaile. New York: Oxford University Press, pp. 494–504.

Guan, W. W., B. Burns, J. L. Finkelstein, and J. Blossom. 2011. Enabling geographic research across disciplines: Building an institutional infrastructure for geographic analysis at Harvard University. *Journal of Map and Geography Libraries* 7(1): 36–60.

Hippocrates. 1886. *The genuine works of Hippocrates*Trans. F. Adams. New York: William Wood.

Hiyashi, A. S., A. Bazemore, and J. McIntyre. 2011. Transforming community health and primary care education using clinical and administrative data and geographic information systems. *Journal of Map and Geography Libraries* 7(1): 61–70.

Jablonksi, J. 2004. Information literacy for GIS curricula: An instructional model for faculty. *Journal of Map and Geography Libraries* 1(1): 41–58.

Kalipeni, E., L. C. Zulu, and V. Escamilla. 2011. Using new geographic methods to map the spread and prevalence of HIV/AIDS in Africa. *Journal of Map and Geography Libraries* 7(3): Forthcoming.

Kalkstein, L. S., and R. E. Davis. 1989. Weather and human mortality: An evaluation of demographic and interregional responses in the United States. *Annals of the Association of American Geographers* 79(1): 44–64.

Langley, S., and J. Messina. 2011. Embracing the open–source movement for the management of spatial data: A case study of African trypanosomiasis in Kenya. *Journal of Map and Geography Libraries* 7(1): 87–113.

Mangan, E. 2007. Cartographic materials: A century of cataloguing at Library of Congress and beyond. *Journal of Map and Geography Libraries* 3(2): 23–44.

May, J. M. 1950. Medical geography: Its methods and objectives. *Geographical Review* 40: 9–41.

Meade, M. S., and R. J. Earickson. 2000. *Medical geography*. New York: Guilford Press.

Olson, J. S. 2004a. Library-based GIS labs: A case study—Syracuse University. *Journal of Map and Geography Libraries* 1(1): 75–88.

Olson, J. S. 2004b. JPEG2000: Ride the wavelet. *Journal of Map and Geography Libraries* 1(1): 137–140.

Paul, B. K. 1985. Approaches to medical geography: An historical perspective. *Social Science and Medicine* 20: 399–407.

Peters, J., and G. B. Hall. 1999. Assessment of ambulance response performance using a geographic information system. *Social Science and Medicine* 49: 1551–1566.

Quest Diagnostics. 2010. HealthTrends. http://www.questdiagnostics.com/brand/business/healthtrends/index.html (accessed September 22, 2010).

Senior, M. L., S. J. New, A. C. Gatrell, and J. Francis. 1993. Geographic influences on the uptake of infant immunisations: 1. Concepts, models, and aggregate analyses. *Environment and Planning* 25(4): 425–36.

Shannon, G. W., and G. F. Pyle. 1993. *Disease and medical care in the United States*. New York: Macmillan.

Smith, T. 2003. End-user issues should have a first class status. *Working paper*, National Science Foundation Post Digital Libraries Workshop. June 15–17, in Chatham, MA.

Strasser, T. C. 1998. Geographic information systems and the New York State Library: Mapping new pathways for library service. *Library Hi Tech* 16(3/4): 43–50.

Suh, H.–S., and A. Lee. 1999. Embracing GIS services in libraries: The Washington State University experience. *The Reference Librarian* 30(64): 125–137.

Theunissen, Y. 2007. Developing and promoting outreach services for elementary and middle schools: Case study of a rare map library at a public university. *Journal of Map and Geography Libraries* 3(2): 5–22.

Vernon, Z. D., and G. H. Ting. 2011. The role of race and ethnicity predictive modeling and spatial analysis in addressing health disparities. *Journal of Map and Geography Libraries* 7(3): Forthcoming.

Walsh, F. 2004. Retrospective cataloguing of maps in a small liberal arts college: A case study. *Journal of Map and Geography Libraries* 1(1): 89–104.

Wennberg, J., E. Fisher, D. Goodman, and J. Skinner. 2008. *Dartmouth Atlas of Health Care: Tracking the Care of Patients with Severe Chronic Illness*. Lebanon, NH: Dartmouth Institute for Health Policy and Clinical Practice, Center for Health Policy Research.

The Role of the Map and Geographic Information Library in Medical Geographic Research

ELLEN K. CROMLEY
University of Connecticut School of Medicine, Farmington, Connecticut, USA

Map and geography libraries play an important role in supporting the work of medical geographers conducting research in the U.S. and other countries. Libraries provide access to three key types of information needed in medical geographic research: geographic data on places including their locations and environmental contexts, spatially-referenced data on population, and spatially-referenced data on health events. There is an important ongoing role for map and geography libraries and librarians in acquiring, cataloging, and making accessible information needed to advance medical geographic research.

INTRODUCTION

Medical geography is a field of study involving the use of geographic data and methods in the study of health. The field is broad in scope, including research on geographical patterns of health and disease and the environmental and social correlates of these patterns, the locations of health services and geographic factors affecting access and utilization, and spatial methods for analyzing health data, often involving the use of geographic information systems (GIS) (Cromley and McLafferty 2002; Meade and Emch 2010). Data for medical geographic research may be gathered from observations made in the field, from secondary data sources, or both. The techniques of medical geography are also used in the design, implementation, and evaluation of prevention and intervention studies.

The connections between geography and health have been recognized for centuries. Although the term "medical geography" is used here, the field has also embraced the term "health geography" to shift the perspective from disease and medical care to wellbeing and broader social models of health and health care (Kearns and Moon 2002). This shift has been accompanied by recognition of the range of theoretical approaches engaged in studying the geographies of health (Gatrell 2002). In this assessment of the role of map and geography libraries in medical geographic research, the positivist approach is emphasized—an approach grounded in "the observable, the measurable, and the generalizable" (Gatrell p. 31). Map and geography libraries play a particularly important role in supporting the work of medical geographers in the U.S. and other countries which focuses on areal patterns of health and disease. Other library collections may be equally valuable for other theoretical approaches to medical geography exploring individual experiences of health and illness and the social, economic, and political forces affecting health and health care provision.

Map and geography libraries provide access to three key types of information needed in medical geographic research: geographic data on places including their locations and environmental contexts, data on populations, and data on health events. Examples are provided citing the library resources supplying each type of information in research projects addressing a wide range of health issues at a variety of geographic scales in the U.S. and other countries. Libraries provide access to published maps and atlases, gazetteers, and other reference materials in their collections and in collections at other institutions, increasingly through the Internet. Map and geography libraries have played an important part in providing online access to many of these resources. The importance of metadata standards for digital spatial databases related to health and the need to improve keywords in metadata are discussed. Even with the shift to the Internet, there is an essential ongoing role for map and geography libraries and librarians in acquiring, cataloging, and making accessible information needed to advance medical geographic research.

GEOGRAPHIC DATA ON PLACES

Medical geographic research is grounded in place. Foundation spatial data are important for defining the locations and areas of interest for studies of human health. Map and geography libraries provide critical support to researchers by making these data accessible. These data help analysts locate points of interest and register existing data to a spatial reference system.

Locations

In order to describe and analyze real patterns of health and disease, observations need to be located or positioned in space. Digital geospatial data are not always associated with reported observations. A doctoral dissertation on contamination from the Chernobyl disaster that affected Belarus (Serebriakova 2005) used data from a published report on observations made at 3,326 settlements in the country (Matyukhin 1992). This report contained data on the annual effective equivalent dose (AEED) of radiation in millisiverts (mSv) from external sources (ground contamination) and from internal sources (food). The widely reproduced official map of Chernobyl contamination in Belarus, *Karta Radiatsionnoy Obstanovki*, an area-class map showing broad contamination patterns in the Soviet Republic at 1:1,000,000 scale, was based on ground contamination from Cesium-137 and other isotopes (ZAP AGP Belgeodezii 1992; Marples 1992). Contamination from food is also important in its effects on human health, and the intent of the research was to use spatial statistical analysis implemented in a geographic information system (GIS) to model AEED from both external and internal sources using AEED data for the villages modeled as points. The report described only the name of the settlement and the *rayon*, the lowest level administrative district, where the settlement was located.

In order to create a digital geospatial database of settlement locations for use in the analysis, the settlements had to be georeferenced. Ideally, spatial coordinates would have been available for all settlements in digital form. Online gazetteers such as the GEONet Names Server (GNS) operated by the National Imagery and Mapping Agency, now the National Geospatial-Intelligence Agency (NGA) (NGA 2010), did not have complete coverage of the settlements. Only five of the settlements could be located using information from GEONet. Many of the places of interest were small agricultural settlements with fewer than 100 residents. Furthermore, place names were not always consistent with names in databases or on maps, due to errors in compiling the original database, differences in the Russian and Belarussian versions of spelling local place names, or changes in village names since the publication of the topographic maps.

Locations of towns and villages were digitized as point data from a set of paper topographic maps of 1:100,000 and 1:200,000 scales in the collection of the Map and Geographic Information Center (MAGIC), Homer Babbidge Library, University of Connecticut. Of ninety topographic maps covering the entire republic, fifty-two were used to digitize the locations where ground and food samples had been collected and analyzed. These maps were published between 1976 and 1999 by one of five mapping agencies: GUGK

USSR, Belgeodezia, and Goskomzem in Minsk; Roskartographia in Russia; and the Soviet general staff. Regional topographic maps of Brest, Gomel, and Mogilev Oblasts published by GUGK USSR in 1979 at 1:400,000 scale were also consulted. The data digitized from these maps were supplemented with data for five of the settlements from the GEONet Names Server and for three of the settlements located in a 1:500,000 scale road atlas published in Minsk (Pejchvasser et al. 2001). The road atlas was obtained through interlibrary loan.

MAGIC allowed the maps to circulate so that they could be used on a digitizing tablet in a laboratory in the geography department at the university. The availability of these resources made it possible to geocode 3,256 of the 3,326 villages listed in the report (Figure 1). For 230 of these places, the spelling of the place name on the map was slightly different from the spelling in the report.

Once the database of the locations of the settlements had been created, a table of digital data compiled from the printed report on AEED from external and internal sources observed at each settlement was joined to the point database in a GIS application. Kriging, a spatial statistical method for interpolating data (Chang 2008), was used to create maps of contaminated areas in Belarus that took into account contamination from internal as well as external sources. The analysis identified Checherskiy, Lel'chitskiy, and Yel'skiy Rayons in Gomel Oblast as areas with villages where the level of contamination from internal sources was high, even though the villages were located in areas classified in the low contamination zone on the official map based only on ground contamination (Figure 2).

In this example, the maps were used to support creation of a digital spatial database of settlement locations so that spatial statistical analysis could be conducted using GIS. Map and geography library resources are also useful for helping researchers describe, communicate, and analyze the geographic contexts of study communities.

Contexts: The Built Environment and Environmental Quality

Even after the study communities of interest have been located and their boundaries defined, it is often important in medical geographic research to investigate the regional context. Individuals circulate in an environment larger than the neighborhood around their residence during the course of daily activities (Sherman et al. 2005), and migration from one residential setting to another is an important process to investigate in analyzing the connections between place and health (Boyle and Norman 2010). Features in the built environment and geographic patterns of environmental quality are important factors influencing human health (Jackson 2003; Jerrett, Gale, and Kontgis 2010).

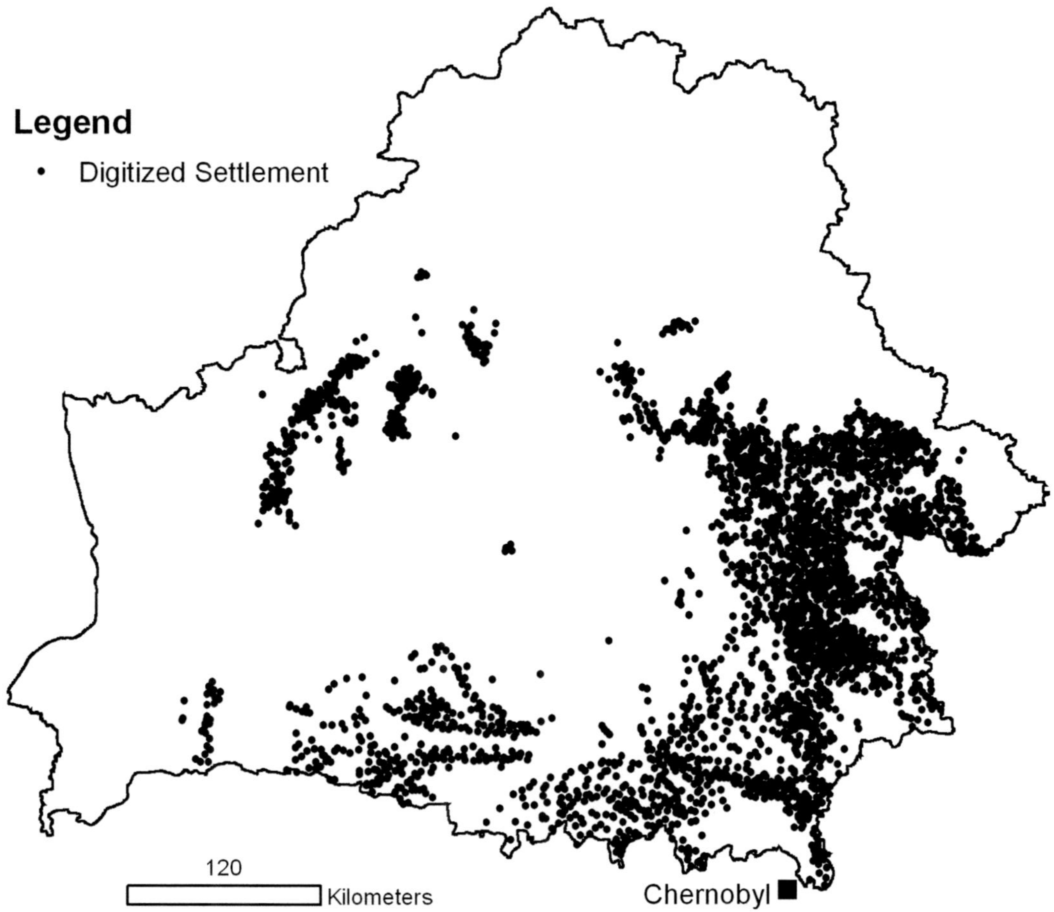

FIGURE 1 Map of Belarus showing 3,256 settlement locations digitized from a variety of sources. Measurements of ground radiation and of food samples were taken at these locations and used to develop estimates of annual radiation dose following the disaster at the Chernobyl nuclear power plant. Data were provided by Tatiana Serebriakova.

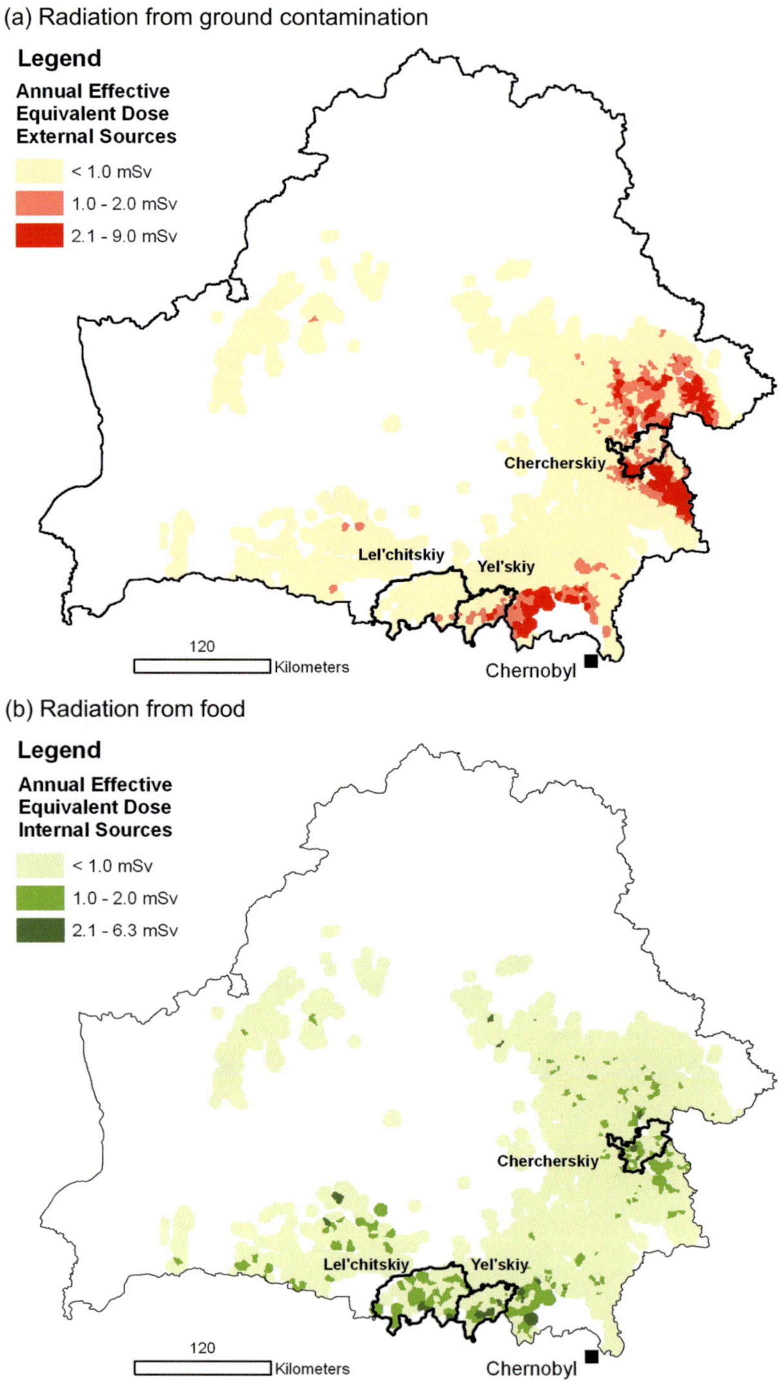

FIGURE 2 Annual effective equivalent dose of radiation from Chernobyl from ground contamination (Figure 2a) was generally low in settlements in Let'chitskiy, Yel'skiy and Chercherskiy rayons but the dose from internal sources (food) was high in settlements in these areas (Figure 2b). Data were provided by Tatiana Serebriakova.

Mapping the Built Environment

A study of alcohol use and sexual risk conducted in three slum communities in the Mumbai metropolitan area gathered data on the places where men drank from a large-scale survey of 1,239 men (Cromley et al. 2010). Spatial ecological models of alcohol use underscore the importance of the places where people drink in explaining drinking behavior (Gruenewald 2007). The boundaries of the study communities were defined based on natural features, elements in the built environment including major roads, and local knowledge the research team gained from formative work in the field. Spatial data describing the built environment of the larger metropolitan region were also important because drinking locations were spread throughout the region. Of the 751 men in the study communities who reported regularly drinking with friends, 16 percent described places located outside one of the three study communities as the location where they usually drank. Understanding these patterns is important for designing interventions to promote healthier behavior (Muhib et al. 2001).

At the time of the study, affordable digital spatial databases were not available for Mumbai. A map of the metropolitan region showing major highways, the regional rail network, and other features of interest in the built environment was purchased as part of a city atlas (Eicher 2002) produced by a diversified company that manufactures automotive equipment and publishes city maps and travel guides. There was no spatial reference information on the map. The MAGIC collection had a series of 1:250,000 scale maps of India and Pakistan produced by the U.S. Army Map Service (U.S. Army Map Service 1955). Two of these maps (NE 43–5 Bombay and NE 43–1 Kalyan) (Figure 3) were used to set up the digitizing tablet so that the map sheet from the road atlas could be properly registered to digitize features of interest from the city atlas map. The digital databases created for the alcohol study were used to map and analyze drinking and other activity sites visited by men in the large-scale survey (Figure 4).

Mapping Environmental Quality

In addition to providing data on features in the built environment, map and geographic libraries provide access to data on environmental quality, also important in studies of human health. The European Commission and the ministries responsible for Chernobyl affairs in Russia, Ukraine, and Belarus collaborated on a research program to study the effects of the Chernobyl disaster. One of the projects involved preparation of an atlas of the deposition of radioactive material released during the Chernobyl disaster over the whole territory of Europe, so that there would be a comprehensive and coherent picture of the impact in the region using data of comparable resolution and quality (De Cort et al. 1998). The atlas contains 65 plates at a variety

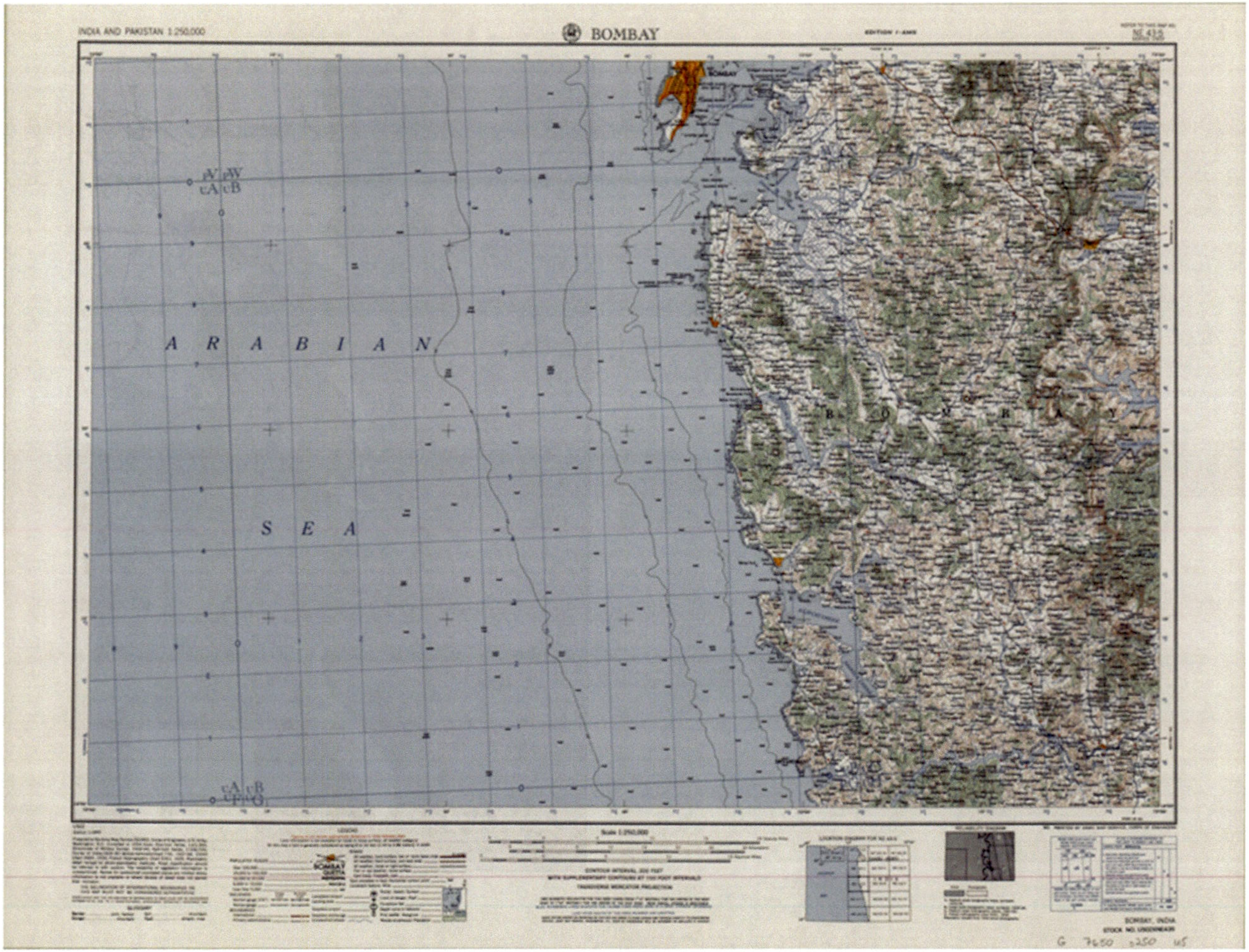

FIGURE 3 Map sheet from a topographic map series covering India and Pakistan produced by the U.S. Army Map Service. This map was used to set up a digitizing tablet to digitize features of the built environment in the Mumbai, India, region. *Source*: Map Collection, Map and Geographic Information Center, Homer Babbidge Library, University of Connecticut.

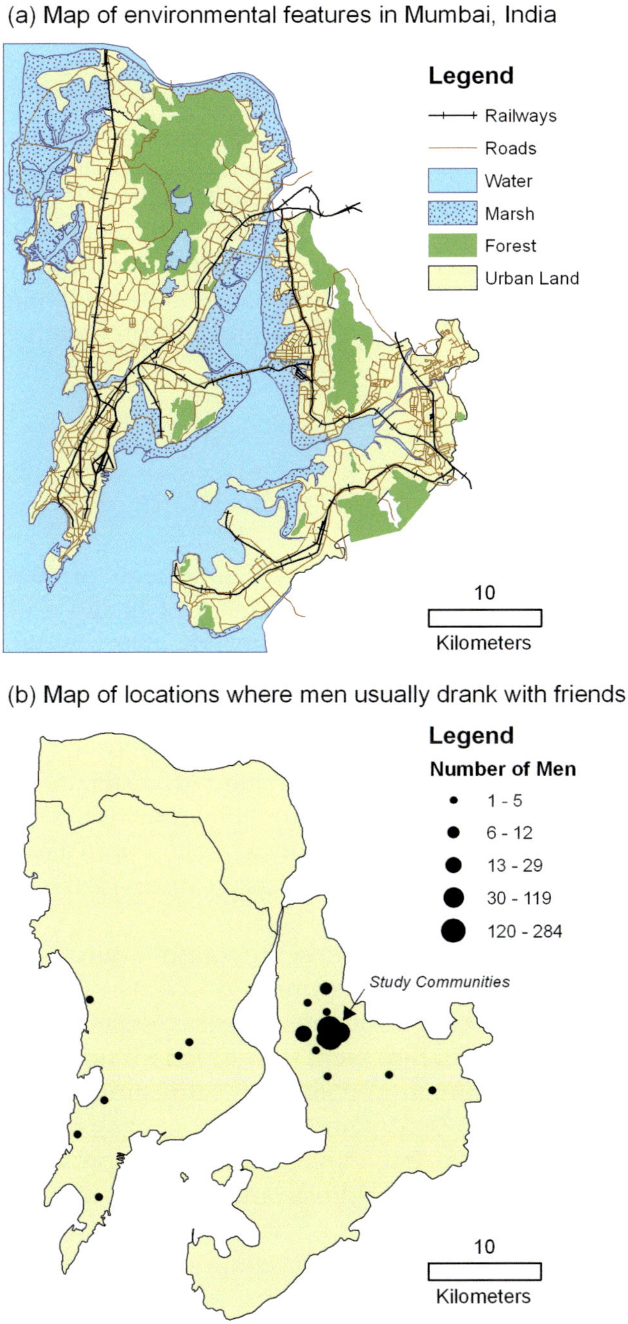

FIGURE 4 A map of Mumbai and Navi Mumbia, India, was digitized and georegistered for use in research on alcohol use among young men in three study communities (Figure 4a). Spatial data and mapping of places where young men reported usually drinking with friends made visual the dispersion of settings, including sites outside the study communities where participants resided (Figure 4b).

of scales, mapping patterns of deposition, meteorological conditions, and demographic patterns.

Health-related atlases are important, not only as sources of data on environmental conditions and health outcomes (as discussed below), but also as sources of information on analytical methods. The *Atlas of Caesium Deposition on Europe after the Chernobyl Accident* includes two appendices describing methods used to prepare the atlas. Appendix C describes geographic information systems and their role within the project. Appendix D provides a detailed explanation of the inverse distance weighting method used to interpolate contamination values and the procedures used to map the interpolated values.

DATA ON POPULATIONS

Data on human populations are also key components of many medical geographic studies. Although explaining patterns of health and disease is an important goal of medical geographic research, many worthwhile studies have been conducted with population data alone. An important body of work in medical geography focuses on modeling contamination or exposure zones associated with environmental hazards (Jerrett, Gale, and Kongtis 2010). Population data are used in this research to estimate how many people live or engage in activities within the contamination zones or potential hazard zones to identify the population at risk. Population data are also used to model access to health care services (Tanser, Gething, and Atkinson 2010).

Census data are perhaps the most important source of data on populations. Census data are usually reported as counts of population for the geographic areas used as reporting units. For the 1980 Census conducted in the United States, GBF/DIME files were developed for urban areas to support the work of the Census Bureau in collecting, tabulating, and reporting data. Geographic base files (GBF) contained census geographic statistical codes and dual independent map encoding (DIME) files provided a schematic map of a city's streets segments, address ranges, and associated geostatistical codes so that population data could be linked to the geography of the census. TIGER (Topologically Integrated Geographic Encoding and Referencing system) was developed for the 1990 Census (Marx 1986); it covers the entire country, and it has been updated over the past two decades (U.S. Census Bureau 2010). The availability of TIGER data for 1990 was an important factor spurring the adoption of GIS in the U.S. (Cromley and McLafferty 2002). It also marked the separation of the census population data from the census geographic data, which has implications for how these data are accessed by researchers.

In addition to their use in medical geographic studies to identify populations at risk and to investigate access to health care services, census population and geographic data are important in analyzing patterns of health events. Population data from the census provide denominators for the calculation of disease rates. A database of death certificates, for example, provides data on health events such as deaths from cancer, but these data must be coupled with population data to derive mortality rates, which can then be mapped and analyzed using spatial statistical methods. Because many health problems occur more frequently in particular age-sex groups, population data by age and sex are particularly important.

A recent trend in mapping population data used in medical geography and other fields is the conversion of population data from census unit areas like census tracts or counties to grids. The LandScan database is a worldwide population distribution dataset based on a 30″ by 30″ longitude/latitude grid (Oak Ridge National Laboratory 2010). Only the most recent LandScan database for 2008 is distributed because the data are not considered adequate to support studies of population change due to natural increase or migration. Unlike TIGER data distributed by the Census Bureau, LandScan data are copyrighted, but a sample database is available for researchers who might be interested in gridded population data (Figure 5).

Geographic data from the census are used to create area boundary files for mapping aggregated health data. They have also made it possible to

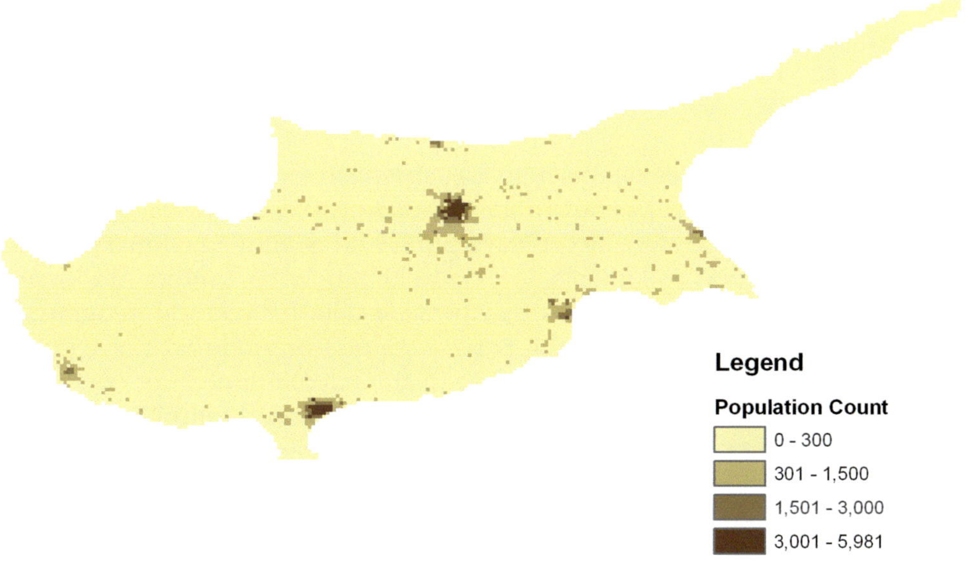

FIGURE 5 A map based on the sample LandScan dataset for Cyprus from the LandScan 2007 Global Population Database, which provides population counts for grid cells. The raster data set uses lon/lat based on WGS 1984.

geocode individual health events, usually by address-match geocoding residential locations using data from disease registries or health care provider databases (Rushton et al. 2006). Parcel databases are also used to geocode health events and to develop more accurate maps of population distribution in medical geographic research (Maantay, Maroko, and Porter-Morgan 2008). Map and geography libraries are also important sources of data on the location of health events for medical geographic research.

DATA ON HEALTH EVENTS

There are strong connections between medical mapping and the development of thematic cartography during the nineteenth century (Gilbert 1958). Maps of health events were important in investigating the causes of diseases at times when their etiologies were unknown. Snow's often-cited map of cholera cases in London (Snow 1855) was not used to discover the source of the disease outbreak, as commonly reported, but was developed as a "visual representation of a deduction from a theory of transmission developed earlier" (Brody et al. 2000, p. 68). Data on health events can be mapped at the individual or area level.

Maps of Individual Health Events

An interesting early example from 1819 of a map showing individual health events plots yellow fever cases near Old Slip in Lower Manhattan in 1819 (Shannon 1981). A copy of this map (Figure 6) is in the National Library of Medicine (NLM 1819), along with earlier yellow fever maps for U.S. cities dating to 1796. The cases on this map are labeled to show the temporal order of "sickening." These maps show highly disaggregated, individual-level data.

Maps of this type were not always published as individual map sheets. Federal government documents and journal articles are other important sources of maps of health events that provide data for medical geographic research. A series of Public Health Service reports on outbreaks of typhoid in Washington, D.C., in the first decade of the twentieth century contained maps of the location of each case (Rosenau, Lumsden, and Kastle 1907; Rosenau, Lumsden, and Kastle 1908; Rosenau, Lumsden, and Kastle 1909; Lumsden and Anderson 1911). A century later, these maps provided the data for a spatial statistical analysis of disease clusters (Figure 7) (Hinman, Blackburn, and Curtis 2006). The Public Health Service investigators reported at the time that cases of the disease appeared to be evenly distributed across the district, but subsequent analysis using Getis and Ord's G_i^* statistic (Getis and Ord 1992) revealed clustering at multiple spatial scales.

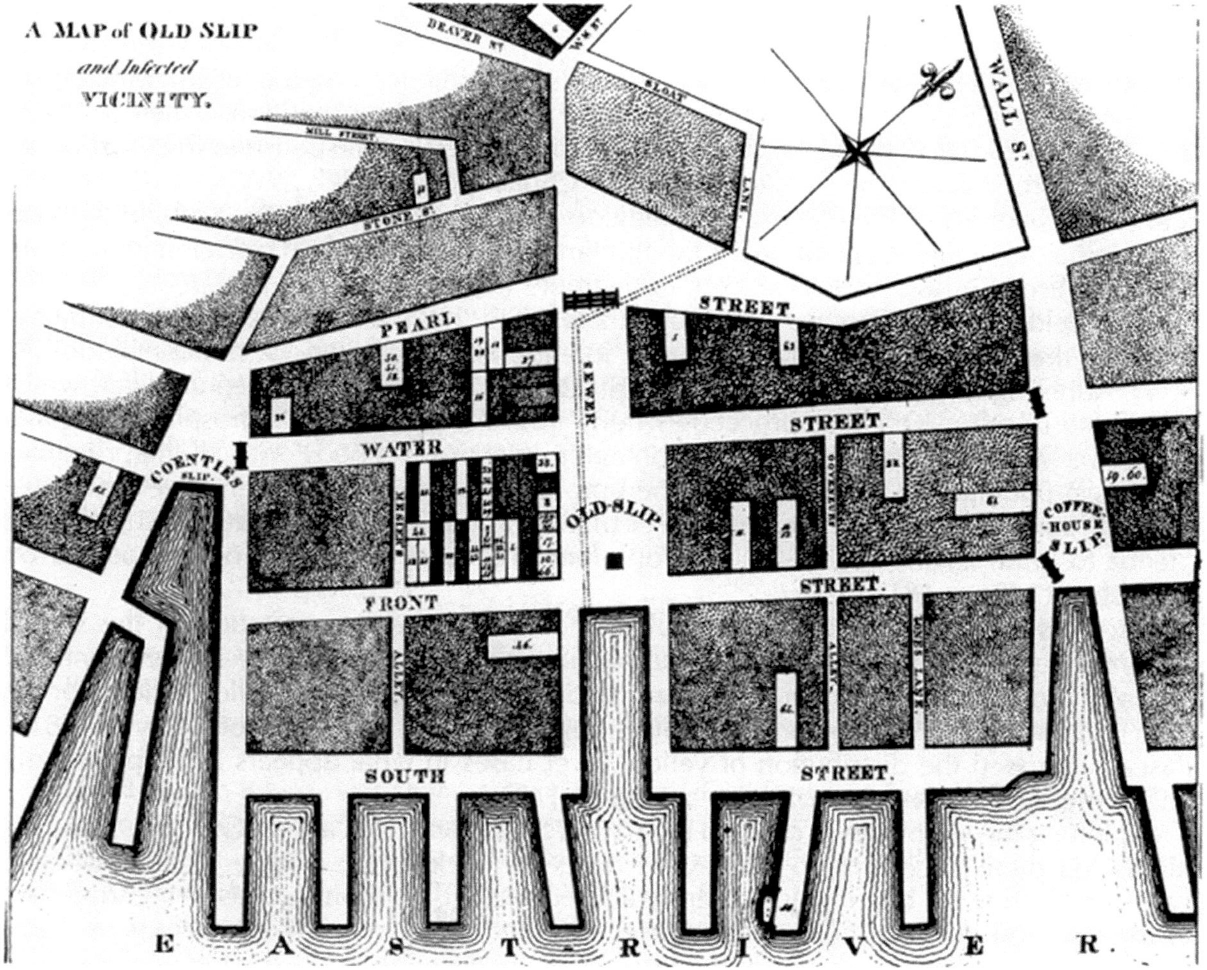

FIGURE 6 Yellow fever cases in Manhattan in 1819. The numbers mapped at the case locations show the order in which people fell ill from the disease. This map is in the public domain. *Source*: Images from the History of Medicine, National Library of Medicine, National Institutes of Health.

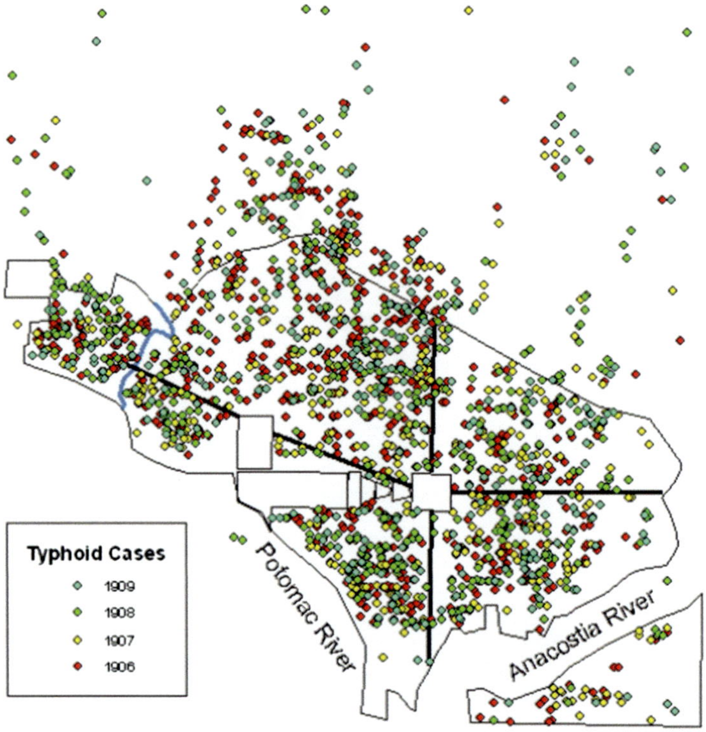

FIGURE 7 The locations of all cases of typhoid with signs of onset between May 1 and October 31, 1906, through 1909 in Washington, D.C. These data were captured from maps published in a series of Public Health Service reports on outbreaks of the disease. *Source*: Originally published by BioMed Central, Open Access, in S. E. Hinman, J. K. Blackburn, and A. Curtis, 2006, Spatial and temporal structure of typhoid outbreaks in Washington, D.C., 1906–1909: Evaluating local clustering with the G_i^* statistic, *International Journal of Health Geographics* 5:13.

Journal articles may also contain maps of health events. Maxcy (1926) published maps showing the locations of individual cases of typhus in Montgomery, Alabama. One map shows the case distribution based on where people who contracted the disease lived and another map shows the case distribution based on where they worked (Figure 8). The concentration of cases in focal areas near the city center suggested that transmission was occurring where people worked.

Today, the ability to scan, register, and screen-digitize features on maps using GIS has made it possible to reverse geocode mapped data on individual health events, posing a threat to privacy and confidentiality (Brownstein, Cassa, and Mandl 2006; Curtis, Mills, and Leitner 2006). The impact of this on the publication of maps of individual health events like those published by Snow or Maxcy is unclear, but it is likely that, in the future, data on individual health events will be mapped for publication using some method

(a) Cases of Brill's disease mapped by residence

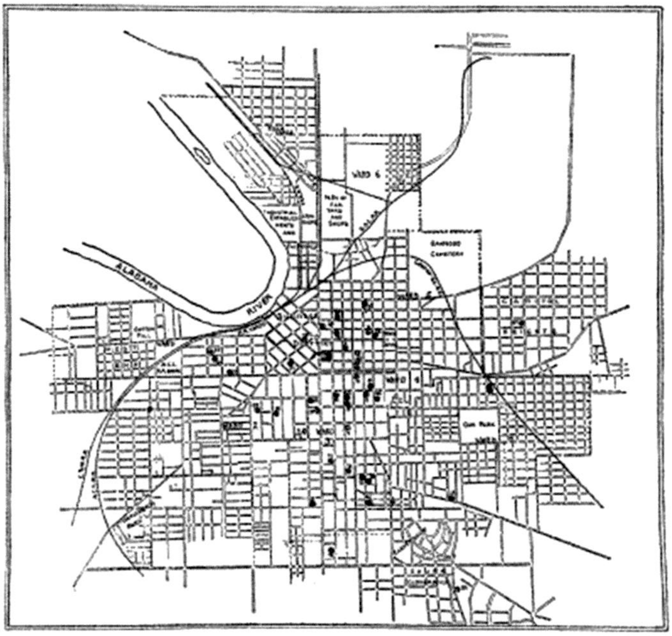

(b) Cases of Brill's disease mapped by workplace

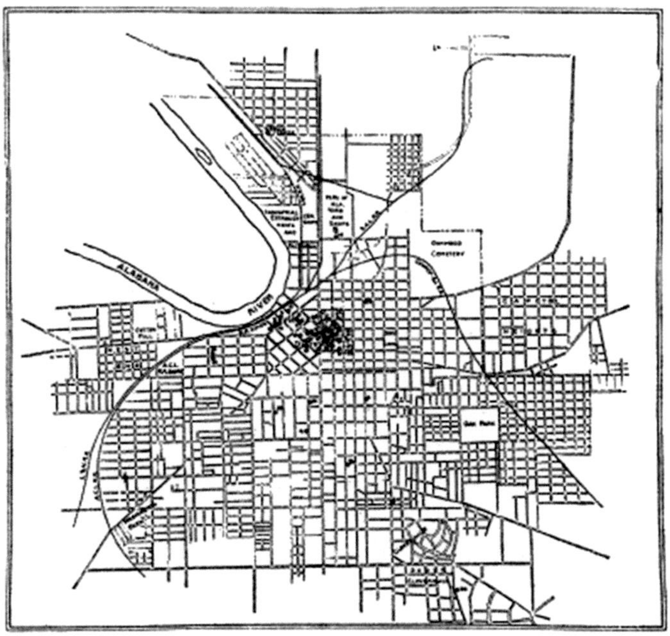

FIGURE 8 Cases of mild typhus (Brill's disease) mapped by residential location (Figure 8a) show no pattern of clustering. When cases were mapped by place of employment or residence if the individual was unemployed (Figure 8b), a cluster of cases is apparent. *Source*: Originally published in K. F. Maxcy, 1926, An epidemiological study of endemic typhus (Brill's disease) in the Southeastern United States with special reference to its mode of transmission, *Public Health Reports* 41(52):2967–2995.

to prevent reverse geocoding of individual data (Wieland et al. 2008) or will be mapped as aggregated data (El Emam, Brown, and AbdelMalik 2009).

Maps of Aggregated Health Data

Atlases of health and disease generally map aggregated data on health outcomes. The *Atlas of Cancer Mortality in the Federal Republic of Germany* (Becker, Frentzel-Beyme, and Wagner 1984) mapped cancer mortality rates for men and women for a wide range of cancers at the *kreise* level, an intermediate administrative level between the state and the local municipality. Cancer rates were mapped using quintiles.

Some atlases publish, in the form of tables, the data from which the maps in the atlas were prepared. This provides analysts with the opportunity to look up specific disease rates for individual areas and to develop other cartographic representations of the same data. In addition to the maps, the tables of data used to prepare the maps were published as part of the West German cancer atlas. Subsequent to its publication and in response to the public's interpretation and use of the *Atlas*, one of the authors proposed an alternative approach to map classification based on absolute scales to make it easier for map readers to compare rates for the same cancers for different sexes and to compare rates over time (Becker 1994). Publication of the data tables also made it possible for other researchers to explore alternative approaches to mapping the data, including using a classification method that maximized spatial similarity among contiguous *kriese* whose cancer mortality rates were in the same class interval (Cromley and Cromley 1996).

Although disease atlases are frequently published as bound volumes, some atlases have been published as individual plates. The *Atlas of Disease* is a series of plates published by the American Geographical Society in the 1950s under the leadership of Dr. Jacques M. May, a physician and medical geographer with expertise in tropical medicine (American Geographical Society, 1944). These plates were published with various issues of the society's journal, *Geographical Review*, from 1950 through 1954 (Martin 2005). In some libraries, these plates might still be shelved with the bound periodicals rather than retained in the collection of the map and geography library. Some digital versions of the articles accompanying the maps accessible through online systems for archiving academic journals such as *JStor* (*Journal Storage*) include the maps (see for example, May, 1952, http://www.jstor.org/stable/211391, Map of the World Distribution of Dengue and Yellow Fever), although the maps were scanned in page-size sections rather than single full-size plates. As these examples illustrate, information used by medical geographers in conducting research can be found in the collections of map and geography libraries, but they may also be found in a wide range of sources held in other library collections or on line.

METADATA, DATA ARCHIVES, AND ONLINE SEARCH

Metadata

The key to finding information is metadata. Metadata or data about data are important in the search for research resources (Green and Bossomaier 2002). In the online environment, three categories of metadata may be important to medical geographers searching for information: metadata describing digital geospatial databases, metadata records used by libraries to describe items in their collections, and metadata used to facilitate online search. These three types of metadata were developed by different communities, using different standards.

For digital spatial databases, the International Organization for Standardization (ISO) has adopted standards for digital geospatial database metadata (International Organization for Standardization 2003). National standards like the standard developed by the Federal Geographic Data Committee in the United States have been brought into conformity with them. One of the nineteen theme keywords in the ISO 19115 standard is "health." This provides a starting point for finding digital spatial databases held in data archives.

Data Archives

Map and geography librarians pioneered the development of online sites from which digital geospatial databases could be downloaded (McGlamery 1995). This approach is now used by a wide range of agencies and state and local governments for making their databases available to the public. Because there is a latency period between exposure to a cause of disease and the emergence of the disease, medical geographic research frequently involves reconstructing past patterns of exposure. Agencies like the U.S. Census Bureau that produce and distribute online data used for medical geographic research—and a wide range of other applications—generally provide access to the most recent version of the data. Older versions of the TIGER data are no longer available for download from the Census Bureau's Web site, although metadata are still available. Users must find these data through other sources. Some data may be available on CD through Federal Depository System institutions or, depending on the institution, in a map and geography library. But it is not clear how users will be able to access the various versions of TIGER data from the 1990s in the future to reconstruct census geography of that era or whether the CD data can be read in its existing format by GIS software systems of the future.

There is recognition of the need to archive digital spatial databases that have been created over the past thirty years (Bethune, Lazorchak, and Nagy 2010; Erwin and Sweetkind-Singer 2010; Morris 2010). Some of these initiatives are taking place at the state level, which is important because many GIS databases are created at the state and local level in the U.S. Geography helps create user communities for these data. These archives are useful for finding digital spatial data but, as this paper has pointed out, many important sources of information for medical geographic research can be found in topographic map sheets, government documents and journal articles in paper or digital image formats. Online search will be the key to finding these materials.

Online Search

The explosion of online information has made finding materials of interest ever more challenging. One recent Web application, HEALTH GeoJunction, attempts to use Web services to extract place-time-content information from bibliographic data describing documents and to query and filter the information (MacEachren et al. 2010). This application relies on place name extraction, disambiguation, and geocoding. Map librarians have been active participants, with information technology professionals and geographers, in searching for more effective georeferences to use in metadata to facilitate search and discovery. Hill (2006, p. viii) advocates unified georeferencing, "where placenaming and geospatial coding are interchangeable to the degree that place-based information retrieval can be expected to work satisfactorily across the vast and dissimilar collections of data, images, library and museum holdings, news, online resources, and so on." This approach overcomes the many query difficulties associated with choosing the right words/terms/place-names to specify a location, expressions in multiple languages, and historical transitions. Because so many geospatial materials have been the province of map and geography libraries or data centers whose collections may not be well-integrated with general collections, little attention has been paid in systems like PubMed to the value of adopting georeferences that would support more powerful place-based information retrieval. Given the importance of maps and data on health events published in the journal literature, it would be particularly useful if metadata for journal articles were structured in such a way that users could easily search for and identify articles containing maps or data. Library catalog entries for reports and monographs generally indicate whether these volumes include maps or tables of data, but most search tools for the journal literature do not.

Standard library cataloging of large topographic maps series even in online cataloging systems does not generally provide sheet-level cataloging. Researchers generally identify map series of interest through the catalog and then explain what is needed to map library personnel who provide assistance in locating specific series and sheets in the collection, often by referring to a map index published as part of the series to show which map sheets cover particular areas within the mapped region. Library and agency Web sites from which users download digital images of map sheets or digital orthophoto images commonly enable users to view and download the map index for a series of topographic maps or orthophotos and to perform queries to find the particular sheets or tiles covering the areas of interest, but these functions are supported outside the standard library cataloging system.

Online data archives and search tools have some important limitations, however, which are not adequately acknowledged. At many health agencies, computer system security configurations prevent health analysts from downloading applications such as GoogleEarth or accessing other sources of online information. Equally important, governments and organizations may block access to some sites.

Reliance on online search and discovery tools has fundamentally changed how the user community searches for and acquires materials. Not so long ago, individuals could search the library collections anonymously with few if any limitations on their ability to access items. Online search tools may make finding resources easier in some ways, but they also raise serious issues. An article in the *New York Times* (Pear 2008) reported that Johns Hopkins University had programmed its computers to ignore the word "abortion" in searches of a large, publicly financed database of information on reproductive health known as Popline. This restriction was later lifted, but it raises the question about how open Open Access really is. Furthermore, online search behavior can be monitored. Although monitored search behavior can be used to provide better information on the user community (McGlamery 1997), the potential for abuse of this information has also been recognized (Angell 2010).

CONCLUSIONS

Medical geographic research involves integrating data on the environment, population, and health events from a wide variety of sources. Map and geography libraries and librarians provide access to a wide range of research materials. Not all these materials are directly related to human health in the sense that they contain data on health outcomes or health care facilities. In many cases, materials are needed to locate features of interest, to georeference data, or to illustrate mapping and spatial analytic methods.

Map and geography libraries have been important in advancing medical geographic research through making gazetteers, atlases, map plates, and other items in their collections available in paper and digital formats. They have also contributed to the development of online systems for accessing digital geospatial data and the metadata records needed to support search and discovery of resources for research. As the field of medical geography moves forward, it is more important than ever to continue to broaden the dialogue between map and geography librarians, librarians who manage health and general collections, and people who use these resources to study and address human health needs.

REFERENCES

American Geographical Society. 1944. A proposed atlas of disease. *Geographical Review* 34(4): 642–652.

Angell, K. 2010. Are we lawyers or librarians? Bibliographical defenders of information. *Library Student Journal* 5: http://www.librarystudentjournal.org/index.php/lsj/article/view/137 (accessed June 10, 2010).

Becker, N. 1994. Cancer mapping: Why not use absolute scales? *European Journal of Cancer* 30A(5): 699–706.

Becker, N., R. Frentzel-Beyme, and G. Wagner. 1984. *Atlas of Cancer Mortality in the Federal Republic of Germany*, 2nd ed. Berlin: Springer-Verlag.

Bethune, A., B. Lazorchak, and Z. Nagy. 2010. GeoMAPP: A geospatial multistate archive and preservation partnership. *Journal of Map & Geography Libraries* 6(1): 45–46.

Boyle, P., and P. Norman. 2010. Migration and health. In *A companion to health and medical geography*, ed. T. Brown, S. McLafferty, and G. Moon. Chichester, UK: Wiley-Blackwell, 346–374.

Brody, H., M. R. Rip, P. Vinten-Johansen, N. Paneth, and S. Rachman. 2000. Map-making and myth-making in Broad Street. *The Lancet* 356(9223): 64–68.

Brownstein, J. S., C. A. Cassa, and K. D. Mandl. 2006. No place to hide—reverse identification of patients from published maps. *New England Journal of Medicine* 355(16): 1741–1742.

Chang, K-T. 2008. *Introduction to geographic information systems*, 4th ed. Boston: McGraw Hill.

Cromley, E. K., and R. G. Cromley. 1996. An analysis of alternative classification schemes for medical atlas mapping. *European Journal of Cancer* 32A(9): 1551–1559.

Cromley, E. K., and S. L. McLafferty. 2002. *GIS and public health*. New York: Guilford.

Cromley, E. K., J. J. Schensul, S. K. Singh, M. J. Berg, and E. Coman. 2010. Spatial dimensions of research on alcohol and sexual risk: A case example from a Mumbai study. *AIDS & Behavior* 14(Suppl. 1): S104–S112.

Curtis, A., J. Mills, and M. Leitner. 2006. Spatial confidentiality and GIS: Re-engineering mortality locations from published maps about Hurricane Katrina. *International Journal of Health Geographics* 5: 44.

De Cort, M., G. Dubois, S. D. Fridman, M. G. Germenchuk, Y. A. Izrael, A. Janssens, G. N. Kelly, et al. 1998. *Atlas of Caesium Deposition on Europe after the Chernobyl Accident*. Luxembourg: Office for Official Publications of the European Communities.

Eicher. 2002. *2002 Mumbai and Navi Mumbai Route Planner*. New Delhi: Eicher Goodearth.

El Emam, K., A. Brown, and P. AbdelMalik. 2009. Evaluating predictors of geographic area population size cut-offs to manage re-identification risk. *Journal of the American Medical Informatics Association* 16(12): 256–266.

Erwin, T., and J. Sweetkind-Singer. 2010. The National Geospatial Digital Archive: A collaborative project to archive geospatial data. *Journal of Map & Geography Libraries* 6(1): 6–25.

Gatrell, A. C. 2002. *Geographies of health: An introduction*. Oxford: Blackwell.

Getis, A., and J. K. Ord. 1992. The analysis of spatial association by use of distance statistics. *Geographical Analysis* 24(3): 189–206.

Gilbert, E. W. 1958. Pioneer maps of health and disease in England. *Geographical Journal* 124 (2): 172–183.

Green, D., and T. Bossomaier. 2002. *Online GIS and Spatial Metadata*. London: Taylor & Francis.

Gruenwald, P. 2007. The spatial ecology of alcohol problems: Niche theory and assortative drinking. *Addiction* 102(6): 870–878.

Hill, L. R. 2006. *Georeferencing: The Geographic Associations of Information*. Cambridge: MIT Press.

Hinman, S. E., J. K. Blackburn, and A. Curtis. 2006. Spatial and temporal structure of typhoid outbreaks in Washington, D.C., 1906–1909: Evaluating local clustering with the G_i^* statistic. *International Journal of Health Geographics* 5: 13.

International Organization for Standardization. 2003. *ISO 19115:2003 Geographic information—Metadata*. http://www.iso.org/iso/catalogue_detail.htm?csnumber=26020 (accessed June 10, 2010).

Jackson, R. J. 2003. The impact of the built environment on health: An emerging field. *American Journal of Public Health* 93(9): 1382–1384.

Jerrett, M., S. Gale, and C. Kontgis. 2010. An environmental health geography of risk. In *A Companion to Health and Medical Geography*, ed. T. Brown, S. McLafferty, and G. Moon. Chichester, UK: Wiley-Blackwell, 418–445.

Kearns, R., and G. Moon. 2002. From medical to health geography: Novelty, place and theory after a decade of change. *Progress in Human Geography* 26(5): 605–625.

Lumsden, L. L. and J. F. Anderson. 1911. *Report No. 4 on the Origin and Prevalence of Typhoid Fever in the District of Columbia (1909–1910)*. Washington, DC: U.S. Government Printing Office.

Maantay, J. A., A. R. Maroko, and H. Porter-Morgan. 2008. Research note—A new method for mapping population and understanding the spatial dynamics of disease in urban areas: Asthma in the Bronx, New York. *Urban Geography* 29(7): 724–738.

MacEachren, A. M., M. S. Stryker, I. J. Turton, and S. Pezanowski. 2010. HEALTH GeoJunction: Place-time-concept browsing of health publications. *International Journal of Health Geographics* 9: 23.

Marples, D. R. 1992. Post-Soviet Belarus and the impact of Chernobyl. *Post-Soviet Geography* 33(9): 419–431.

Martin, S. L. 2005. *Cartography, discourse, and disease: How maps shape scientific thought about disease. Master's thesis*. Atlanta: Georgia State University. http://digitalarchive.gsu.edu/anthro_theses/2/ (accessed September 30, 2010).

Marx, R. W. 1986. The TIGER system: Automating the geographic structure of the United States Census. *Government Publications Review* 13(2): 181–201.

Matyukhin, V. 1992. *Katalog doz oblucheniya zhiteley naselennikh punktov respubliki Belarus'* (Catalog of Radiation Dose of Citizens of Populated Places in the Republic of Belarus). Minsk: Institute of Radiation Medicine, Academy of Medical Science of Belarus (In Russian).

Maxcy, K. F. 1926. An epidemiological study of endemic typhus (Brill's disease) in the Southeastern United States with special reference to its mode of transmission. *Public Health Reports* 41(52): 2967–2995.

May, J. M. 1952. Map of the world distribution of dengue and yellow fever. *Geographical Review* 42(2): 283–286.

McGlamery, P. 1995. Identifying issues and concerns: The University of Connecticut's MAGIC—A case study. *Information Technology and Libraries* 14(2): 116–121.

McGlamery, P. 1997. MAGIC transaction logs as measures of access, use, and community. *The Journal of Academic Librarianship* 23(6): 505–510.

Meade, M. S., and M. Emch. 2010. *Medical geography*, 3rd ed. New York: Guilford.

Morris, S. P. 2010. The North Carolina Geospatial Data Archiving Project: Challenges and initial outcomes. *Journal of Map & Geography Libraries* 6(1): 26–44.

Muhib, F. B., L. S. Lin, A. Stueve, R. L. Miller, W. L. Ford, W. D. Johnson, D. J. Smith, and Community Intervention Trial for Youth Study Team. 2001. A venue-based method for sampling hard-to-reach populations. *Public Health Reports* 116: 216–222.

National Geo-Spatial Intelligence Agency. 2010. *NGA GEONet Names Server (GNS)*. http://earth-info.nga.mil/gns/html/index.html (accessed June 10, 2010).

National Library of Medicine. 1819. *Images from the History of Medicine [Yellow fever: A map of Old Slip and infected vicinity]*. http://ihm.nlm.nih.gov/luna/servlet/view/search?q=A012623 (accessed June 10, 2010).

Oak Ridge National Laboratory. 2010. *LandScan*. http://www.ornl.gov/sci/landscan/ (accessed June 10, 2010).

Pear, R. 2008. Database set to ignore "abortion" in searches. *New York Times*. Saturday, April 5, p. A9.

Pejchvasser, V. et al. 2001. *Atlas Avtomobil'nych dorog: ot Baltiki do Sibiri* (Road Atlas from the Baltic to Siberia). Minsk: Trivium (In Russian).

Rosenau, M. J., L. L. Lumsden, and J. H. Kastle. 1907. Report on the origin and prevalence of typhoid fever in the District of Columbia. Washington, DC: U.S. Government Printing Office.

Rosenau, M. J., L. L. Lumsden, and J. H. Kastle. 1908. Report No. 2 on the origin and prevalence of typhoid fever in the District of Columbia (1907). Washington, DC: U.S. Government Printing Office.

Rosenau, M. J., L. L. Lumsden, and J. H. Kastle. 1909. Report No. 3 on the origin and prevalence of typhoid fever in the District of Columbia (1908). Washington, DC: U.S. Government Printing Office.

Rushton, G., M. P. Armstrong, J. Gittler, B. R. Greene, C. E. Pavlik, M. M. West, and D. L. Zimmerman. 2006. Geocoding in cancer research: A review. *American Journal of Preventive Medicine* 30: S16–S24.

Serebriakova, T. N. 2005. Mapping radiation from the external and internal sources in Belarus after the Chernobyl disaster: Implications for epidemiological analysis.

Doctoral dissertation. Storrs, CT: University of Connecticut, Homer Babbidge Library.

Shannon, G. W. 1981. Disease mapping and early theories of yellow fever. *The Professional Geographer* 33(2): 221–227.

Sherman, J. E., J. Spencer, J. S. Preisser, W. M. Gesler, and T. A. Arcury. 2005. A suite of methods for representing activity space in a healthcare accessibility study. *International Journal of Health Geographics*, 4: 24.

Snow, J. 1855. *On the mode of communication of cholera*, 2nd ed. London: John Churchill.

Tanser, F., P. Gething, and P. Atkinson. 2010. Location-allocation planning. In *A Companion to Health and Medical Geography*, ed. T. Brown, S. McLaffery, and G. Moon. Chichester, UK: Wiley-Blackwell, 540–566.

United States Army Map Service. 1955. *India and Pakistan 1:250,000, Series U502*. Washington, DC: Army Map Service.

U.S. Census Bureau. 2010. *Tiger, Tiger/Line, and Tiger-related products*. http://www.census.gov/geo/www/tiger/ (accessed June 10, 2010).

Wieland, S. C., C. A. Cassa, K. D. Mandl, and B. Berger. 2008. Revealing the spatial distribution of a disease while preserving privacy. *Proceedings of the National Academy of Sciences of the United States of America* 105(46): 17608–17613.

ZAP AGP Belgeodezii. 1992. *Karta Radiatsionnoy Obstanovki*. Minsk: ZAP AGP Belgeodezii.

Enabling Geographic Research Across Disciplines: Building an Institutional Infrastructure for Geographic Analysis at Harvard University

WEIHE WENDY GUAN
Harvard University Center for Geographic Analysis, Cambridge, Massachusetts, USA

BONNIE BURNS
Harvard Map Collection, Cambridge, Massachusetts, USA

JULIA L. FINKELSTEIN
Harvard School of Public Health, Boston, Massachusetts, USA

JEFFREY C. BLOSSOM
Harvard University Center for Geographic Analysis, Cambridge, Massachusetts, USA

Founded in 1818, the Harvard Map Collection (HMC) is the oldest map collection in America, holding 400,000 maps, more than 6,000 atlases, and thousands of reference books. HMC has a strong commitment to digital resources, and it manages the Harvard Geospatial Library, a foundation for geospatial data service at Harvard. The Center for Geographic Analysis (CGA) at Harvard University was founded in 2006, independent of the library system, to serve the entire university. This article presents the history, organizational structure, and operational model of CGA and HMC, reviews achievements, lessons learned, suggests future improvements, and reviews GIS-related medical research at Harvard.

HISTORICAL BACKGROUND

Harvard lost its geography department in 1948 (Smith 1987) and the Computer Graphics and Spatial Analysis Lab in 1991 (Chrisman 2006). Support for maps and geographic analysis for medical research and much of the rest of the university fell on the Harvard Map Collection (HMC)[1] alone, which had limited resources. By the early 2000s the university recognized that it was missing out on the potential contributions the new geography—the approach to geospatial analysis that combined geographic information systems (GIS) technology with quantitative analysis—could make to disciplines across the university, from medicine to epidemiology to sociology to history to trade policy. The question the university faced was How effectively and quickly can we make it possible for students and faculty to bring geospatial to bear on research and teaching (Guan and Bol 2010)? The Center for Geographic Analysis (CGA)[2] was established to do just that (Gehrman 2006), with a mandate to collaborate closely with administrators of the map collection and the ongoing digital library project, the Harvard Geospatial Library[3] (HGL; Siegel, et al. 2004).

HISTORY OF THE HARVARD MAP COLLECTION

The HMC, a unit under the Harvard College Library, was founded in 1818 with the gift of the Ebeling Collection of 10,000 maps and books, presented to the university by Israel Thorndike (Figure 1). The collection has grown consistently since that time. With the transfer of maps after the dissolution of Harvard's Institute for Geographic Exploration, the HMC became one of the largest map collections in North America. Visiting the HMC is an opportunity to see some of the cartographic treasures of the world, because the stacks contain not just paper but also digital materials (Figure 2).

The HMC began its GIS activities in earnest in 1992. More and more cartographic materials were being made available in digital form, but at that time the HMC had only a single PC and it was dedicated to browsing the library catalog. There were data but no methods for library patrons to access them, because the library had no GIS workstations and the staff had minimal GIS experience. There was no support on GIS outside the library, either. The Harvard Graduate School of Design[4] had a strong GIS presence, but support was limited to students in that school. For undergraduates and graduate students in other programs, there were very few options.

At that time, the Association of Research Libraries (ARL)[5] launched the GIS Literacy Project, an effort "to introduce, educate, and equip librarians with skills needed to provide access to spatially referenced data in all formats and to provide effective access to selected electronic information resources in library collections" (Adler 1995). ARL solicited donations and support from the GIS industry to achieve its goals of increased GIS presence in academic libraries. The HMC was in the first wave of libraries to be awarded such support, and it began to build up the infrastructure and staff needed to

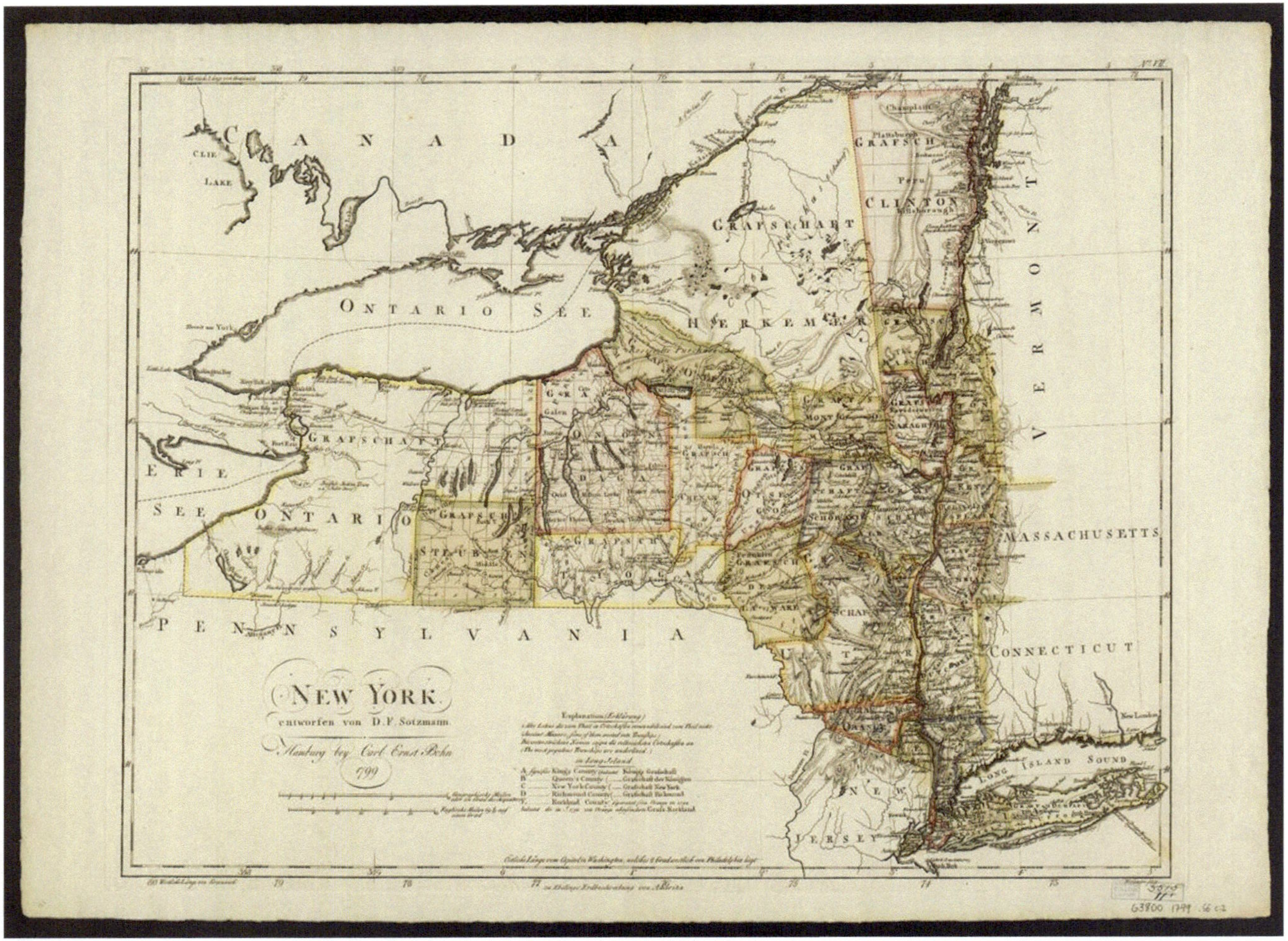

FIGURE 1 New York State by D.F. Sotzmann 1799. From the Ebeling Collection, Harvard Map Collection.

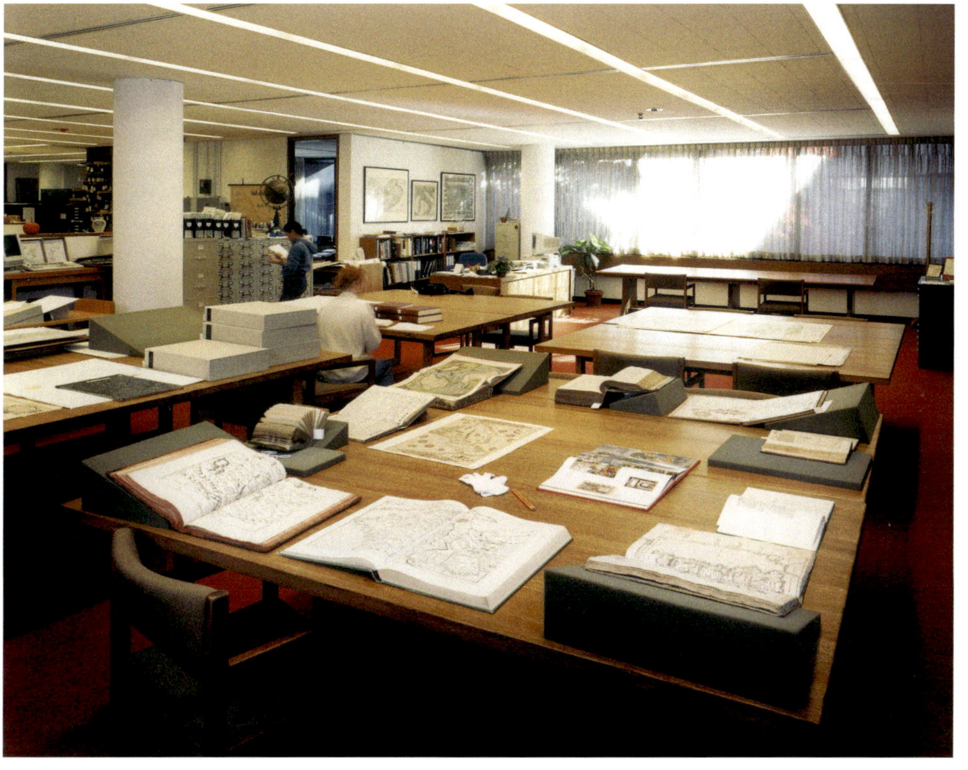

FIGURE 2 Harvard Map Collection reading room, photograph by Peter Vanderwarker, courtesy of Harvard College Library.

provide the research community with a place to go for GIS data, software, and help.

The first step was to provide access to the materials on the HMC shelves. Computers in the reading room were installed with a variety of GIS and cartographic software programs for general use. Staff were trained in ArcView, and they started to answer requests from patrons for simple custom map requests. Students and researchers soon saw the value of GIS, and requests for assistance became more and more complex, to the point where in 1999, a GIS specialist was hired in the HMC to assist with GIS data creation, analysis, and programming.

In addition to creating an infrastructure for GIS support in the library, the HMC began, in 1995, to bring GIS to the Internet via the Massachusetts Electronic Atlas (MEA). Hosted by the HMC and created by Harvard, UMass Boston, and the Metropolitan Area Planning Council, the MEA allowed users to map over 200 variables for the state, including extensive health data, as well as crime statistics and natural resources information (Cobb 1995). The site proved to be quite popular and useful, but did not allow for data downloading; also, it covered only Massachusetts, and therefore did not include data of interest to most students.

A new project was envisioned in 1998, a system that would allow patrons to have access to the rich collection of data in the Harvard libraries at all hours via the Internet (Siegel et al. 2004). This system would not only serve data for download but include a robust search engine, allowing users to quickly find relevant data without having to browse a file system. By 2001, the Harvard Geospatial Library (HGL) was live and receiving 300 hits per day.

HGL currently holds over 6,000 data layers that are ready for use in GIS (Figure 3). These layers are at a variety of scales—from global (VMAP 1) to local (cadastral data for Boston)—covering many different areas of the world and ranging in age from current to 400-year-old historic maps. The catalog is based on detailed Federal Geographic Data Committee[6] Content Standard compliant metadata records that allow for finely tuned searches of the repository. Users can display and download these layers for use in their desktop software.

In addition to current library holdings, HGL is also a distribution mechanism for researcher-created datasets. When GIS projects lead to the creation of new data, those files can be sent to the HMC for inclusion in the repository and catalog. This ability to accept GIS data for distribution led to further collaborations with the CGA since 2006.

ESTABLISHMENT OF THE CENTER FOR GEOGRAPHIC ANALYSIS

The field of geographic analysis underwent a series of revolutions in the past half century. The quantitative revolution brought quantitative analysis into geography in the 1950s, which inspired a new generation of students and scholars (Dutton 2006). The birth of GIS in the 1960s equipped geographic analysis with computers (Niemann and Niemann 1998). Computer cartography and analysis of remotely sensed images in the 1970s presented new dimensions to the discipline. The integration of geographic analysis with numerical models gained much ground in the 1980s, especially in the field of environmental studies. The information technology (IT) boom in the 1990s gave geographic analysis a swift push into the IT mainstream, complete with relational and object-oriented database management systems, programming platforms, client server architectures, and Web-based implementations. Completion of the Global Positioning System (GPS) and the ever-increasing earth surveillance satellites resulted in an exponential increase of spatial data in native digital format, feeding content to, and at the same time putting pressure on, the GIS. By the middle of this century's first decade, Google released Google Maps and Google Earth, which generated a heightened public interest in geographical issues and expanded awareness of geography in

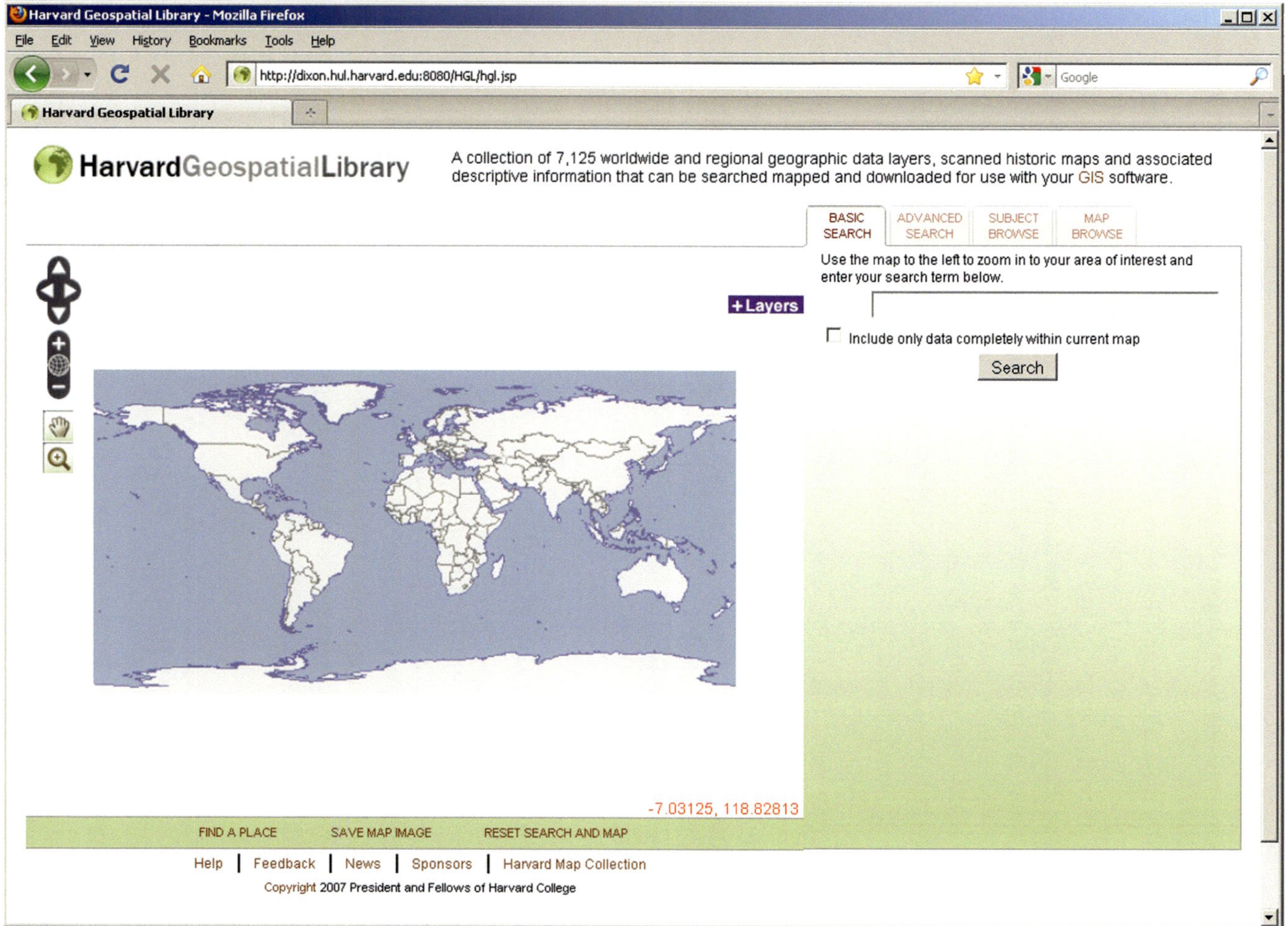

FIGURE 3 The Harvard Geospatial Library entry page.

other disciplines. The geo-technological revolution is still ongoing, pushing geographic analysis up to computing clouds and down to mobile devices, into the hands of people from all walks of life. Its continued growth has expanded the job market for geographers, increased enrollment in geography departments, and brought improvement in geography education at all levels (Murphy 2007).

In 2003, a faculty committee on spatial analysis was formed at Harvard University, led by Professor Peter Bol, a prominent historian and a pioneer in applying GIS to the study of history. The committee was set to find a solution for the increasing concerns from faculty and students on improving access to spatial data, supporting research in geospatial analysis, and developing curricula. Two years of investigation and discussion led to the decision by the university president and the provost to establish the Center for Geographic Analysis (CGA). Inauguration of the center was held May 5, 2006 (Gehrman 2006), a day some called "a new dawn for geography at Harvard" (Waters 2006).

From day one, the CGA has been focused on research and education in the field of spatial analysis and geographic information. Building on the foundation established by the HMC and HGL, the CGA was expected to create a more substantial infrastructure to support a wide range of scholarly research projects designed to apply, improve, or study geospatial analysis techniques. One of the largest and most advanced user groups is Harvard's medical and public health research community.

MULTIFACETED MEDICAL RESEARCH AT HARVARD UNIVERSITY

Medical research is conducted at a number of institutions at Harvard University, including the Harvard School of Public Health, the Harvard Medical School (see Figure 4) and affiliated hospitals, the Harvard Humanitarian Initiative, the Harvard Initiative for Global Health, and the Faculty of Arts and Sciences. The following section describes the application of geographic analysis and GIS to the medical research being conducted at Harvard University.

APPLICATION OF GEOGRAPHIC ANALYSIS TO MEDICAL AND PUBLIC HEALTH RESEARCH

Early applications of geographic analysis to medical research can be traced to the small Soho district in London in 1854. John Snow, a British physician, identified the Broad Street water pump as the source of one of the most severe cholera epidemics in history by using observational data and a series of maps. Based on this work, he is considered the father of modern epidemiology, one of the cornerstones of public health (Singer and de Castro 2001). John Snow's study was a transformative event in the history of medical geography and public health. The handle of the Broad Street pump has become a symbol, marking the integration of medicine, geographic analysis, and public health research.

Over 150 years since John Snow's cholera outbreak investigation, geographic analysis remains intricately linked to medical research. The application of spatial analytic techniques to understand the distribution of disease and determinants of health is at the core of medical and public health research. During the past two decades, advances in technologies have made it possible to examine spatial and temporal trends in large-scale epidemiological data with enhanced precision and speed.

GIS techniques are ideally suited for public health surveillance and infectious disease control, as transmission of infectious diseases is closely related to geographic proximity. This includes locating cases; identifying clusters; and mapping epidemic dynamics, disease burden, and response. More recently, geographic analytic methods have been applied to the fields of environmental health and chronic disease epidemiology to link proximity to exposure with incidence of noncommunicable diseases. Application of GIS methods and collaborative data sharing has also contributed to the emerging fields of crisis mapping and response to natural disasters and infectious disease outbreaks, to inform timely targeted emergency responses, resource allocation, and health care delivery strategies.

Understanding spatial and temporal distribution of disease is central to targeting health problems. Using GIS facilitates exploration of a broad range of determinants—such as demographic, socioeconomic, geographic, and environmental factors—from a diverse array of disciplines that influence disease transmission patterns in a single environment.

Geographic analysis provides a unique interface between health data and a map to effectively present information to key decision makers. GIS methods enable summation and presentation of large amounts of data for disease surveillance and health reporting, and they can identify new cases, map at-risk populations, stratify risk factors, and quantify distribution of risk and transmission patterns. Optimal summary and visual presentation of complex medical and scientific health data can be used to communicate abstract quantitative data and inform health care policy, program planning, and health resource allocation. Geographic analysis also informs evidence-based policy and program planning, such as the design, implementation, and monitoring of targeted interventions, and it examines patterns of disease burden and health care delivery. Selected examples of applying geographic analysis to medical research at Harvard University are presented in Table 1.

EXAMPLES OF GIS IN MEDICAL RESEARCH AT HARVARD

Geographic analysis and examining medical research questions spatially have helped to integrate medical and public health research across disciplines and

TABLE 1 Selected Medical Research Projects at Harvard University

Faculty	Department/Program	Selected GIS-related Projects
Harvard School of Public Health	Dept. of Environmental Health, Exposure, Epidemiology and Risk Program	• Worcester Heart Attack Study • Eastern Massachusetts Pollution Study • Normative Aging Study • ACCESS Study • Investigating Local Air Pollution Sources in Dudley Square, Boston
	Occupational Health	• Taiwan Petrochemical Study
	Society, Human Development and Health Dept.	• Public Health Disparities Geocoding Project • Socioeconomic trends in breast cancer incidence • Objective measures of outdoor recreational areas • Neighborhood and school environments and youth physical activity • Play Across Boston** • Human Development in Chicago Neighborhoods
	Global Health and Population	• Spatial Aspects of Contraceptive Use in Malawi • Spatial Patterns in Malaria Transmission • Health, Poverty and Place: Modeling Inequalities in Accra Using RS and GIS • Human rabies focusing on dog ecology in Sri Lanka
	Biostatistics	• Integrating ground monitoring data and satellite observations to estimate PM2.5 concentrations in the eastern United States
	Nutrition	• Nurses Health Study • Ecological covariates of infections in children in KwaZulu-Natal, South Africa
Brigham and Women's Hospital*	Channing Laboratory	• Trucking Industry Particle (TrIP) • Nurses Health Study: Spatio-temporal estimation of particulate matter exposure • Physical Activity and the Built Environment • Home Allergens and Asthma Study • Safe Surgery Saves Lives Web Map • Youth Tobacco Initiative—School and Retail Outlet Analysis
	Div. of Rheumatology, Immunology and Allergy	• Roxbury Lupus Project
Children's Hospital, Boston*	Informatics Program	• The Automated Epidemiologic Geotemporal Integrated Surveillance System • HealthMap.org (Live Disease Outbreak Mapping)
Massachusetts General Hospital*		• Edmap.org (Emergency Dept. Mapping) • Physical Activity in the Built Environment Study
Dana Farber Cancer Institute*		• Organ Transplant Proximity Study • Community Health Center / Public Housing Distance Analysis
Harvard Humanitarian Initiative		• Crisis Mapping and Early Warning Project • Incubator Implementation Tracking

Note. *Harvard affiliated Hospital; **http://www.hsph.harvard.edu/prc/proj_play.html

departments at Harvard University. For example, the Exposure, Epidemiology and Risk Program at the Harvard School of Public Health brings together the departments of environmental health and epidemiology to explore environmental and occupational determinants of health and disease and to inform evidence-based policy.

Researchers have applied novel GIS techniques and cutting-edge statistical methods to longitudinal epidemiological studies to answer unanticipated research questions not envisioned at the study onset. The Nurses Health Study, inaugurated in 1976 in the Department of Nutrition, is among the largest and longest running investigations of factors that influence women's health. This study of over 238,000 nurses has led to many new insights into health and disease. Researchers in the Exposure, Epidemiology and Risk Program and the Departments of Environmental Health, Nutrition, and Epidemiology have applied GIS techniques to analyze data from the Nurses Health Study. They used semiempirical models to predict spatially and temporally resolved long-term average outdoor concentrations of particulate matter (PM) (Yanosky, Paciorek, et al. 2008). They have also successfully predicted chronic fine and coarse particulate exposures using spatio-temporal models for the northeastern and midwestern United States (Yanosky, Paciorek, et al. 2009). Spatial methods are also being incorporated into new research designs for longitudinal studies; in fact, the third Nurses Health Study is currently under way over three decades later, examining environmental and lifestyle exposures of women.

Similarly, researchers have applied GIS methods to examine long-term, ambient multipollutant exposures (PM10, PM2.5, nitrogen dioxide, and sulfur dioxide) in 53,814 men in the U.S. trucking industry and found that residential ambient air pollution exposures were associated with significantly increased mortality (Hart, Garshick, et al. 2010). GIS methods have also been applied to the Harvard Six Cities Study, one of the most influential, innovative, and long-running studies to address the health effects of air pollution in America; this landmark study has led to the regulation of airborne particulate matter and the development of the Clean Air Act.

Geographic analysis has also been used in medical research to target advocacy and social justice in resource-limited settings. In an example of geographic analysis bringing together the university with the community, researchers examined the influence of traffic on air quality in an urban neighborhood (Buonocore, Lee, et al. 2009). In this project in the Mission Hill neighborhood of Boston, Massachusetts, GIS methods were used to examine spatial and temporal patterns of traffic-related air pollutants to determine factors contributing to elevated concentrations and to inform environmental justice concerns. In another project in Malawi, Africa, investigators used GIS methods and data from the Malawi Health Facility Inventory and the Malawi Demographic and Health Survey to identify disparities in access to modern reproductive health services (Heard, Larsen, et al. 2004).

Geographic analysis has been transformative in international medical research at Harvard University. GIS technologies have allowed researchers to send portable GPS units to remote field settings to monitor conflict zones, urban slums, and remote villages, and provide precise health data in areas with limited infrastructure. GIS and remote sensing technologies have also been used to identify host habitats and clusters of cases, examine infectious disease transmission patterns, and inform targeted interventions. For example, researchers in the Department of Nutrition at the Harvard School of Public Health used GIS methods to examine ecological determinants of parasitic infections in school children of rural KwaZulu-Natal, South Africa, including *Ascaris lumbricoides* and hookworm (Saathoff, Olsen, et al. 2005). Researchers in the Department of Global Health and Population also obtained complete coverage of larval control to suppress malaria vector mosquitoes through comprehensive spatial coverage with community-derived sketch maps in Dar es Salaam, Tanzania (Dongus, Nyika, et al. 2007). Researchers also used spatial and temporal analysis of malaria risk to inform policies for disease control in the Amazon region of Brazil (Singer and de Castro 2001).

Geographic analysis has also emerged with increasingly important humanitarian projects. In the aftermath of natural disasters, such as the 2010 earthquake in Haiti, GIS technologies have played a critical role in rapid and efficient response to crises and in conducting public health research to develop and monitor evidence-based programs. GIS also plays an important role in crisis-mapping initiatives and developing early warning systems to mitigate the effects of natural disasters, avert mass atrocities, strengthen international aid coordination, inform resource allocation, and develop evidence-based humanitarian interventions.

The Harvard Humanitarian Initiative (HHI) is a university-wide center formed by multiple entities within the Harvard community. It provides expertise in public health, medicine, social science, management, and other disciplines to respond to complex humanitarian emergencies. In the Humanitarian Crisis Mapping and Early Warning project, GIS methods and mapping technologies are used to promote evidence-based approaches to humanitarian assistance, and to advance the science and practice of humanitarian response worldwide. For example, in the Incubator Implementation project in Indonesia, GPS devices were used to map remote areas where incubators were placed. Within the HHI and the Harvard medical community at large, researchers understand the utility of GIS technology in their research, and they use it for a diverse range of projects.

COLLABORATION BETWEEN CGA AND HMC

To effectively support the diverse needs for geographic analysis from the Harvard medical community as well as the university at large, CGA established a governing structure that includes faculty members from the medical school and the School of Public Health in its faculty steering committee and key GIS professionals from the library and the medical campus in its technical advisory committee. The faculty committee meets once per semester to guide the center in its strategic development, while the technical advisory committee meets three times per semester to advise the center in its technical operation, such as service level and distribution, technology adaptation, outreach event coordination, and feedback from the user community. Staff of HMC and HGL serve on the CGA technical committee, while CGA staff serve on the HGL standing committee. This cross-organizational structure provides a forum for regular checks and balances of the shared responsibilities between the CGA and the HMC in optimizing user support.

DATA ACQUISITION, DEVELOPMENT, AND SHARING

Data is usually the first thing a user asks for when considering geographic analysis. Using each organization's strength, the HMC focuses on systematically acquiring geospatial data, making them available, and helping users find the appropriate data precisely and quickly from the Harvard Library holdings. The CGA often refers users to the HMC for data-related questions, such as data availability, source, cost, and format. Patrons interested in historical data are often forced to create that data on their own by digitizing paper maps, and HMC has a larger format scanner that can be used to create an image of any material in the collection. Those images can be georeferenced with assistance from either CGA or HMC, and the relevant information can be digitized. When users receive their data, they can return to CGA for help in analyzing and visualizing the data. If the patron requires less complex analysis or straightforward cartography, he or she can get that help at HMC.

Many research projects require unique data not yet acquired by the library but that are available from well-known public data sources, such as international data, high resolution images, or data custom-created by a researcher or a research institution. CGA facilitates the identification of such data sources; helps define and clarify the data properties and quality; serves as liaison between Harvard data users and some data companies and institutions; manages data development service and cross-institutional, data-sharing contracts; and assists the users in submitting their unique data to the HGL with proper permission. The HMC takes on the responsibility of geospatial data stewardship alone, freeing the CGA to focus on analysis services.

Whether data is acquired by CGA or HMC, the goal is to hold on to it and make it available to future researchers. Although licensing restrictions sometimes prohibit data sharing, whenever possible new data are deposited into the HGL. For that the data are delivered to HMC and translated into the HGL-accepted format (ArcSDE layers). Metadata that is compliant with the FGDC standard is created by the Harvard College Library geospatial resources cataloger, and the data is published via HGL. Many layers are restricted to Harvard affiliates only, but all metadata is publically searchable so that non-Harvard researchers can at least discover that a data set exists and get information on how to obtain the layer for themselves. Every effort is made to license data for use by the entire Harvard community. However, sometimes that is just not possible, and only a single user is allowed access at any time. In those cases, metadata is still created and placed in the HGL catalog with information on where to access the data set on campus. By collaborating in this way, CGA and HMC have increased the size and value of the HGL collections as well as the usefulness of the system to patrons.

SOFTWARE LICENSES AND LABS

The CGA manages all university-wide geospatial software license contracts and equips computer labs across the university with updated versions of GIS, image processing, spatial data conversion, visualization and geostatistical analysis software packages from multiple companies, as well as some freeware and open-source GIS tools. Most of these software licenses are managed through a centralized license server, with one or two backup servers to maintain uninterrupted availability. The HMC maintains a small lab of PCs equipped with GIS software distributed by CGA, as well as powerful desktop publishing applications that can be used to create professional-quality illustrations.

The Harvard medical community has unique license requirements because of its geographically distributed nature. Many Harvard Medical School and HSPH faculty members also work in the various hospitals in Boston. The CGA provides special assistance to them, making sure that their research and teaching needs are supported by the university floating licenses, while these licenses are not mistakenly used in the hospitals' operation, which would be a violation of the university site license agreement.

TRAINING PROGRAMS

Before the establishment of the CGA, the HMC GIS staff offered hands-on training in both GIS and remote sensing, which were converted into online tutorials. These tutorial materials continued to be available online through the HMC Web site. In addition, the CGA offers a multifaceted GIS training program both on the main campus and on the Longwood medical campus. This includes a number of credit courses at the introduction level, senior thesis level, and graduate student level, tailored to meet the different needs of students in different disciplines such as social sciences, environmental sciences, engineering, and public health. It also includes noncredit courses and a series of hands-on training seminars of geographic analysis tools and methodologies open to all Harvard affiliates every Friday during the academic year. Since 2009, the CGA has added a 10-day intensive training program called the Harvard GIS Institute, for faculty and graduate students who wish to learn GIS during the winter or summer breaks. The program is so popular that some applicants must wait a year to obtain a seat in it. Software-specific, self-learning tutorials are easily accessible from the CGA Web site as well.

These training programs and the CGA's technical consultation services feed and back each other up, and, combined with the HMC's data service, they form a balanced support network to users with different needs. Some researchers come to CGA for technical consultation first, but as their projects develop, they realize that it would be more efficient if they themselves could do some hands-on GIS work, thus they sign up for the training and gradually become more independent in designing and conducting their geographic analysis. On the contrary, some researchers at first have unrealistic goals in their geographic analysis project. After taking the training courses, they realize that GIS is not as simple as just learning to use a piece of software. Their time would be better spent focusing on their disciplinary topics, leaving the geographic analysis work to the CGA staff. Thus they become more frequent users of the CGA analytical services after the training.

Many students who have taken these courses or training programs have gone on to apply geographic analysis to their thesis or dissertation. In the past five years, one of the authors who served on the review committee for the Howard T. Fisher Prize in GIS[7] has witnessed significant improvement in the complexity and quality of GIS work among the award applicants. This observation is shared by all members of the review committee.

CONSULTATION AND HELP DESKS

The CGA has designated office hours when users can walk in and ask for help (Figure 5). Questions addressed at the CGA help desks include where to find certain data, how to do certain analyses, which software tool is most appropriate for certain projects, how much to budget for geographic analysis in certain grant proposals, which GPS model meets certain field work needs, how to design the database or Web service for certain projects, how to quickly learn certain GIS skills, and many more. The CGA help desks on the main campus and the medical campus, together with the virtual help desk (24 hour response time by e-mail or phone) serves over 100 inquires per month on average. Users include faculty members, research associates, postdoctoral fellows, graduate and undergraduate students, staff, and visiting scholars. Among them, graduate students are the most numerous help-desk users.

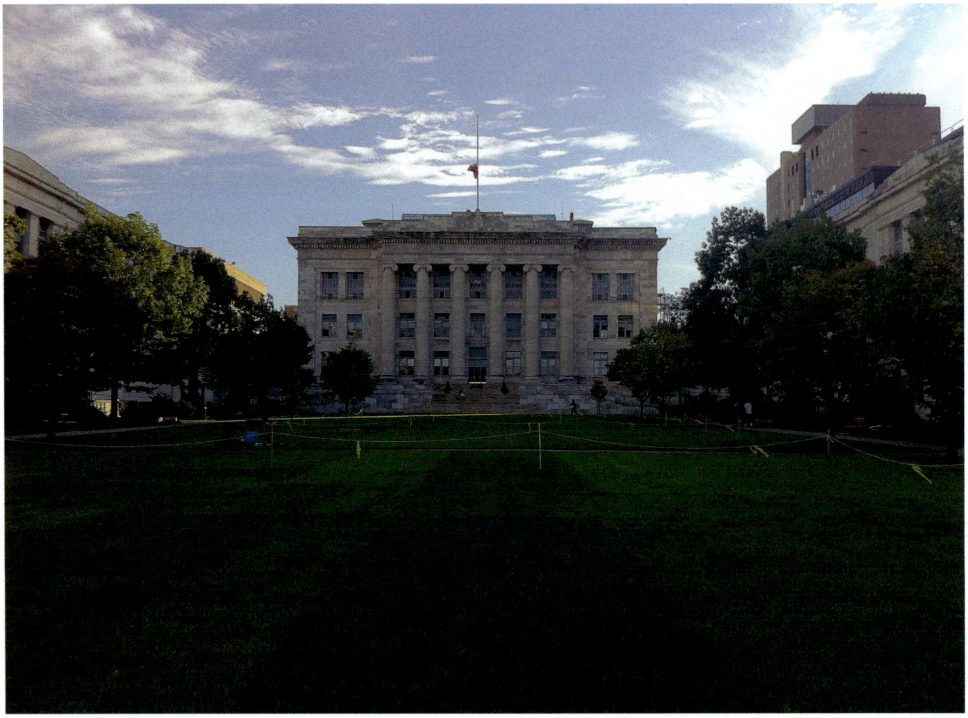

FIGURE 4 The Harvard medical campus.

The HMC reference desk gets GIS and digital data requests daily, and the questions tend to be from patrons who may not even know what GIS is or how it can help them. There are no set hours for GIS-related questions, because patrons are just as likely to be looking for a road atlas as for GIS help. Patrons with time-consuming requests are often asked to schedule an appointment, and complex projects are referred back to CGA. Most GIS interactions are with undergraduates, but there are also many graduate students being introduced to GIS for the first time at the HMC reference desk.

ANALYTICAL SERVICES

In some cases, a help-desk visit could lead to a follow-up consultation session, which could lead to a more dedicated service project. At this capacity, the CGA operates like an internal consulting firm, working with the users to define project scope, specify deliverables, estimate risks and uncertainties, plan alternatives, set schedules and milestones, and calculate service costs. Most of such service projects are completed internally by CGA staff, but a portion of them involves outsourcing services, too. For those cases, the CGA staff identify appropriate external service providers, negotiate service

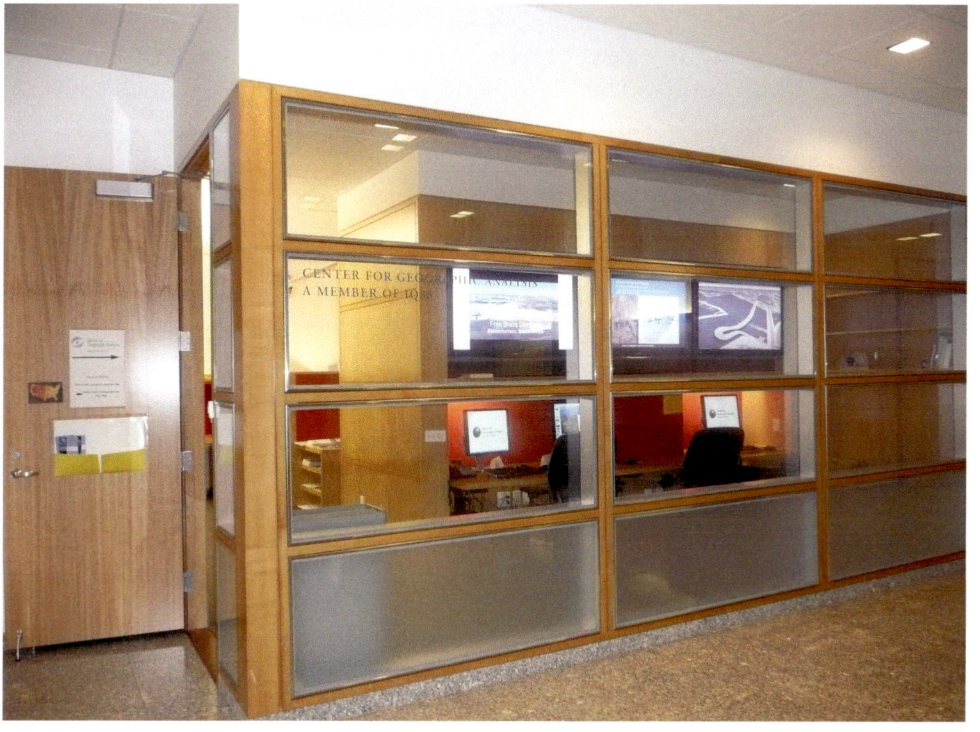

FIGURE 5 The CGA front office and help desk.

contracts, communicate technical requirements, perform quality assessment and quality control on their deliverables, and manage the external contracts for the end users. Work requiring external services are usually labor-intensive (such as digitizing features from historical maps), or highly specialized (such as developing a software module to plug into certain CGA systems). Another type of CGA service supports teaching directly, where the CGA staff would develop and deliver a customized GIS training module for a non-GIS class or research team. Such training is usually followed up by more hand-holding when the students or researchers start to use what they have learned to apply geographic analysis in their course work or research project. The authors will discuss more specific geographic analysis service cases in support of medical research at Harvard in the next issue of this publication.

TECHNOLOGY MONITORING

With the rapid evolution of geospatial technology, many faculty and students find that even after investing significant time learning the GIS tools, it is still very hard to keep their skills and knowledge up-to-date with the changes. They could be proficient with one version of a popular software program or one model of popular equipment, but after a couple of years they are again at a loss when facing the new versions, new models, new data formats, or new visualization trends. The CGA staff serves as the geospatial technology steward for the Harvard GIS user community, monitoring, evaluating, reporting, selectively acquiring new technology products, and introducing new methodologies, standards, architectural platforms, and technology services. They attend the major geospatial conferences periodically, subscribe to the popular technical newsletters and journals, and remain active in the geospatial professionals' circle. In return, they publish a monthly newsletter for over 1,000 readers and maintain the CGA Web site that averages over 1,000 hits daily.

The CGA also hosts annual conferences, providing a forum for Harvard users to exchange ideas and experiences with invited scholars on geospatial technology and its application in designated fields. Conference themes include GIS, remote sensing, geocoding/georeferencing, spatial-temporal modeling, technology applications in the study of religion, global temporal gazetteer development, and Web mapping. Another technology forum is cosponsored by the CGA and the Harvard grassroots technology group called ABCD-GIS.[8] The monthly brown-bag seminars bring out speakers from the Harvard GIS professional community and other universities, companies, and government agencies. It is open to the GIS community at Harvard and beyond.

WEB MAP SERVICES

Anyone who has kept an eye on the geospatial technology trend in recent years would not have missed the wave of Web services. In addition to the HGL discussed earlier, the CGA has developed and continues to enhance a number of Web-mapping applications, engaging in a variety of technology platforms from ArcGIS Server (ESRI 2008) to GoogleMap API to complete open-source systems built on OpenLayers, MapServer, and PostgreSQL (Lewis and Guan 2010). Among them are several applications in support of medical research, such as the Surgical Safety Web Map and the Emergency Department Web Map. These applications will be discussed in detail in the next issue of this publication.

The WorldMap is an example of collaboration between the CGA and the HMC at the system development and collections levels. It was built to assist academic research and teaching as well as the general public with an open-source system that allows for discovery, investigation, analysis, visualization, communication, and archiving multidisciplinary, multisource and multiformat data, organized spatially and temporally. The first instance of WorldMap was focused on Africa, called AfricaMap (Lewis and Guan 2010).[9] Since its beta release in November 2008, the framework has been implemented in several different locations with different research focuses, including metro Boston, East Asia, Vermont geological sites, Harvard Forest and the city of Paris. These Web mapping applications are used in courses and by individual researchers. Figure 6 shows the Malaria seasonal variation overlaid on population density in AfricaMap.

Some data layers presented in the WorldMap systems are contributed by the HMC, and some data layers acquired by these systems are in turn submitted to the HMC for long-term archiving. Moreover, critical data layers in these systems are included in HGL, and the download function calls an HGL download service directly. This cross-system integration avoids the duplication of data storage and system development, offering the users a seamless experience utilizing both systems behind the scenes. Further integration is under development that will allow cross-serving of data layers between the two systems as Web map services (WMS) and Web feature services (WFS).

CONCLUSION

The HMC, with a history of nearly two centuries, and the CGA, with merely 5 years of existence, form the core components of the infrastructure in support of geographic analysis at Harvard University today. Their success relies on collaboration, not only between each other, but also with various research support organizations in the schools and departments throughout the university (Figure 7). The CGA's Technical Advisory Committee includes members from not only the libraries, but also the Harvard-MIT Data Center, the Institute for Quantitative Social Sciences, the Instructional Computing Group of the Faculty of Arts and Sciences, the Computer Resources Group of the Graduate School of Design, the Harvard School of Public Health, the Harvard Planning and Allston Initiative, the FAS Department of Earth and Planetary Science, and the School of Engineering and Applied Sciences. Each of these organizations provides infrastructure support to their department, school, or the university at large, and covers different technology domains, such as statistical analysis, database management, Web design and development, computer-aided design, three-dimensional visualization, and system engineering. Geospatial technology intertwines with these technology domains, and the CGA receives support from these organizations while providing support to them at the same time. The CGA staff could be an end user of their service in one project, a collaborative partner in another project, and a subject matter expert offering consultation service to them in yet another project. For example, the CGA is an end user of the Dataverse Network (DVN) for data archiving and dissemination; the CGA staff and the DVN development team are working together to explore methodologies for mapping the study cased in the DVN; and the CGA has built a geographic location finder tool for

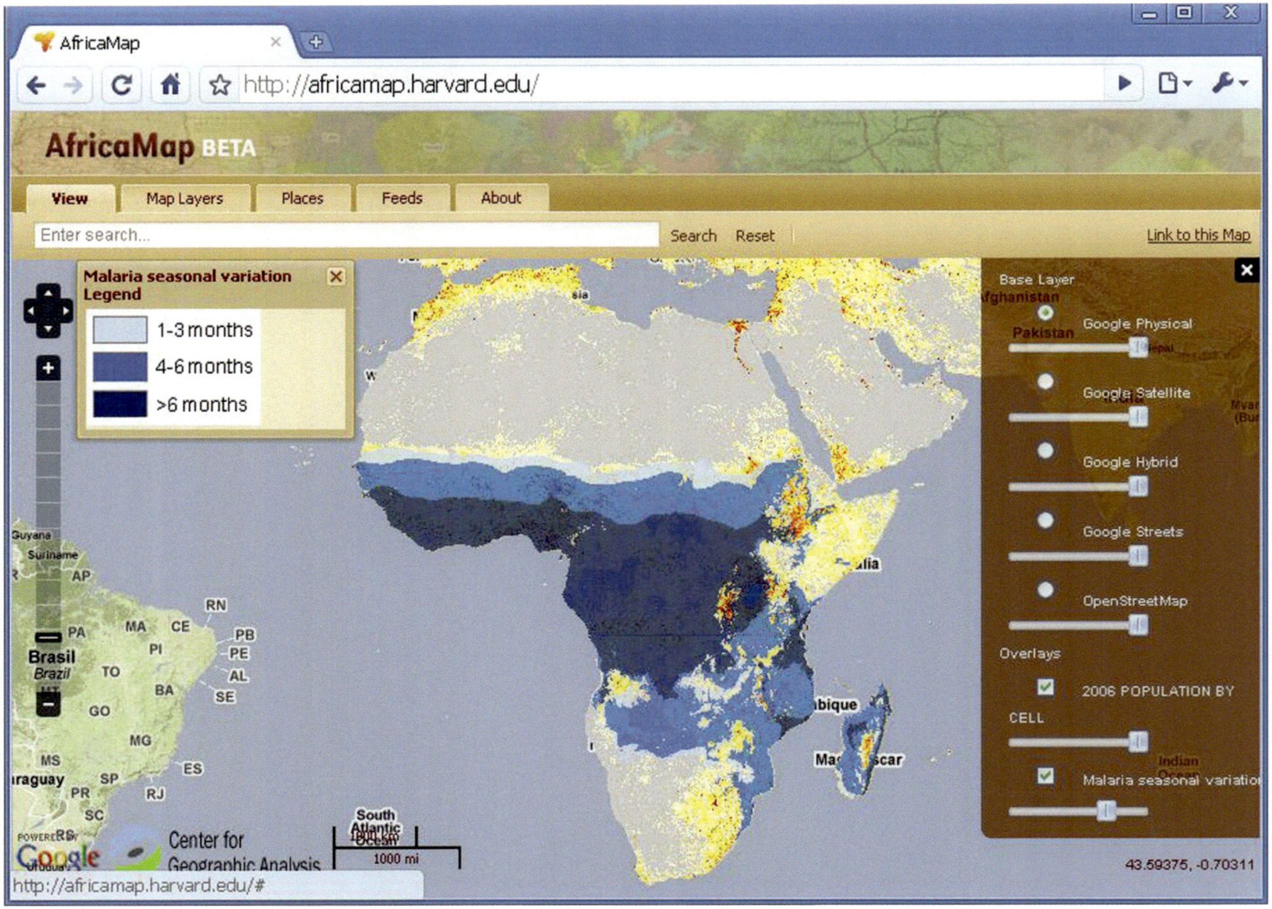

FIGURE 6 Malaria seasonal variation overlaid on population density in AfricaMap.

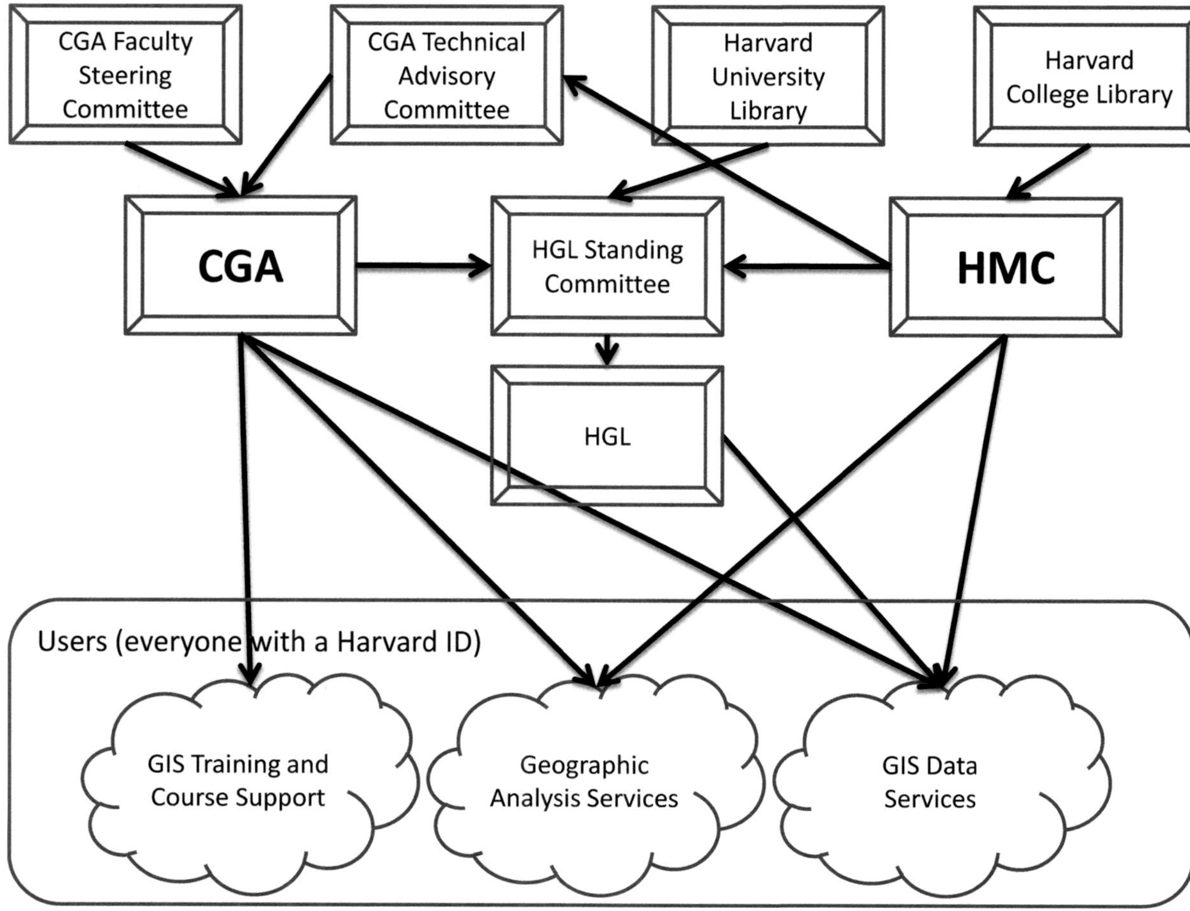

FIGURE 7 The institutional relationship among CGA, HMC, and other organizations.

the DVN users to populate the latitude and longitude fields in the metadata when they submit data to the DVN.

These multidimensional collaborations form a support web, providing many places and methods for patrons to start their projects with the proper technology support, and to be guided to geographic analysis if their projects call for it. This support web also ensures that the people in each place work together, each according to their own strengths, to get the patron the help he or she needs. It avoids redundant capacity building, which is critically important in the current financial decline. For example, the CGA does not invest in long-term data repository. All geospatial data that are worth archiving are handed over to the HMC to be properly cataloged, loaded into HGL for user download, and archived in the Harvard Digital Repository Service.

Such a collaborative infrastructure is not without challenges. Harvard University has the tradition of being a distributed system, with each organization operating under autonomous terms, described as "every tub has its own bottom." Many excellent support teams have been focused on supporting their own department or school only, with no mandate or capacity to provide support across the administrative boundaries. The CGA's operational model broke this tradition. It was established to serve the entire university from the beginning. But five years into its operation, the CGA has yet to reach out to all potential users. The demand on CGA's service is still growing exponentially, almost doubling every year (Figure 8). Outreach and coordination continue to be major tasks for CGA, competing for limited resources with technical projects.

Moreover, for users familiar and satisfied with CGA services, CGA became their "one-stop shop" for technology support. It is often hard for end users to clearly define their project's need for the different technical domains. Oftentimes one project needs data acquisition, database design, Web development, geographic analysis, and statistical modeling. Researchers may not be familiar with all the specialty support teams for each of these components. They may rely on CGA or whichever team they are most familiar with, to help them define their project scope, identify technology needs, and establish initial contact with the other specialty teams.

The CGA's operational model has not only bridged among the technical support teams, but has also made cross-disciplinary and cross-school connections. People from all parts of the university come to CGA for assistance in finding data, making maps, selecting analytical tools, or receiving training. The broad user contacts have put CGA staff in a unique position to help make cross-disciplinary connections for scholars. An epidemiologist from the Harvard School of Public Health might be looking for the same census data as a political scientist from the Harvard Kennedy School of Government studying violence, and an entomologist from the Harvard Museum of Comparative Zoology may be interested in building the same digital

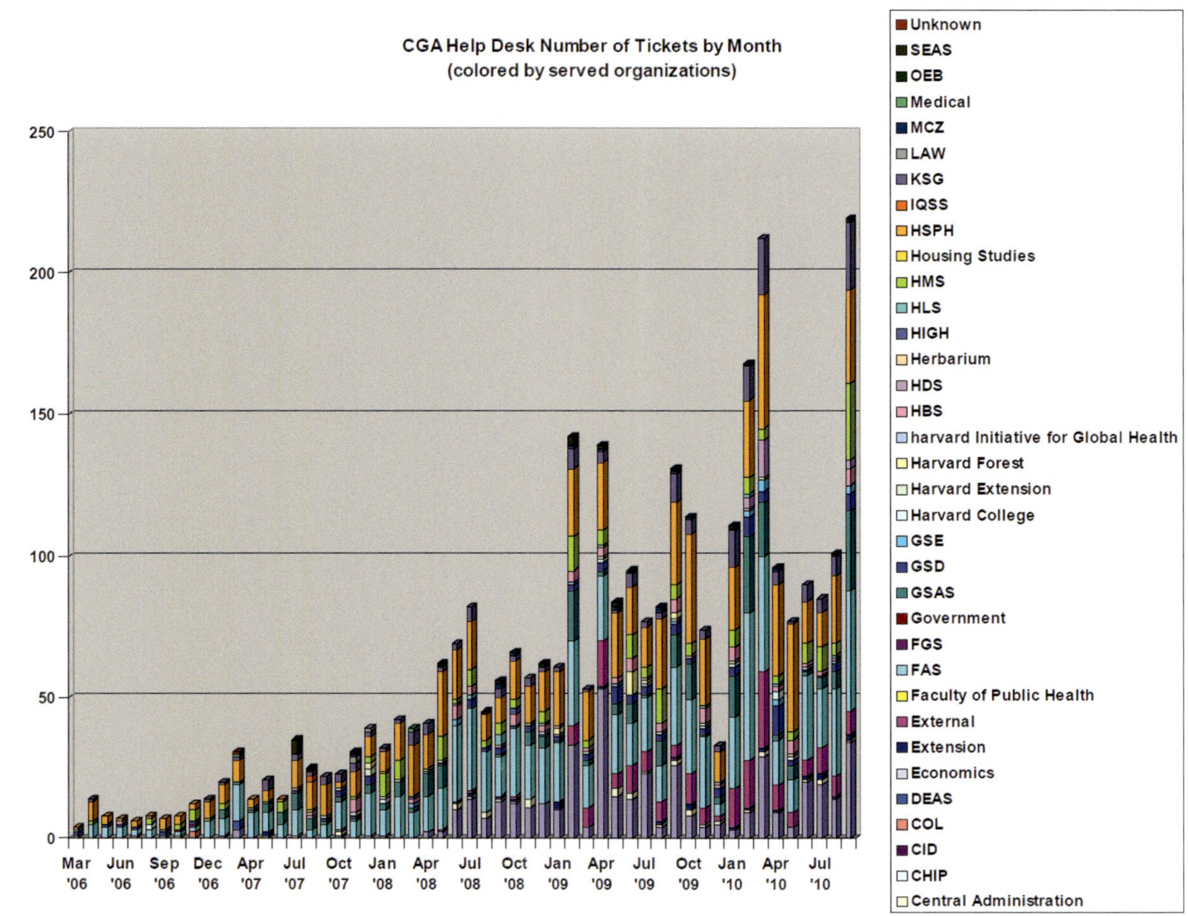

FIGURE 8 CGA help number of tickets (2006–2010).

elevation model and hydrologic network as a historian or archaeologist studying ancient trade routes. Through the CGA, some of them have become aware of others' work in the same region of the world, made contacts with each other, shared base data and local data sources, coordinated equipment usage (such as GPS), and some have even found other's work inspiring to their own research (Guan and Bol 2009).

The CGA started with a humble beginning of three FTEs and a two-room office. By the fifth year, it has doubled its annual budget, tripled its staff, and quadrupled its office space. The core funding from the provost office has allowed for the CGA to offer basic services free of charge to anyone with a Harvard ID, including help desk, noncredit training, and initial consultation service. An educational endowment supports the GIS Institute, and income from service projects, grants, and gifts makes up the rest of the operational budget. By focusing on serving everybody else across the university, the CGA has gradually advanced its own status despite the financial hardships of the past year.

The HMC and the CGA share the same mission of enabling geographic research across disciplines. The quest to build an institutional infrastructure for geographic analysis at Harvard University has just begun. As the geospatial technology evolves and people's awareness and expectations increase, both the HMC and the CGA will continue to adapt and adjust in order to improve efficiency and effectiveness, to better serve research and teaching at Harvard University.

NOTES

1. Harvard Map Collection Web site: http://hcl.harvard.edu/libraries/maps/
2. Center for Geographic Analysis Web site: http://cga.harvard.edu/
3. Harvard Geospatial Library Web site: http://hgl.harvard.edu
4. Harvard GSD Web site: http://gsd.harvard.edu
5. ARL Web site: http://www.arl.org/
6. FGDC Web site: http://www.fgdc.gov
7. The Howard T. Fisher Prize in GIS website: http://gis.harvard.edu/icb/icb.do?keyword=k235&pageid=icb.page190018
8. The ABCD-GIS group Web site: http://www.abcd.harvard.edu/harvard/groups/abcd-gis/
9. AfricaMap Web site: http://africamap.harvard.edu

REFERENCES

Adler, P. S. 1995. A special issue of geographic information systems and academic libraries: An introduction. *Journal of Academic Librarianship* 21(4): 233–235.

Buonocore, J. J., H. J. Lee, et al. (2009). The influence of traffic on air quality in an urban neighborhood: A community-university partnership. *Am J Public Health* 99(Suppl 3): S629–635.

Chrisman, N. 2006. Charting the unknown: How computer mapping at Harvard became GIS. Redlands, CA: ESRI Press.

Cobb, D. A. 1995. Developing GIS Relationships. *Journal of Academic Librarianship* 21(4): 275–277.

Cobb D. A., and A. Olivero. 1997. Online GIS Service, *Journal of Academic Librarianship* 23(6): 484–497.

Dongus, S., D. Nyika, et al. 2007. Participatory mapping of target areas to enable operational larval source management to suppress malaria vector mosquitoes in Dar es Salaam, Tanzania. *Int J Health Geogr* 6: 37.

Dutton, G. 2006. Everything is where it is having moved there. A memoir on the occasion of the dedication of the Harvard Center for Geographic Analysis. http://isites.harvard.edu/fs/docs/icb/topic39008.files//Dutton_Memoir.pdf (accessed November 23, 2010).

ESRI. 2008. China earthquake Geospatial Research Portal launched by Harvard University. ArcNews Online, Fall 2008. http://www.esri.com/news/arcnews/fall08articles/china=earthquake.html (accessed November 23, 2010).

Gehrman, E. 2006. Geography center launched—Center for Geographical Analysis to explore "vast intellectual territory." *Harvard Gazette*. May 11 2006. http://www.news.harvard.edu/gazette/2006/05.11/05-geography.html

Guan, W. W., and P. Bol. 2009. Harvard revisited: Geography's return as GIS. *In The Geography Teacher* 6(2).

Guan, W. W., and P. Bol. 2010. Embracing geographic analysis beyond geography—Harvard's Center for Geographic Analysis enters its 5th year. *International Journal of Applied Geospatial Research* (in press).

Guan, W. W., and G. Huang. 2009. Bringing operational GIS into university classrooms. *Geomatica—Special Issue on Higher Education in Geomatics* 63(2).

Gudrais, E. 2010. Harvard Center's maps help Haiti effort. *Harvard Magazine*, January 19 2010. http://harvardmagazine.com/breaking-news/harvard-center-hosts-haiti-map-portal (accessed November 23, 2010).

Hart, J. E., E. Garshick, et al. 2010. Long-term ambient multi-pollutant exposures and mortality.*Am J Respir Crit Care Med. PMID*: 20656944.

Heard, N. J., U. Larsen, et al. 2004. Investigating access to reproductive health services using GIS: Proximity to services and the use of modern contraceptives in Malawi. *Afr J Reprod Health* 8(2): 164–179.

Kaplan, R. M. 2006. Medical geography—Who gets the goods? More may not be better. In *Optimizing Health: Improving the Value of Healthcare Delivery*, ed. F. Porzsolt and R. M. Kaplan. New York: Springer US.

Lewis, B., and W. W. Guan. 2011. Jump starting the next level of online geospatial collaboration: Lessons from AfricaMap. In *Advances in Web–based GIS, Mapping Services and Applications*, ed. S. Li, S. Dragicevic, and B. Veenendaal (in press).

Murphy, A. B. 2007. Geography's place in higher education in the United States. *Journal of Geography in Higher Education* 31(1): 121–141.

Niemann, B. J. Jr., and S. S. Niemann. 1998. GIS innovator—Allan H. Schmidt: GIS journeyman. *GeoInfoSystems*, May and October 1998.

Reed, C. 2006. Hello, Geotech—"Modeling our world," geography returns to Harvard. *Harvard Magazine*, November/December 2006. http://harvardmagazine.com/2006/11/hello–geotech.html (accessed November 23, 2010).

Saathoff, E., A. Olsen, et al. (2005). Ecological covariates of Ascaris lumbricoides infection in schoolchildren from rural KwaZulu-Natal, South Africa. *Trop Med Int Health* 10(5): 412–422.

Saathoff, E., A. Olsen, et al. (2005). Ecologic covariates of hookworm infection and reinfection in rural Kwazulu-Natal/South Africa: A geographic information system-based study. *Am J Trop Med Hyg* 72(4): 384–391.

Siegel, D., B. Burns, and T. Strawn. 2004. HGL: A Web-enabled geospatial digital library. ESRI International Conference Proceedings 2004. http://proceedings.esri.com/library/userconf/proc04/docs/pap1024.pdf (accessed November 23, 2010).

Singer, B. H., and M. C. de Castro (2001). Agricultural colonization and malaria on the Amazon frontier. *Ann N Y Acad Sci* 954: 184–222.

Smith, N. 1987. Academic war over the field of geography: The elimination of geography at Harvard 1947–1951. *Annals of the Association of American Geographers* 77(2): 155–172.

Sui, D., and Z. Sui.2007. Geographic information systems and medical geography: Toward a new synergy. *Geography Compass* 1(3): 556–582.

Waters, N. 2006. Harvard, geography and GIS: A race to the top, M2MEDIA360. http://www.geoplace.com/uploads/FeatureArticle/0609_EDGENODES.asp (accessed November 23, 2010).

Yanosky, J. D., C. J. Paciorek, et al. (2008). Spatio-temporal modeling of chronic PM10 exposure for the Nurses' Health Study. *Atmos Environ* 42(18): 4047–4062.

Yanosky, J. D., C. J. Paciorek, et al. (2009). Predicting chronic fine and coarse particulate exposures using spatiotemporal models for the Northeastern and Midwestern United States. *Environ Health Perspect* 117(4): 522–529.

Youngblood, D. 2009. A case study in proactive development: David Cobb, Harvard University's curator of maps. *Journal of Map and Geography Libraries* 5(2): 187–197.

Transforming Community Health and Primary Care Education Using Clinical and Administrative Data and Geographic Information Systems

ARTHUR SEIJI HAYASHI

Health Resources and Services Administration, Bureau of Primary Health Care, Washington, DC, USA

ANDREW BAZEMORE

The Robert Graham Center for Policy Studies in Family Medicine and Primary Care, Washington, DC, USA

JESSICA McINTYRE

Georgetown University, Providence Hospital Family Medicine Residency Program, Washington, DC, USA

Community-oriented primary care (COPC), a common model used for integrating the principles of primary care and public health, has been taught in family medicine residency programs to create community-responsive providers. As the initial step in a comprehensive COPC curriculum for a family medicine residency program, we used GIS maps, graphs, and tables to introduce new interns to the community served by the residency clinic. A fourteen-question pre/post test showed that interns' knowledge and understanding of the community improvement overall were deficient. Using practice-based administrative data combined with population-based data can efficiently and effectively improve interns' knowledge of the communities they serve.

INTRODUCTION

Described initially by Sydney and Emily Kark, community-oriented primary care (COPC) integrates primary care practice with public health principles in an effort to improve population health (IOM 1983; Rhyne et al. 1998). COPC assures community responsiveness through community participation and the use of epidemiological methods. These methods are employed to define and characterize the community, assess its needs, and incorporate participatory processes, especially for setting priorities and conducting interventions (Smilkstein 1990). Variants on the original COPC models exist, but most use some or all of the following steps: (1) defining and characterizing the community; (2) prioritizing its health problems; (3) assessing in detail the priority problem; (4) developing, implementing, and evaluating the intervention; and (5) reassessing adherence to its principles (IOM 1983; Nutting 1999; Mullan et al. 2004). Hand-drawn maps were often used in the community definition and characterization steps. COPC has been implemented in varying degrees throughout the world; in the United States, federally qualified health centers and other safety net clinics have developed systems of care around these principles (Geiger 2002; Mullan and Epstein 2002).

Creating a community-responsive practice, however, is challenging, and it requires training, experience, and commitment to adapt clinical practices to the needs of populations and make judicious use of existing resources (Mullan et al. 2004; Oandasan 2004; Steiner et al. 1999). Acknowledging this, many primary care residency programs in the U.S., especially in family medicine, incorporate COPC teachings in residency education to develop the knowledge and skills required for community-responsive primary care practice. These residency-based curricula vary greatly in content and methods that range from sporadic community-based experiences to complete implementation of the COPC process (Brill, Ohly, and Steams 2002; Plescia, Conan, and Lindcourt 2002; Dobbie, Kelly, and Sylvia 2006; Gavagan 2008). Furthermore, few curricula apply key public health approaches, such as the systematic use of databases or the use of regional, state, and national morbidity and mortality databases, to understand and articulate a community's health issues (Brill, Ohly, and Steams 2002; Cashmen et al. 1999; Longlett, Phillips, and Wesley 2002).

Recognizing the importance of residency training in community medicine and the need to create benchmarks, the community medicine curriculum area for the 2007 Accreditation Council for Graduate Medical Education (ACGME) expanded its program requirements for graduate medical education in family medicine. The new residency review committee (RRC) requirements incorporate basic public health concepts such as epidemiology and the interpretation of public health statistical information; community-based disease screening, prevention, and health promotion; experience in community health assessments; understanding factors associated with

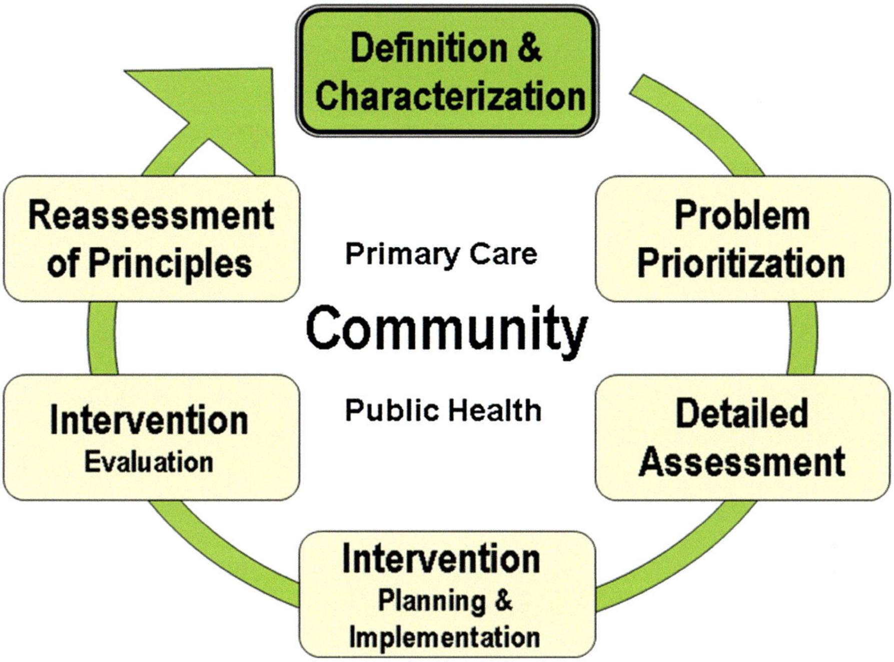

FIGURE 1 COPC Cycle.
Source: Hayashi, A. S. 2008. "Introduction to COPC." George Washington University School of Public Health and Health Services, Washington, DC.

differential health status among subpopulations; and the role of family physicians in reducing such gaps (ACGME 2007).

To make the most of limited time for nonclinical curricula and capture the power of COPC and geographic information systems (GIS), we developed a process for residency educators and learners to use available data through the clinic and the Internet displayed in simple tables, graphs, and—specifically—maps. We hypothesized that such a process would facilitate earlier and efficacious acquisition of information about the practice and community. This approach built on the strengths of information conveyed by combing detailed and specific practice-based data with broad and generalizable population-based data.

This paper describes a pilot process of orienting recently graduated, new family-medicine interns to their patient population and practice service area as the initial part of a three-year community medicine curriculum based on the COPC model described and used by the Masters of Public Health Program in COPC at George Washington University (Mullan et al. 2004). The residency curriculum has three major components: (a) Didactic learning through lectures and seminars in postgraduate years (PGY) 1, 2, and 3, (b) experiential learning through site visits and service-learning activities in PGY 2 and 3, and (c) community-based learning through a longitudinal COPC project in PGY 3. This intern-orientation seminar conducted within the first month of starting residency addresses the initial steps of a COPC cycle that includes community definition and characterization and identification of priority problems (see Figure 1).

Project Description

As educators in family medicine with particular expertise in COPC, we sought to better understand the feasibility of improving training in community health using administrative data from the residency clinic using GIS. The steps in the process were to (1) obtain clinical data and convert them into a usable format; (2) geocode, analyze, and combine clinical and relevant population data using GIS software; (3) incorporate the seminar into the existing curriculum for community medicine; and (4) evaluate the process.

The intern-orientation seminar had three main learner-centered objectives: (1) understand and describe the types of clinical and administrative data available at the residency clinic and in publicly available databases, (2) define and characterize the residency clinic's patient population and service area, and (3) describe the most common health issues encountered by patients and the community.

METHODS

We obtained institutional review board (IRB) approvals from three affiliated hospitals and universities and obtained data on each patient visit to the residency clinic from January 1, 2002, to December 31, 2005. Data fields included year of visit, date of birth, gender, race, insurance information, complete address, and up to five diagnoses associated with each visit. The International Classification of Disease (ICD-9) codes were used for the diagnoses.

Summary and descriptive statistics of patient characteristics were generated and spatial analyses conducted using ArcView 8.3 (ESRI, Redlands, CA). Patient addresses were geocoded and analytic maps created through the integration of existing clinic data, U.S. census data, and publically accessible geographic data. Graduated chloropleth maps and dot maps were created to demonstrate the clinic's service area and population penetration rates (number of patients/total population) using established methods for geographic retrofitting (Mullan et al. 2004). All socio-demographic variables and ICD-9 codes were then plotted as a function of address. Population-based, socio-demographic information from the U.S. Census Bureau was used to create the map's base layer for comparison with patient characteristics. County- and Zip Code–level health data and maps were generated from Behavioral Risk Factor Surveillance System data.

Information gathered for the seminar was presented in three sections. The first section discussed data types, availability, and their uses. The second section described community characteristics and patient visit patterns using tables, graphs, and maps (Figure 2), and the last section discussed the relevance and uses of the information to the practice of medicine. The principles and methods of COPC were reviewed, providing the framework and longitudinal process for uses of the information.

A fourteen-item, multiple-choice pretest and posttest (identical) were administered to assess seminar effectiveness.

RESULTS

Seven interns participated in the seminar and completed the pretest and posttest. All seven were women with an average age of twenty-nine. Of the seven interns, three were new to the area, one had attended medical school in the area (four years), and three had resided in the area for more than five years prior to medical school. Five out of seven interns had some formal public health coursework or community health experience. Thirteen questions tested the interns' knowledge of the residency practice and community served (Table 1). The average percentage of correct responses for the pretest

TABLE 1 Test Questions and Number of Residents Who Answered Questions Correctly (N = 7)

Test Questions	Pretest	Posttest
In what county is the clinic located?	6 (86%)	7 (100%)
Do most clinic patients live within a mile of the clinic?	4 (57%)	5 (71%)
Where do most Hispanic patients live?	3 (43%)	5 (71%)
The racial and ethnic distribution of patients mirrors that of the surrounding communities	2 (29%)	2 (29%)
Which of the following most closely approximates the gender makeup of clinic patients?	1 (14%)	6 (86%)
Appox. what% of the patient population is comprised of African Americans according to clinic data?	2 (29%)	5 (71%)
Approx. to what degree has the percentage of Hispanic patients grown since 2002?	5 (71%)	6 (86%)
What is the most common type of insurance used by patients?	5 (71%)	7 (100%)
Of the following, what is the most common reason for a child younger than 18 to visit the clinic?	0 (0%)	3 (43%)
What is the most frequent reason (diagnosis) for all patient visits?	3 (43%)	3 (43%)
Approx. how many individual patients does the clinic serve annually?	0 (0%)	5 (71%)
On average, how many times does each patient visit the clinic?	4 (57%)	6 (86%)
Which age group visits the clinic the most?	4 (57%)	6 (86%)
Overall Mean	3 (43%)	5.1 (72.8%)

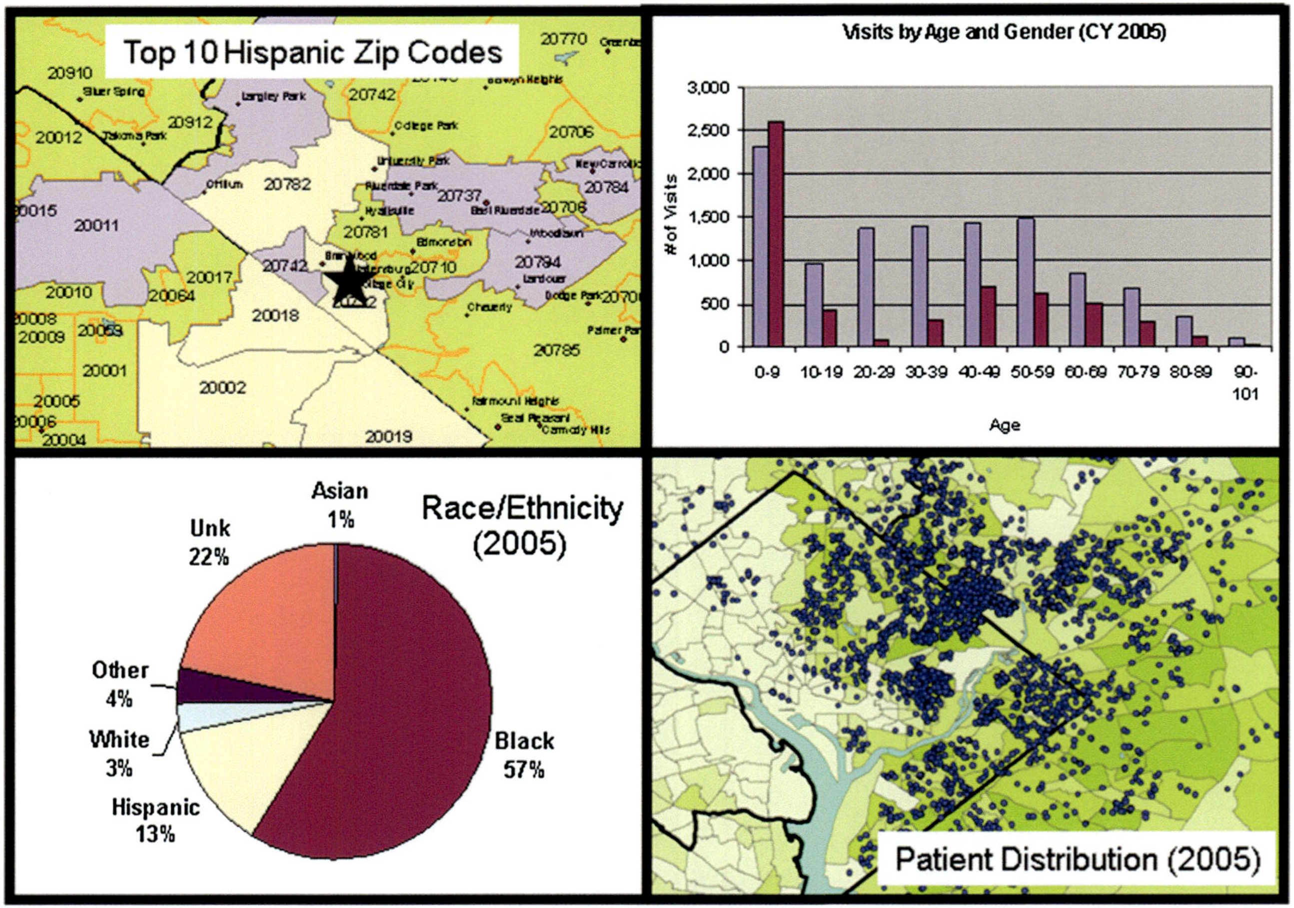

FIGURE 2 Examples of maps and graphs used in intern orientation.

and posttests were 43 percent and 73 percent, respectively, showing a 30 percent increase in overall score. When the interns were asked, "Is the use of maps helpful to you as a clinician in understanding the patients and community served by the clinic?" before the seminar, three interns responded, "Marginally helpful," three responded, "Fairly helpful," and one responded, "Very helpful." After the seminar, all seven answered, "Very helpful."

CONCLUSIONS AND LIMITATIONS

In a time of health system reform and primary care practice transformation, it is essential that the new generation of primary care trainees possess the skills necessary to provide care for individuals in a population-based context. The results of this pilot project show that improvement in the interns' knowledge of the patient population and that of the clinic's service area can be accomplished quickly and effectively. The posttest average score of 73 percent reveals the need for improvement in the curriculum as well as in content delivery. It may also reveal the learner's unfamiliarity with the topic or types of information. One intern did not know the county where the clinic sits, and as a group, learners revealed inadequate understanding of local geography and political boundaries. Certain topics such as the racial and ethnic distribution of patients and the most frequent reasons for patient visits did not improve after the seminar, suggesting the need for refining the approach. Although compared with the other topics, learners were most able to identify the insurance type for their patients, there are still opportunities for educators to link insurance status to other population health indicators.

This study does not assess retention of knowledge over time nor does it assess eventual use of the information in the interns' clinical practice. Feedback from the seminar revealed that maps of community resources would be helpful if presented together with the health conditions. Overall, participants agreed that the information would be helpful during patient visits.

DISCUSSION AND NEXT STEPS

The capacity of GIS tools paired with administrative and population data to inform community-based primary care has been demonstrated (Mullan, Phillips, and Kinman 2004). Additionally, its potential impact in a time of primary care transformation that emphasizes patient-centered medical homes, the meaningful use of health information technology, and sweeping health reform is considerable. Providing family medicine residents with the basic knowledge and skills to conduct analytic mapping of their clinic and community improves community medicine curricula by placing the data within

TABLE 2 Curriculum Content Covered to Meet RRC Requirements and Data Sources Used

RRC Requirements	Content Covered to Meet RRC Requirements	Data Sources Used
(9a) Reportable communicable disease	Prevalence and distribution of diseases including hepatitis, TB, and STIs	CAD, BRFSS
(9c) Population epidemiology, and the interpretation of public health statistical information	Top 20 diagnoses cared for in the clinic, regional epidemiology of diabetes, hypertension, asthma	CAD, BRFSS, Local public health data, US Census
(9d) Environmental illness and injury	Prevalence and geographic distribution of patients with elevated lead levels and injuries	CAD, US Census, BRFSS
(9f) Disease prevention through immunization strategies	Reviewed and discussed pediatric patient age distribution and service utilization patterns	CAD
(9h) Factors associated with differential health status among subpopulations, including racial, geographic, or socioeconomic health disparities	Disease prevalence, service utilization patterns, geo distribution based on socio-demographic variables (age, race/ethnicity, gender, language, insurance)	CAD, US Census
(9j) Experience in using community resources appropriately for individual patients who have unmet medical or social support needs	Disease prevalence and geographic distribution, clinic service area analysis, community resource distribution	CAD, US Census, health services directory
(9k) Structured interaction with the public health system	Public health data sources, health department role, and scope of work	Local public health Web site and database
(9m) Experience in community health assessment	COPC (comm. Definition, characterization, problem prioritization), prevalence and distribution of disease	CAD, US Census, local public health database, BRFSS
(9n) Experience in developing programs to address community health priorities *and* (9m) Community-based health education of children and adults	COPC (Problem prioritization), identifying best- practices for priority health issues. Incorporation of quality improvement processes to address community health priorities.	Various Internet-based sties

BRFSS: Behavioral risk factor surveillance system; CAD: Clinic administrative data.

the community context. Placed within a health promotion framework such as COPC, such curricula can serve as a tool for community-based interventions (Mullan et al. 2004; Mullan and Epstein 2002).

In addition, the process used in this pilot can serve a vital function toward fulfilling the Residency Review Committee (RRC) for Family Medicine requirements for community medicine (Table 2). The content covered in the seminar such as disease prevalence and distribution align well with RRC requirements. Data sources necessary to create the content are available to most clinical residency programs through their own databases and public Internet portals.

The overall goals and objectives of the project were accomplished; however, more-than-expected time and effort were necessary. IRB approvals were obtained from two university medical centers and from a community hospital where the clinic data was stored. Two residents and a master of public health (MPH) student facilitated the IRB approval process. This process took six months to complete due to the number of institutions involved and the community hospital staff's unfamiliarity with the process. The IRB approval process was a challenge, but the hassle can be avoided if the data are used internally as part of an educational or quality improvement process.

Data collection took nearly two months to complete due to nonresponse from the information systems administrator and the need for revised data requests. Three revised data requests were necessary before a data set with appropriate variables was delivered. Data analysis was completed by a residency faculty member (who was also on the faculty of a local school of public health) with prior knowledge and experience using administrative data and GIS software. The presentation was developed by the faculty and an MPH student.

Understanding the limitations of a discrete and brief educational intervention, the residency is developing sessions to train residents in data collection, analysis, and presentation. Chief residents in their third year of training have begun creating processes to streamline data requests to the information systems personnel. In partnership with researchers, the residency program has begun training residents to use an online GIS application.

In order to allow residents to generate maps themselves, recent clinical and administrative data have been uploaded to an online GIS application, Health Landscape (www.healthlandscape.org). All residents will be trained in the use of the software. Residents will use Health Landscape for their COPC projects as well as their senior quality improvement project.

Disclaimer

The views expressed here are those of the authors, and do not represent the position of the Health Resources and Services Administration or the Department of Health and Human Services.

REFERENCES

Accreditation Council for Graduate Medical Education. 2007. Program requirements for residency education in family medicine. (Section IV.A.5.b.[9]). Available at www.acgme.org (accessed February 15, 2008).

Brill, J. R., S. Ohly, and M. A. Stearns. 2002. Training community-responsive physicians. *Academic Medicine* 77(7):747.

Cashman, S., R. Anderson, J. Weisbuch, M. Schwarz, and H. Fulmer. 1999. Carrying out the Medicine/Public Health Initiative: The roles of preventive medicine and community–responsive care. *Acad Med* 74(5):473–483.

Dobbie, A., P. Kelly, E. Sylvia, and J. Freeman. 2006. Evaluating family medicine residency COPC programs: Meeting the challenge. *Fam Med* 38(6):399–407.

Gavagan, T. 2008. A systematic review of COPC: Evidence for effectiveness. *J Health Care Poor U* 19(3):963–980.

Geiger, H. J. 2002. Community-oriented primary care: A path to community development. *Am J Public Health* 92(11):1713–1716.

Institute of Medicine. 1983 *Community Oriented Primary Care: New Directions for Health Services Delivery*. Washington, DC: National Academy Press.

Longlett, S., D. Phillips, and R. Wesley. 2002. Prevalence of community-oriented primary care knowledge, training, and practice. *Fam Med* 34(3):183–89.

Mullan, F., C. Focht, A. S. Hayashi, J. Gofin, R. Gofin, Y. Neumark, and L. Epstein. 2004. *Community Oriented Primary Care: An Implementation Guide*. Washington, DC, and Jerusalem, Israel: George Washington University School of Public Health and Health Services and Braun School of Public Health and Community Medicine, Hebrew University of Jerusalem.

Mullan, F., and L. Epstein. 2002. Community-oriented primary care: New relevance in a changing world. *Am J Public Health* 92(11):1748–1755.

Mullan, F., R. L. Phillips, and E. L. Kinman. 2004. Geographic retrofitting: A method of community definition in community-oriented primary care practices. *Fam Med* 36(6):440–6.

Nutting, P. A. 1999. *Community Oriented Primary Care: From Principle to Practice*. Albuquerque: University of New Mexico Press,

Oandasan, I., R. Malik, I. Waters, and A. Lambert-Lanning. 2004. Being community-responsive physicians: Doing the right thing. *Can Fam Physician* 50:1004–1010.

Plescia, M., J. Konen, and A. Lincourt. 2002. The state of community medicine training in family practice residency programs. *Fam Med*; 34(3):177–82.

Rhyne, R., R. Bogue, G. Kukulka, and H. Fulmer. 1998. *Community-Oriented Primary Care: Health Care for the 21st Century*. Washington, DC: American Public Health Association 1998.

Smilkstein, G. 1990. Designing a curriculum for training community-responsive physicians. *J Health Care Poor U* 1(2):237–242

Steiner, B. D., D. E. Pathman, B. Jones, E. S. Williams, and T. Riggins. 1999. Primary care physicians' training and their community involvement. *Fam Med* 31(4):257–62.

Harnessing Geographic Information Systems (GIS) to Enable Community-Oriented Primary Care

ANDREW BAZEMORE and ROBERT L. PHILLIPS
The Robert Graham Center, Washington, DC, USA

THOMAS MIYOSHI
University of Arkansas, Fayetteville, Arkansas, USA

Background: *Despite growing acceptance and implementation of geographic information systems (GIS) in the public health arena, its utility for clinical population management and coordination by leaders in a primary care clinical health setting has been neither fully realized nor evaluated.*

Methods: *In a primary care network of clinics charged with caring for vulnerable urban communities, we used GIS to (1) integrate and analyze clinical (practice management) data and population (census) data and (2) generate distribution, service area, and population penetration maps of those clinics. We then conducted qualitative evaluations of the responses of primary care clinic leaders, administrators, and community board members to analytic mapping of their clinic and regional population data.*

Results: *Practice management data were extracted, geocoded, and mapped to reveal variation between actual clinical service areas and the medically underserved areas for which these clinics received funding, which was surprising to center leaders. In addition, population penetration analyses were performed to depict patterns of utilization. Qualitative assessments of staff response to the process of mapping clinical and population data revealed enthusiastic engagement in the process, which led to enhanced community comprehension, new ideas about data use, and an array of applications to improve their clinical revenue. However, they also revealed barriers to further adoption, including time, expense, and technical expertise, which could limit the use of GIS and mapping unless economies of scale across clinics, the use of web technology, and the availability of dynamic mapping tools could be realized.*

Conclusions: *Analytic mapping was enthusiastically received and practically applied in the primary care setting, and was readily comprehended by clinic leaders for innovative purposes. This is a tool of particular relevance amid primary care safety-net expansion and increased funding of health information technology diffusion in these settings, particularly if the hurdles of cost and technological expertise are overcome by harnessing new advances in web-based mapping technology.*

Primary care clinics and the patients they serve are bound to one another by geography. In the case of community health centers (CHCs), policies tie clinics to geography via the federal designations of medically underserved areas (MUAs) or health professional shortage areas; financial incentive is provided to clinics located within these areas. However, planners and clinicians often assume or ignore the characteristics of these primary care geographies, fail to use utilization data to evaluate their assumptions, and rarely study or use them in the process of planning clinical services by CHCs or other private outpatient providers. To efficiently plan new clinic locations and improve access to care for vulnerable populations, it is critical to understand existing clinical service areas and patterns of service utilization, particularly amid three concurrent national trends: growing numbers of uninsured, rapid expansion of CHCs, and the likelihood of a mandated insurance requirement increasing the burden on existing primary care providers.[1,2] One potential tool for understanding access to and utilization of care is geographic information systems (GIS), which permit the combination of many data sources into dynamic analytic maps; these are increasingly implemented in the public health sector.[3] However, although GIS has been used by health services researchers and epidemiologists to study populations to better understand cancer epidemiology, disease outbreaks, and even the impact of distance on care, there is little known about GIS applications using clinical data or measuring access to and utilization of care at a community level. Specifically, few studies have demonstrated the ability of GIS to better understand access to primary health care.[4–7]

Although combining CHC data with existing population data using GIS has been reported, its usefulness and barriers to, and means of, expanding the use of GIS among clinical and community leaders of CHCs has not been thoroughly evaluated.[8–10] We applied qualitative methods to investigate in depth the perspectives and responses to mapping clinical and population data in a real community health setting, exploring with CHC leaders the barriers to and opportunities for implementation of this powerful technique.

METHODS

This study used informant interviews and focus group techniques to evaluate a collaborative community-based project between Baltimore Medical System, Inc. (BMSI) and the Robert Graham Center for Policy Studies in Family Medicine and Primary Care. It was approved by the Georgetown University Medical Institutional Review Board.

Study Setting, Community Project Description, and Data Sources

We extracted from practice management software a comprehensive dataset of the nearly 30,000 patients who had visited a system of seven federally qualified CHCs in 2003. At the time, the system of clinics employed more than forty primary care providers in the service of indigent patients in urban and periurban Baltimore, Maryland. We cleaned and geocoded all clinical data representing unique patients during a single year period, achieving an 80% geocoding match rate. Using ArcView GIS software (ESRI, Redlands, CA), we integrated the geocoded clinical data with U.S. Census data and other publicly accessible spatial information to create simple analytic maps and outputs in a variety of formats. To reveal neighborhood utilization patterns for each clinic and to create individual clinic and system-wide service area maps, we reviewed possible spatial techniques, selected a modified Griffith's commitment index and evaluated methods previously described in the limited primary care literature on the subject (see Figure 1).[11] The index measures the degree of patient utilization of a clinic from individual geographies—in this case all census block groups or tracts containing patients from the clinics that were studied. Tracts were ranked by index in descending order and were included in the overall clinic or system-wide service area only until 60% of all patient data were included. Maps of the designated MUA for a clinic were also generated (Figure 2) to demonstrate differences between federally-intended and utilization-derived (actual) service areas. We additionally plotted patient and subpopulation distribution maps and calculated area penetration rates for each clinic (see Figure 3), which were defined by the number of yearly clinic users per total population in each census tract according to the 2000 Census. Our methods are described in greater detail elsewhere.[10] These maps were then presented to BMSI clinicians and leaders as a series of focus groups and in-depth interviews designed to evaluate the utility of analytic mapping in a primary care setting and the potential for and barriers to broader application.

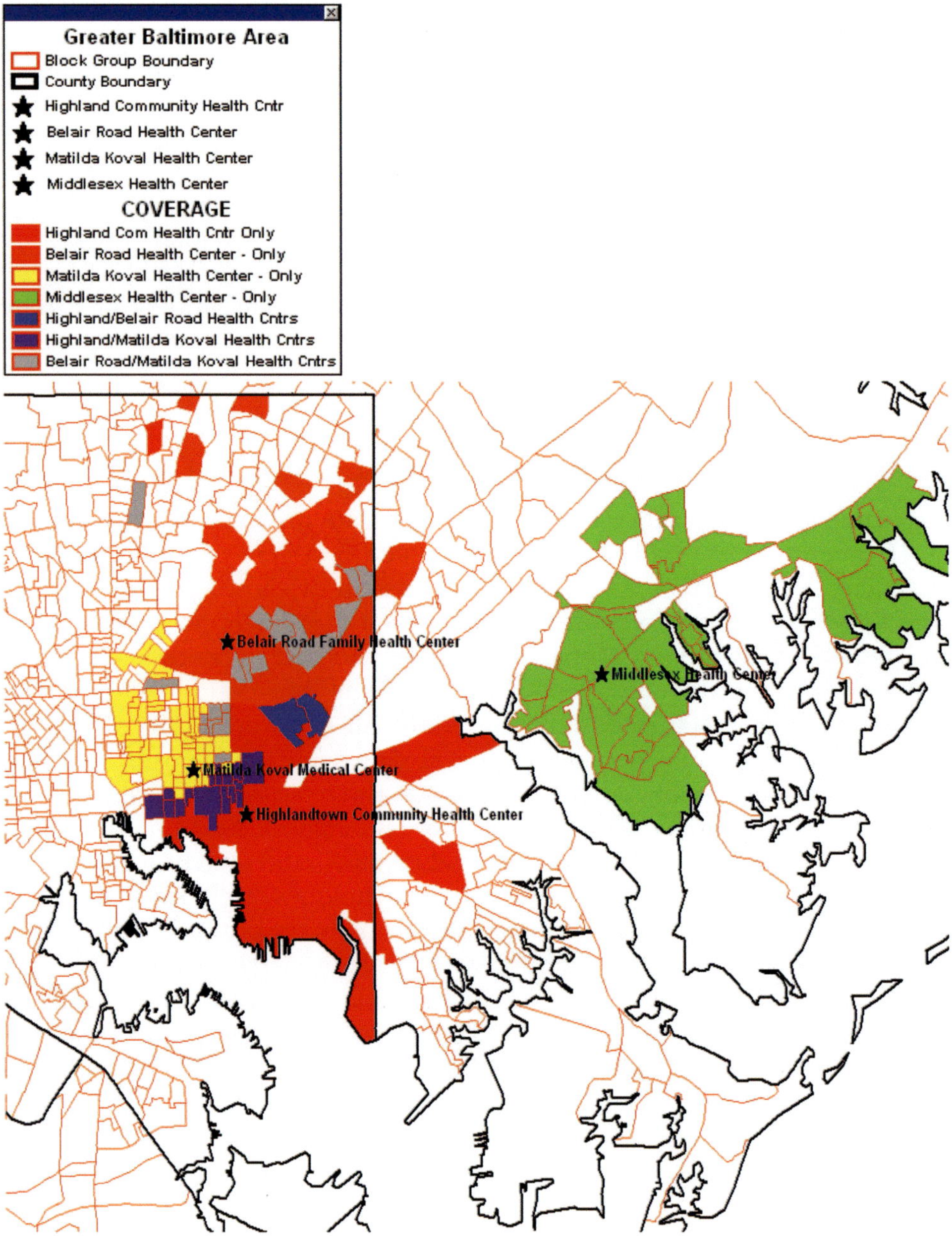

FIGURE 1 Baltimore Medical Systems, Inc.'s aggregate service area. Using billing and administrative data assigned to clinic, this map shows the service area (census tract) of 4 BMSI clinics and their overlap.

Qualitative Data Collection and Analysis

With the help of BMSI administrative staff, we assembled our sample from the leadership of BMSI, including clinicians, administrators, staff representing

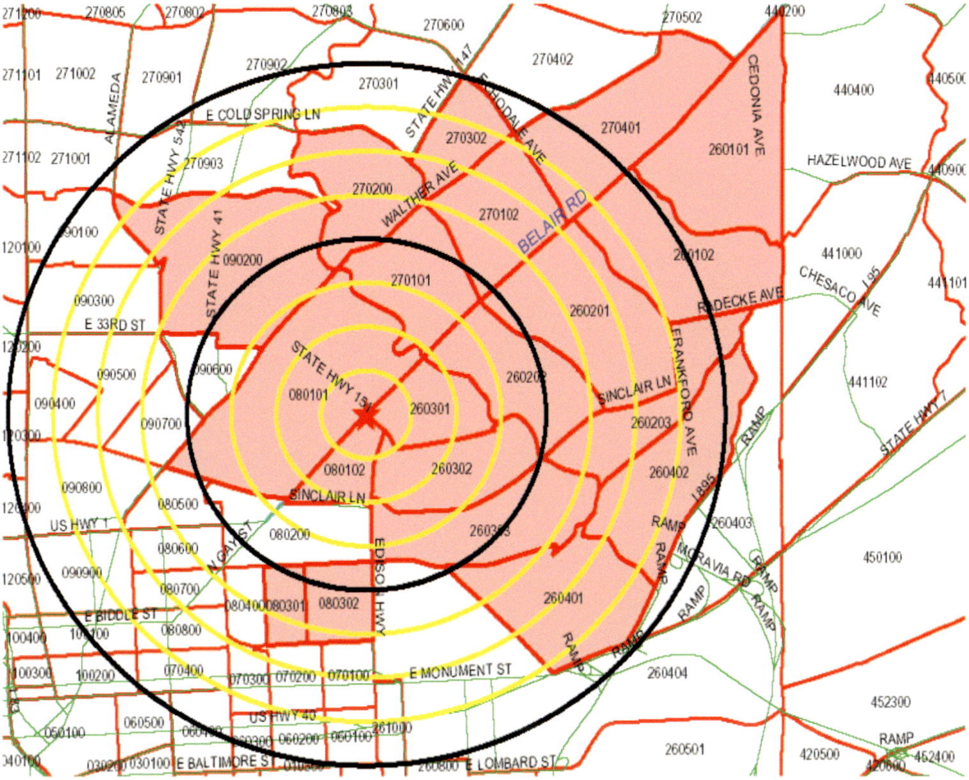

FIGURE 2 This map demonstrates the federally designated medically underserved area that a single Baltimore Medical Systems, Inc. clinic receives federal funding to serve, with quarter-mile radii from clinic marked out to 2 miles. Discrepancies between maps of these "ideal" service areas and the actual service areas (such as that in Figure 1) were cited by BMSI executives as informative and surprising; they later used the actual service area information to change a relocation decision based previously on medically underserved area alone.

potential constituents of mapped data, and community board members. The organizational knowledge of an investigator who had previous knowledge of BMSI as a clinician, coupled with queries of network leaders, was used to ensure that leadership from all BMSI divisions and the community it served were represented when key informants and group participants were selected.[12] Data were assembled using three qualitative methods: (1) as participant observers in a longitudinal interaction with BMSI and its staff, (2) through key informant interviews with selected clinicians and administrators most involved with the management of the organization, and (3) through focus groups with those most involved in the strategic planning and operations of BMSI. Participant observation was used to capture participant reactions to our mapping project and to gather comments about how an organizational culture views and embraces or rejects a new technology such as this.[13] Key informant interviews helped us understand the perspectives of individuals

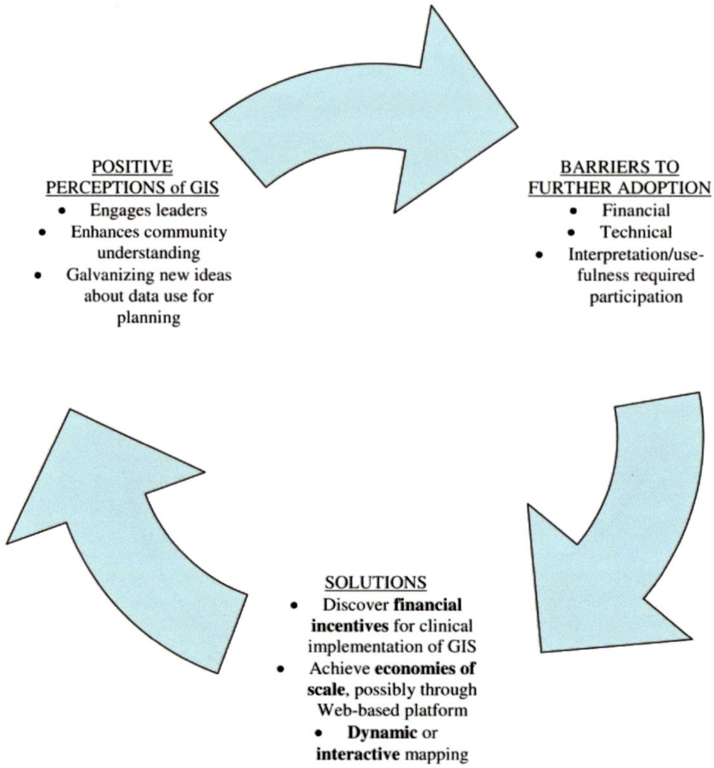

FIGURE 3 Census tract population penetration rate for a single Baltimore Medical Systems, Inc. clinic. Revealing dense utilization (as high as 30% of the population) by persons in the census tracts most proximal to this clinic, these maps were cited as critical to strategic planning for future expansion and service delivery.

with essential but distinct roles within the organization, in this case the Chief Executive Officer, the Chief Medical Officer, the Chief Operating Officer, and the Director of Community Outreach. Focus groups provided a broad array of perspectives from clinician leaders (e.g., the physician directors of pediatric and adult medicine), nursing leaders, ancillary services leaders, community liaisons, administrators, and representatives of the communities directly served by BMSI. They also permitted capture of group responses to, spontaneous conversations and discussions about, and interactions over analytic mapping. The small sampling frame of BMSI leaders limited our focus groups to two: one with members of the Clinical Operations Committee (10 attendees) and the other with members of the Community Advisory Board for BMSI (5 attendees).

Each session began with a short summary presentation of project background, maps, and details of the collaboration to date, followed by a semi-structured query to assess four domains of interest: (1) understanding of the analytic mapping process, (2) interpretation of the data presented, (3) perceived usefulness of analytic mapping for strategic planning and delivery of improved services in the primary care outpatient setting, and (4) barriers to and enablers of continued use of these methods. Clarifying and additional questions were asked based on participant responses. Key informant interviews were similarly structured, with additional questions tailored to the informant's position within the organization. All information was recorded and later transcribed. In each interview and focus group, one interviewer recorded responses while the other guided the presentation and interview. Investigators alternated between presentation/querying and note taking to ensure a more robust set of observations and information recording. Thematic analysis of transcriptions and interview notes were reviewed by two of the investigators (AB and RLP) and then discussed until consensus was reached regarding common themes. The project was approved by the Georgetown Institutional Review Board.

RESULTS

With minimum explanation and a brief iterative exchange, BMSI administrators and their information technology support team were able to produce a comprehensive, one-year, patient-level database for analysis. Geocoding yielded an 80% first-pass match. Service area maps revealed previously unrecognized range and overlap of individual clinical services (Figure 1), whereas MUA/service area match and area penetration densities varied widely by clinic (Figures 2 and 3). As qualitative reporting revealed (below), dynamic mapping and static maps—such the samples seen in the figures—helped BMSI leaders identify and strategize around unrecognized patterns of clinic use, including unexpected use by remote populations. They also revealed the geographic dimensions of BMSI's primary care services and the extent to which the communities they served depended on their clinics for primary care services.

Initial qualitative analysis revealed the following seven central themes and perceptions:

1. Mapping and spatial analysis of clinical data resulted in engagement of busy administrators and clinicians. Responses were enthusiastic regarding the potential of analytic mapping to help guide CHC strategic planning and resource allocation.
2. Participants reported enhanced community comprehension as a result of analytic mapping and were, in fact, better suited to interpreting their mapped clinic data than the investigators; interviewees stated a ready understanding of health service area and penetration maps. Many offered suggestions about how to make the maps more easily interpretable that neither presenting investigator had considered. Both investigators also

noted that participants could easily grasp the limitations of mapped data and were quick to recognize the perils of overinterpretation of map data in isolation. Participants from the Clinical Operations Committee were visibly engaged in the presentation portion of the focus group, interrupting the authors repeatedly with queries and suggestions. Both investigators noted that committee members had visible epiphanies ("a-ha moments") when they saw certain maps. After presenting aggregate BMSI service area maps (Figure 1), the presenters were interrupted by multiple participants at once, as if the maps had unveiled a mystery. During the six months after our interviews, participants requested a number of additional maps to support a BMSI application to expand that clinic.

3. Participatory interpretation of mapped clinic data was essential and was deeply enriched by provider and administrator knowledge of their patient population. Participant knowledge was essential to and revealed through the analytic map interpretation process. As noted above, interviewees applied their experience and local knowledge to interpret service areas. However, multiparty interaction between technical staff, administrators, clinicians, and community members allowed the unique knowledge and expertise of each—whether in data, neighborhood geographies, community history, or other areas—to capture the real power of mapped data. Energy was highest in the group settings, and investigators were struck by how essential local knowledge was to interpreting clinical and community maps relative to tables, graphs, and other forms of data frequently reviewed in these settings. In both focus groups, considerable and far-ranging knowledge of socioeconomic status and social capital among participants was revealed amid animated discussions of why maps showed variable service penetration by African-Americans in specific neighborhoods.
4. Mapping existing and previously dormant practice management data in this fashion galvanized new ideas about data use for strategic planning and population management. CHC leaders and staff quickly and enthusiastically generated a list of additional spatial analyses that they desired to improve their operations. Further, this phenomenon was not limited to selected individuals; staff from each administrative and clinical unit of the CHC network was able to identify a potential analytic mapping project of value to them. The participatory process generated numerous practical applications for analytic mapping that the investigators had not considered.
5. Mapping was identified as having the capacity to support clinic financing and resource allocation. Leaders and clinicians were most enthusiastic about using analytic mapping to support the expansion of grant applications and clinical operations and to impact the effectiveness of patient outreach.

6. Financial and technologic issues were perceived barriers to project sustainability. Many participants cited concerns that the expense and manpower involved in analytic mapping at the desktop would limit their long-term use of this technology without continued outside assistance. Specifically, they lamented their limited information technology infrastructure and staff expertise in the use of analytic mapping software.
7. Achieving economies of scale across clinics and with foundation or federal support and capturing the power of dynamic mapping through web technology were reported as the best ways to overcome the barriers mentioned above. Participants noted that their likelihood of using clinical data mapping would be far greater if overworked staff had immediate access to their data and the power of GIS when they had a specific question related to mapping. Participants also noted that such a tool should be flexible enough to incorporate other community and population data and to expand into other mapping applications useful to the primary care enterprise.

Investigators further sorted these themes into three principal domains of findings: (1) perceptions of primary care implementation of GIS (mostly positive), (2) barriers to further implementation, and (3) possible solutions (see Table 1 for examples and Figure 4 for a summary schematic).

DISCUSSION

The profound effects of neighborhoods and community on health are well documented.[14] Despite this and continuing calls to understand their patients in the context of community and place,[15–18] most clinicians lack the tools to evaluate and display that community context. In this study we tested novel GIS use in an urban primary care network and demonstrated and categorized the value of analytic mapping to primary care outpatient leaders in identifying community context. Readily available primary care clinical data were easily combined with population data within a GIS environment to understand communities, and clinical leaders affirmed the value of this process for population-based care and planning. Outpatient clinic leaders, clinicians, and community board members in our study were engaged and galvanized by the power of mapped data to enhance community care, and they easily identified applications of analytic mapping that would improve their clinical operations.

Any primary care setting or clinical enterprise could potentially benefit from the techniques described here and previously, in particular the expanding primary care safety net.[19,20] Clearly articulated statements about the value of these tools to clinic and community leaders were couched against the need

TABLE 1 Key Domains Related to Primary Care Adoption of Geographic Information Systems from Community Health Center Key Informants

Key Domains	Perceptions of Primary Care Clinical Applications of GIS	Key Informant Comments, Responses, and Results
Positive perceptions	The process resulted in enthusiastic engagement	"I'm just excited ... We're doing this expansion grant for [clinic A] and there [are] two key questions in the grant being asked: 'Why do you guys think you need to expand?' and 'Tell us who is not being served in your MUA that you need to expand [for].' Now I've got these maps. Look at all of these people in my clinic area that are not being served and we need to expand. And now I have to get some outreach persons [to explain this]."
	Maps enhanced community comprehension	Operations committee members and one administrator were "stunned" by the fact that they were serving more than 1-in-4 people in some blocks around a clinic that was "so close to [other primary care safety net service providers]."
		After seeing the overlapping service areas of 3 of their clinics, 3 participants stated (verbatims intertwined): "We thought [clinic A] was losing business to [a nearby provider network] ... not filling their pediatrics appointments ... but it looks like their kids are going to [sister clinics B and C, also within BMSI]."
	Mapping galvanized new ideas about data use	Gauging the impact of a proposed site move on access for vulnerable patient populations, in follow-up to the focus groups leadership of the network elected not to move a clinic because maps revealed that clusters of 2 vulnerable populations served would have their access threatened.
		Improving the efficiency and effectiveness of existing community health outreach and marketing activities, such as breast cancer awareness among African-American women older than 40. In follow up, this proposal led to a research project to explore this question.
		Merging clinic data with regional Medicaid managed-care data to guide unassigned Medicaid recipients to appropriate safety net facilities for primary care.
		Supporting expansion grant funding for new clinical services, both as new sites and through expansion of high utilization clinics.
		Assessing the success of 2 new clinics in reaching local vulnerable populations targeted in their federal grant applications.
		Leaders pointed out how GIS applications could improve clinical revenue.
		Penetration maps for one clinic generated enthusiastic discussion among clinic leaders. The maps showed that, despite a wealth of nearby safety-net options, as many as 20% to 25% of individuals from the 4 census-block groups adjacent to their clinic were using their services (see Figure 3). These maps confirmed leaders' suspicions that they were the principal provider in a particular neighborhood and served as the impetus for pursuing grant funding to expand that clinic.

Negative perceptions	Participatory interpretation required	Understanding any single static map was best done through discussion, and exploration of the data in a desktop GIS "on the fly."
		In one focus group, a single participant's insight helped the group understand why 2 census-block groups distant from BMSI clinics had unexpectedly high user penetration: "There is a deaf community there that takes advantage of [our hearing impaired services] at [clinic A]."
Barriers to further implementation	Financial and technical	Desktop GIS software use was seen as too expensive and technically challenging to overcome for primary care implementation, even in a large, multisite practice with substantial information technology support.
Possible solutions	Security and workflow	Multiple informants noted the importance of HIPAA-compliance and data security and the need for access across multiple settings.
	Demonstrate financial impact	Demonstrating usefulness in grant writing, defending contracts, and reimbursements with payers, hospitals, and community stakeholders is key to driving adoption.
	Achieve economies of scale through web-based platform	Internet-based solutions that would allow accessibility of data able to be mapped for multiple locations—such as at the point of care—during advocacy efforts or in administrative meetings were cited as the best way to "increase the likelihood of using [clinical data mapping] regularly."
	Ensure a dynamic or interactive mapping process	Focus groups and individuals preferred dynamic mapping that allowed them to turn layers on and off, zoom in and out, filter data, and change data attributes to static maps.

Note. GIS, geographic information systems; MUA, medically underserved area; BMSI, Baltimore Medical System, Inc.; HIPAA, Health Insurance Portability and Accountability Act.

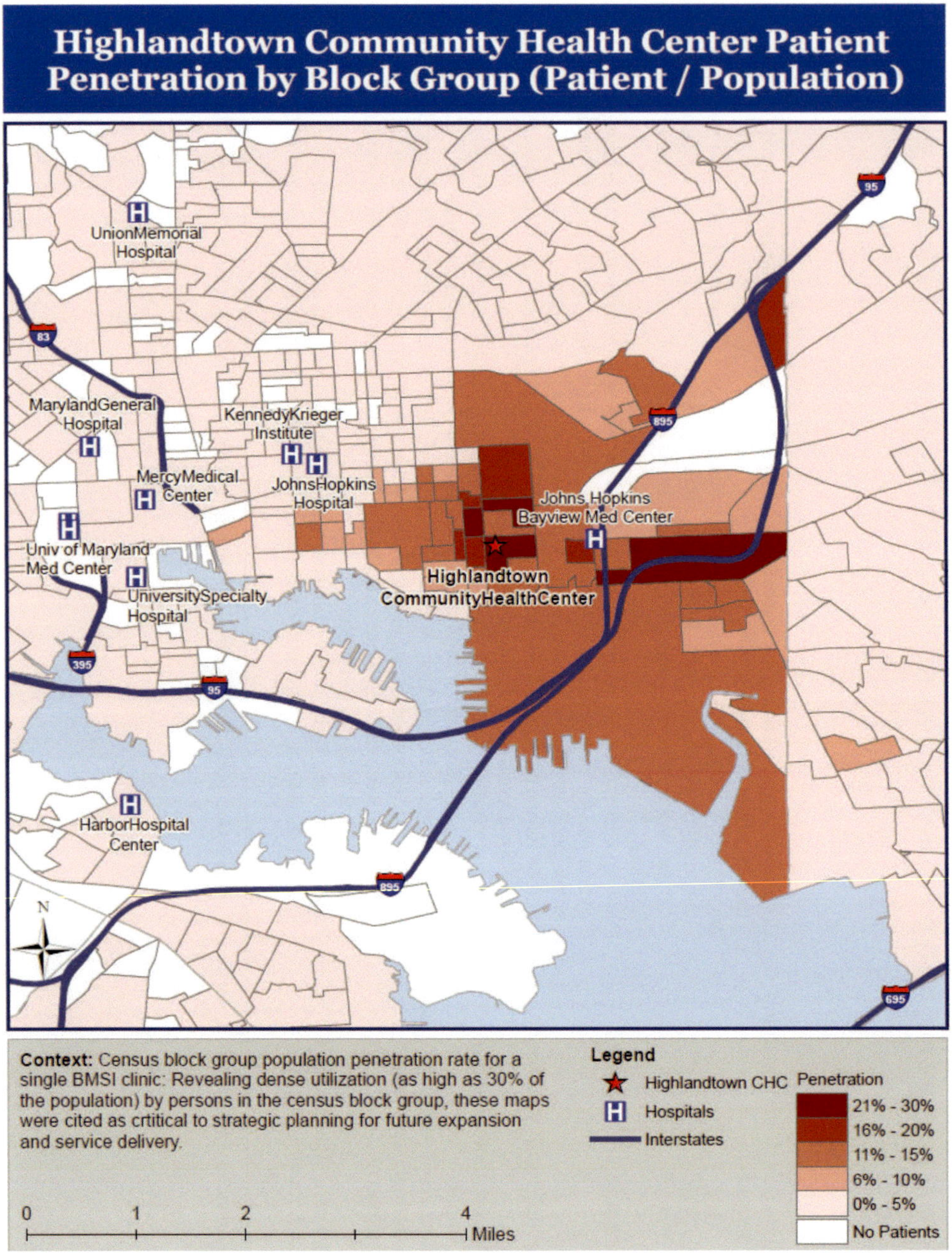

FIGURE 4 Perceptions, barriers, and possible solutions to increase primary care geographic information systems adoption.

BMSI, Baltimore Medical System, Inc.; CHC, community health center.

for less technical and time-intensive processes—processes that could permit secure, interactive queries of mapped clinic and population data, because there is a dearth of tools able to inform primary care leaders about access and utilization patterns at the practice and community levels. On a national level, federal funding initiatives to expand health information technology, regional health information organizations, and uniform dataset collection in primary care safety nets are encouraging opportunities for diffusion of analytic mapping in the primary care setting.[21] Tools are needed more than ever to guide the continued expansion of federally qualified health centers and to identify gaps in safety-net coverage A secure, web-based mapping tool that is broadly implemented in outpatient health centers would complement Health Resources and Services Administration efforts to offer all Americans a "medical home" through projects such as the Models That Work campaign and the Primary Care Service Area project.[22,23]

Whether findings of our exploratory evaluation of a single, large, multi-clinic network that provides primary care to an ethnically and racially diverse population represent broader perspectives merits further study, but our early work with an array of primary care sites has yielded similar results. Although we cannot claim to have represented all clinical and administrative leaders from the organization used for our interviews and focus groups, purposeful and strategic sampling was used to ensure breadth. Additional studies in other settings (e.g., rural, suburban, single-practitioner practices, multispecialty practices) are needed to confirm the usefulness of these techniques in a wide array of clinical settings. Finally, as we learned from the tendency of our informants in this study, it is essential to understand the pitfalls and limitations of mapped data, which risks misinterpretation similar to and often beyond other forms of data display. Expanded use of GIS to inform planning and policy in the clinical setting will require users to consider issues such as data quality, geocoding match rate, the choice of appropriate scale and areal units, as well as issues of causality versus association, and will probably benefit from additional training or partnership with spatial methodologists.

CONCLUSION

Our longitudinal experience with this CHC network since conducting these interviews includes continued requests for new maps, request for a contractual relationship to continue their production, and specific application of mapping in planning future service delivery and expansion, clinic moves, and community outreach. Leaders at BMSI have expressed the opinion that this exercise would be measurably more valuable if all safety-net services were similarly mapping their communities and could collaborate on regional planning. However, broader application of these methods is limited by the lack of financial and technical capacity in CHCs and other primary care settings, a theme identified by CHC leaders as a barrier to sustainability of our collaborative mapping project. Commercially available technologies now permit geocoding and housing of outpatient clinical data in a Health Insurance Portability and Accountability Act-compliant (HIPPAA) fashion; user-friendly internet mapping software have improved substantially in recent years. Such software may offer the ability to overcome the barriers to GIS use cited by clinic leaders and to realize GIS economies of scale for a large body of health centers or primary care clinics, expanding the reach of clinical analytic mapping to CHCs nationwide. Healthy People 2010 calls for an "increase in the proportion of all major national, state, and local health data systems ... to promote nationwide use of GIS at all levels," with a goal of 90% use in such systems.[24] Policy makers and regional planners supporting CHCs should consider policies and incentives that broaden GIS implementation at the clinical level.

ACKNOWLEDGEMENT

We gratefully acknowledge the assistance of Baltimore Medical Systems, Inc. staff, in particular that of Michael Barr and Jay Wolvowsky, as well as Imam Xierali for his assistance in map production and Lisette Dunham for her help in preparing this manuscript for submission.

REFERENCES

1. DeNavas-Walt, C., B. D. Proctor, and C. H. Lee, US Census Bureau. Income, poverty, and health insurance coverage in the United States: 2004. August 2005. Available at www.census.gov/hhes/www/hlthins/hlthin05.html. Accessed 30 October 2009.
2. U.S. Department of Health and Human Resources, Health Resources and Services Administration. The Health Center Program: the President's health center initiative. Available at http://bphc.hrsa.gov/presidentsinitiative./ Accessed 24 October 2009.
3. Miranda, M. L., J. M. Silva, M. A. Overstreet Galeano, et al. 2005. Building geographic information system capacity in local health departments: lessons from a North Carolina project. *Am J Public Health* 95:2180–5.
4. Fryer, G. E., J. Drisko, R. D. Krugman, et al. 1999. Multi-method assessment of access to primary medical care in rural Colorado. *J Rural Health* 15:113–21.
5. Andrews, J. W., C. G. Hames, J. C. Metts, Jr, L. Waters, J. M. Davis, and R. Carpenter. 1980. Relationships between selenium and other parameters in drinking water and blood of subjects from high and low cardiovascular disease rate areas of Georgia. *J Environ Pathol Toxicol* 4:313–8.
6. Farley, E. S. Jr, V. Boisseau, and J. Froom. 1977. An integrated medical record and data system for primary care. Part 5: Implications of filing family folders by area of residence. *J Fam Pract* 5:427–32.

7. Guagliardo, M. F. 2004. Spatial accessibility of primary care: concepts, methods and challenges. *Int J Health Geogr* 3:3.
8. Phillips, R. L. Jr, E. L. Kinman, P. G. Schnitzer, E. J. Lindbloom, and B. Ewigman. 2000. Using geographic information systems to understand health care access. *Arch Fam Med* 9:971–8.
9. Phillips, R. L., A. Bazemore, and T. J. Miyoshi. 2003. *Tools for Monitoring the Health Care Safety Net. Mapping Tools for Monitoring the Safety Net.* Rockville, MD: Agency for Healthcare Research and Quality.
10. Bazemore, A., R. L. Phillips, and T. J. Miyoshi. Using geographic information systems to define healthcare access in an urban community health center network. Available at http://proceedings.esri.com/library/userconf/health03/papers/pap3037/p3037.pdf. Accessed 30 October 2009.
11. Simpson, K., S. DesHarnais, A. Acobs, and A. Enapace. 1994. "Methods for Defining Medical Service Areas". In *Geographic Methods for Health Services Research*, Ricketts T. C., Savita L. A., Gesler W. M., Osborne D. N., and Lanham M. D. (Eds.), 207–32. Lanham, MD: University Press of America.
12. Johnson, J. C. 1990. *Selecting Ethnographic Informants*. Newbury Park, CA: Sage Publications.
13. Crabtree, B. F., and W. L. Miller. 1992. "The Analysis of Narratives from a Long Interview". In *Tools for primary care research*, Stewart M. (Ed.), 209–20.Newbury Park, CA: Sage Publications.
14. Kawachi, I., Berkman, L. F. eds. 2003. *Neighborhoods and health*. New York, NY: Oxford University Press, USA.
15. Gofin, J., and R. Gofin. 2005. Community-oriented primary care and primary health care. *Am J Public Health* 95:757.
16. Kark, S. L. 1974. *Epidemiology and Community Medicine*. New York, NY: Appleton-Century-Crofts.
17. Donaldson, M., K. D. Yordy, K. N. Lohr, and N. A. Vanselow. 1996. *Primary Care: America's Health in a New Era*. Washington, DC: National Academy Press.
18. Institute of Medicine. 2001. *Crossing the Quality Chasm: A New Health System for the 21st Century*. Washington, DC: National Academy Press.
19. Phillips, R. L., F. Mullan, and E. Kinman. Geographic retrofitting: a method for community definition. Presented at the 130th Annual Meeting of the American Public Health Association, Philadelphia, PA, 9–13 November 2002.
20. Phillips R. L., M. L. Parchman., and T. J. Miyoshi. Using geographic information systems to understand health care access. Available at http://proceedings.esri.com/library/userconf/health01/papers/hc01_p01d/hc01_p01d.html. Accessed 24 October 2009.
21. US Department of Health and Human Services. HHS continues health care safety net expansion. Awards $4.9 million to create new or expand existing health centers. Available at http://www.dhhs.gov/news/press/2002pres/20021004.html. Accessed 30 October 2009.
22. Crump, R. L., M. H. Gaston, and G. Ferguson, 1999. HRSA's models that work program: implications for improving access to primary health care. *Health Rep* 114:218–24.
23. US Department of Health and Human Services, Health Resources and Services Administration. HRSA Geospatial Data Warehouse. Primary care service

areas-2006 edition. Available at http://datawarehouse.hrsa.gov/pcsa2006.aspx. Accessed 30 October 2009.

24. US Department of Health and Human Services. *Healthy People 2010: understanding and improving health*, 2nd ed. Available at http://www.hhs.gov/news/press/2000pres/20000125a.html. Accessed 24 October 2009.

Embracing the Open-Source Movement for Managing Spatial Data: A Case Study of African Trypanosomiasis in Kenya

SHAUN A. LANGLEY and JOSEPH P. MESSINA
Michigan State University, East Lansing, Michigan, USA

The past decade has seen an explosion in the availability of spatial data, not only for researchers, but the public as well. As the quantity of data increases, the ability to effectively navigate and understand the data becomes more challenging. Here we detail a conceptual model for a spatially explicit database management system that addresses the issues raised with the growing data management problem. We demonstrate utility with a case study in disease ecology: to develop a multiscale predictive model of African trypanosomiasis in Kenya. International collaborations and varying technical expertise necessitate a modular open-source software solution. Finally, we address three recurring problems with data management: scalability, reliability, and security.

1. INTRODUCTION

The transdisciplinary nature of modern research in disease ecology often requires and generates vast quantities of data varying thematically and in structure. The data management challenge is considerable and often prohibitively costly. Data arise from a multitude of sources and occur in spatially explicit or aspatial forms with concomitant structures. Rarely are these data accompanied by the ontologically coherent metadata necessary to facilitate cooperation and collaboration. Recent discourse in studies of infectious disease ecology have suggested a need to emphasize the role of the changing dynamics of space and land cover in describing the interactions of diseases with environmental processes (Ostfeld, Keesing, and Eviner 2008). Therefore, effective engagement in disease ecology research requires the ability to correctly access, interpret, and integrate these highly diverse data (Shekhar and Chawla 2003; Watson 2004; Longley 2005).

In the early 1990s there was a great deal of research concerning the expansion of traditional database management systems (DBMSs) to incorporate functionality for handling spatially explicit data types (Stonebraker and Moore 1996; Shekhar and Chawla 2003). Traditional DBMSs are self-describing in that the definitions of data are stored in a catalog, along with the raw data, without the need to store separate descriptive files. This is an extremely efficient means for managing and accessing large quantities of data. Databases improve our abilities to interact with data through the construction and querying of indexes, which serve as a data road map stored on the physical media. Early database frameworks rarely interacted directly with spatial data (Egenhofer 1994; Stonebraker and Moore 1996). Yet with technological advances, particularly the development of satellite platforms for remote sensing, great quantities of data were being generated, necessitating the development of DBMS capabilities specifically to facilitate handling of spatial data.

SQL, standard query language, was formally adopted in 1986 by the American National Standards Institute as SQL-86, and it is the most widely used database-querying language (Lans 2007). The SQL framework provided a logical structure for querying information stored in DBMSs. The first versions of SQL, however, could not explicitly handle spatial data structures. Several extensions of SQL were proposed including GEOQL, SAND, GEO-Kernel, and PSQL; however, the extension that proved most influential—and eventually adopted—was Egenhofer's Spatial SQL (Egenhofer 1994; Adam and Gangopadhyay 1997). Spatial SQL extended the domain to include spatial operators and attributes. Egenhofer further defined the graphical presentation language (GPL), a set of tools in which the results of a spatial query could be manipulated. The Open GIS Consortium (OGIS) promoted spatial functionality by recommending a set of critical reforms in SQL, mainly the adoption of Egenhofer's spatial abstraction model, which introduced Geometry as a base class for spatial objects (Egenhofer 1994; OGIS 1999; Shekhar and Chawla 2003).These recommendations were fully adopted in 1999 with the release of SQL3 (OGIS 1999; Lans 2007).

Data sharing is a critical consideration for our research group, as we collaborate with institutions and researchers throughout much of the United States and East Africa; yet the biggest problem we face as a group is the ability to share data and analysis. We require a new medium that facilitates this flow of information without the need to physically carry the data between institutions. Internet-based GIS and data servers are one solution we employ to allow for simultaneous interaction and analysis of the data. Internet-based GIS emerged with the release of two projects, GeoChange

(Drew and Ying 1996) and the Alexandria Digital Library (Smith and Frew 1995). GeoChange, in particular, set the standard in terms of functionality and usability with interface-supporting, batch-processing, import/export, automatic metadata generation capabilities (Adam and Gangopadhyay 1997). The Alexandria Data Library, though spare in relation to GeoChange, became widely adopted by the University of California system for in-house sharing of proprietary spatial data. Today, despite improvements in functionality, most spatial databases still lack the ability to efficiently handle the raster data structure. Two ongoing projects promise to bring this functionality into spatial DBMSs in 2010. Of particular interest to us is the WKTRaster project, a community supported, open-source project by the Open Source Geospatial Foundation (OSGEO). WKTRaster extends the functionality of the PostGIS library to implement the Raster-type class in the same way Geometry was done in order to support spatially explicit handling of vector data (Stonebraker and Moore 1996). WKTRaster, when fully implemented, will facilitate consistency in data handling of all spatial and nonspatial data types, similar to the manner in which spatial data are managed with the GeoRaster loader included in the Oracle Spatial 11g package.

Although advances in scientific understanding and new technologies have helped to curb the spread of infectious diseases in the developed world, the same cannot be said about the developing world. As the incidence of infectious diseases decreased in the developed world, fewer resources and less attention was devoted to combating those diseases in the developing world, contributing to an increase in the prevalence of many illnesses there (Cohen 2000). In order to develop better strategies for combating disease, we need to enhance our understanding of the underlying ecological conditions that contribute to the emergence of diseases and deliver solutions practicable in developing world contexts (Ostfeld et al. 2008). Disease ecology is generally not considered a discipline in itself but it rather seeks to understand the relationship between disease epidemiology and the landscape (climate, physical, and human) (Sutherst 2004; Keesing et al. 2006; Tatem et al. 2006; Johnson and Thieltges 2010). The transdisciplinary nature of the field creates a unique set of problems, many of which pertain to the use of data while maintaining the rigorous standards mandated by institutional review boards, Health Insurance Portability and Accountability Act (HIPAA), and international research and privacy standards. Very little has been published that directly explores these types of management problems within the disease ecology literature. Routinely, issues of scalability, reliability, and security emerge that hinder the effective dissemination of federally funded data and models. Storage of large quantities of data must at a minimum facilitate the range of applications necessitated by the questions posed in disease ecology. Data *scalability* speaks to the ability of researchers to address questions at multiple scales of spatial or temporal resolution, depending upon the question being asked; the storage of such data must facilitate the rapid, concurrent access and integration of the data across varying resolutions (Shekhar and Chawla 2003). *Reliability* requires mechanisms to ensure that data mismatches or inappropriate analytical methods are identified or prevented (Shi et al. 2002; Devillers and Jeansoulin 2006). Furthermore, data reliability, particularly with concurrent usage and modification of the data, necessitates mechanisms for ensuring the integrity of the underlying data over time (Shi et al. 2002; Olson 2003). Finally, *security* issues arise when interacting with individually identifiable human data or sensitive community data stored or generated within the DBMS (Olson 2003). Though institutional guidelines and privacy laws may restrict access of the data to preapproved users, the limitations should not preclude nonprivileged users from asking broader questions that might interact with the underlying data when aggregated to remove identifiable data or other information that may be restricted by institutional guidelines or laws (e.g., ethnic identity at low densities in census block group data). Finally, privacy restrictions should be scalable, changing dynamically with the user and scale of resolution requested.

In collaboration with the International Livestock Research Institute in Kenya (ILRI), we have accumulated an extraordinary volume of data for that country. Irrespective of theme, international collaborations often present unique problems in terms of the management, sharing, and dissemination of data necessary to carry out analyses. Our framework for a data management system is a novel solution for spatial modeling in disease ecology, and the use of open-source software makes this an inclusive cost-effective solution for sharing with international collaborators and organizations with limited budgets. The entire suite of data and models is designed to be packaged electronically or on a portable drive to facilitate electronic transfer and physical transportation.

A framework for data management geared to these issues and flexible in the use of restrictions is an ideal solution for working with data types characteristic of research in disease ecology. As part of the National Institutes of Health (NIH) Roadmap program and with the NIH General Medical Sciences support, we are developing a multiscale predictive model that defines the relationship between climate change, land use and land cover change, social systems, and the distribution of tsetse flies and sleeping sickness across Kenya (Messina et al. 2007). Here we present a case study for the implementation of a generalizable disease ecology DBMS framework that provides scalability, reliability, and security to optimize interactions between users and data.

1.1. Case Study: A Model for African Trypanosomiasis in Kenya

African trypanosomiasis (AT), or sleeping sickness, is a major threat to human health across Africa, particularly among impoverished peoples (Brun et al. 2010; Gyapong et al. 2010). Typically considered a disease of the past, its prevalence has increased in recent years, particularly in East Africa, due to the declining emphasis on trapping and control, climate, and anthropogenic factors (Bauer et al. 1992; WHO 2005; Batchelor et al. 2009). Although monitoring has improved, the extent to which AT impacts East Africa is largely unknown. Recent contributions by foreign countries and aid organizations directed toward addressing AT have declined dramatically in contrast to the increased attention toward AIDS, malaria, and other diseases (WHO 2001; Siringi 2003). The World Health Organization (WHO) has responded by designating AT a neglected tropical disease (Kennedy 2005; WHO 2006; Brun et al. 2010). Not fully understanding the ecological processes that contribute to the spread of AT may result in the inefficient application of control regimes and misallocation of resources, thus retarding the efforts of the African Union to combat and control AT (Cox 2004). As trypanosomiasis has increased in prevalence, the impact on human and animal populations has been considerable, resulting in severe economic hardship for rural families throughout East Africa (Campbell et al. 2000; Campbell et al. 2004).

Tsetse flies (*Glossinidae* family) are the primary vectors for the cyclical transmission of AT. The general distribution of tsetse has been demonstrated in terms of the biophysical extent and the presence of suitable hosts (KETRI 1996; Cecchi et al. 2008). However, the precise limits, historical and contemporary, have not been formalized experimentally (Wint 2001). Furthermore, the current distribution belts reflect outdated data and methodologies (FAO 1979; Wint 2001; Muriuki et al. 2005). Through prior studies, our research group has been able to describe the inaccuracies of these distribution limits, particularly in terms of seasonal changes (DeVisser and Messina 2009; Moore and Messina 2010). Furthermore, global climate change is shifting tsetse habitats, though the degree to which this is occurring is unknown (Sutherst 2004).

To adequately understand the mechanisms behind the increasing incidence of AT, it is important to consider a diverse range of inputs from social, physical, climatic, and even political dimensions. The range of scientific disciplines and methodologies required necessitates an extensive volume of data to be created, collected, and maintained. The management of the volumes and types of data, physically and logistically, has proven to be a significant challenge and the one which we address in this paper. Thus we present a conceptual model for a comprehensive open-source, computing environment that promotes efficient organization, storage, and retrieval of disparate data. Furthermore, we extend the discussion of spatial databases by presenting a model framework for a spatial DBMS that rigorously and consistently manages both spatial and nonspatial data.

1.2. Data Holdings and Acquisitions

We have collected all publicly available data and a significant portion of the known privately held relevant AT disease ecology spatial data for Kenya.

TABLE 1 A Summary of Our Data Library Grouped by Major Theme

Biophysical	Social	Geographical
Precipitation totals	Population density	Land use/Land cover
Monthly temperatures	Population predictions	Land use projections
Evapotranspiration	Historical population	Satellite imagery
Temperature scenarios	Town locations	Lakes
Precipitation scenarios	District census data	Rivers
Historical climate data	Livestock	River basins
Agro-climatic zones	Wildlife	Roads
Agro-ecological zones	Agricultural production	National parks
Lithology	Poverty	Railroads
Soils	Various cadastral data	National boundaries
Landforms	Entomological	Administrative districts
Forest range	Tsetse distribution	Elevation
Wetlands	Tsetse habitat suitability	Topographic maps (countrywide)

The data fall into a classification scheme, defined by topography, soils, vegetation, climate, ecological diversity, water resources, and anthropogenic factors known to control or influence the ecological processes driving tsetse distributions over time and space (see Table 1 for a summary). Nonspatial data consist primarily of governmental and intra-agency reports obtained through private libraries in Kenya. The reports collected focus on policies and governmental and community control and eradication programs. Currently, these reports are neither catalogued nor indexed, limiting efficient use of any information they may contain.

Remotely sensed image data comprise the majority by physical file size of our data collection. We possess most of the known publically available aerial imagery for Kenya from the Landsat, MODIS, PALSAR, and ASTER platforms; including a number of image products summarizing land use classification (MODIS types 1–5 for 2001 to 2005 and Landsat MSS– derived 1 km for 1980), land surface temperature (MODIS LST), precipitation (WorldClim 30-y average at 1 km), and vegetation indexes[1] (NDVI for 2001 to 2008 every 16 d, 250-m resolution). Additional sources of land use and land cover information are provided with Africover as vector or raster data types, GLC2000, CLIP cover,[1] and UMD Global Land Cover. We have elevation data from ASTER, SRTM, and digitized topographic maps (30-m, 90-m, and 250-m spatial resolutions, respectively). Regarding the distribution of tsetse, we possess vector and raster digitized distributions of fly belts for Kenya for 1967, 1973, 1996, and 2000.[2] Finally, there are rasterized estimates of livestock densities (#/km^2) for 2007 (ILRI[3]). Utilizing these data, DeVisser et al. (2010) developed the TED model to predict the distribution of tsetse in Kenya (see Figure 1). To effectively and efficiently recover and maintain the value of the data, we require a solution that not only provides for efficient storage and retrieval of the data, but that also allows for automated metadata generation.

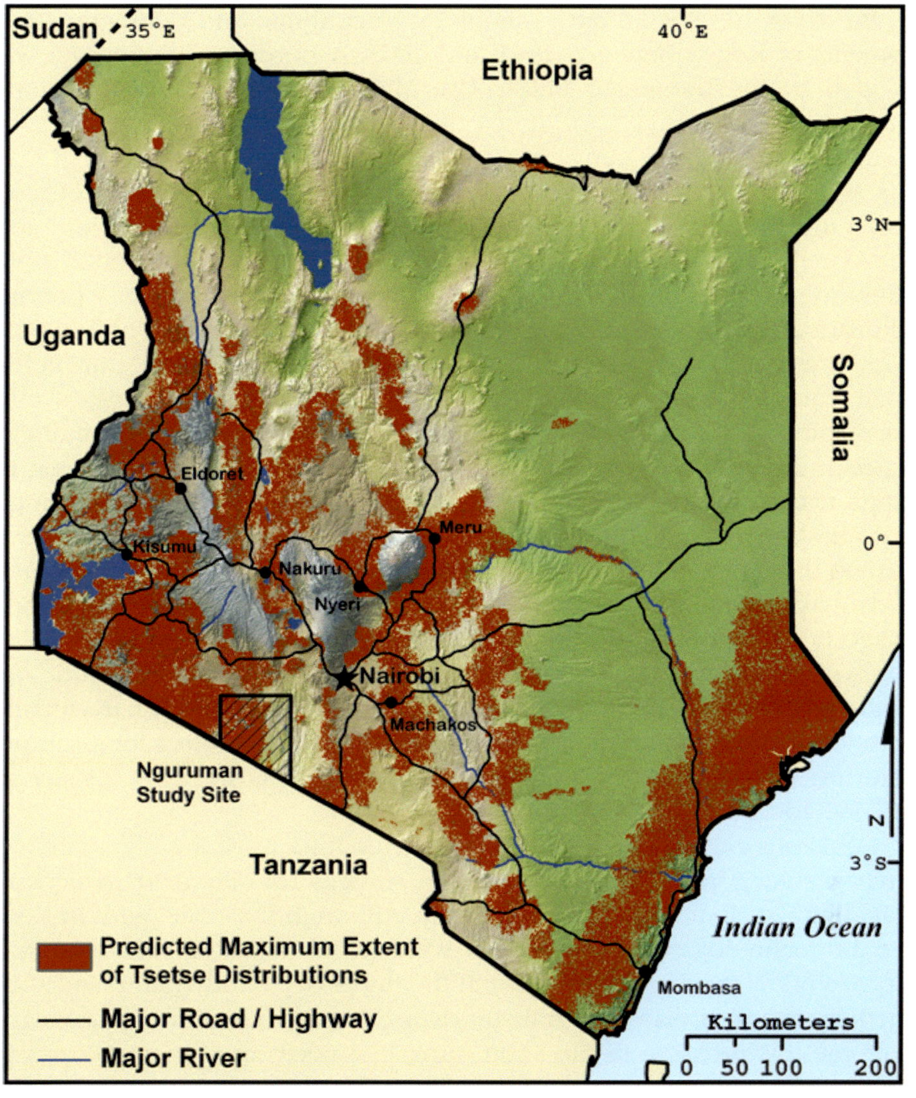

FIGURE 1 Maximum extent of tsetse distribution predicted by the TED Model between the beginning of 2002 and the end of 2009. As described by DeVisser et al. (2010), the TED Model uses five scenes of MODIS 1km annual land cover, 207 scenes of MODIS 250 m Normalized Difference Vegetation Index (NDVI), and 207 scenes of MODIS 1km day/night Land Surface Temperature (LST) products to predict the fundamental niche of tsetse in Kenya, and a fly movement model to predict tsetse distributions or realized niche of the tsetse species of interest. The TED Model is written in Python scripting language and is run within ArcGIS 9.2 (or later versions of ArcGIS). Other data sets used to construct the map include shapefiles of Kenyan major roads, highways, cities, rivers, Kenyan water bodies, lakes, and African country political boundaries. To construct the background topographic relief map, the Shuttle RADAR Topographic Mission (SRTM) 90 m Digital Elevation Model (DEM) was used to create a gridded hillshade product, and a dry season NDVI scene was combined with the SRTM DEM to create an elevation/vegetation color scheme.

We have 103 spatial data sets of socioeconomic and demographic assessments of Kenya between 1971 and 2008. A portion of these data were provided by the Integrated Public Use Microdata Series (IPUMS) International data set for Kenya,[4] and they originate from the Kenya 1989 and 1999 census collected by the Kenya National Bureau of Statistics. The IPUMS data are a systematic sample of every twentieth household; these data represent a sampling fraction of 5 percent and expansion factor of 20. A long-form questionnaire was implemented to survey individuals within households. Location data for each individual are limited to the respondent's province and district, first and second administrative levels respectively, of five possible levels each at an increasingly finer spatial scale of resolution. Data at finer spatial scales are not available as part of the Kenya Bureau of Statistics' effort to maintain privacy. A further complication was a change in the number of districts in Kenya from forty-two in 1989 to sixty-nine in 1999; however, this change was made by subdividing existing districts allowing rough comparisons between associated regions. The IPUMS sample provides ninety-seven household and individual variables, most importantly geographic information (urban/rural status, province, district), utility (electricity, water supply, sewage type, and type of cooking fuel), and dwelling (number of rooms, toilet type, floor, wall, and roof material). Other relevant data include individual variables describing household position, demographic characteristics, education, employment, migration, and disability (see Table 2 for a sample). There are a total of 1,074,048 individual entries for the 1989 census and 1,407,597 for the 1999 census samples.

Decisions on data management often conflict during collaborative research, resulting in the lack of a cohesive strategy for data management and the inability to share such data effectively. Although our colleagues in Kenya have the technological skills to work with spatial data, the telecommunication network is insufficient to provide the necessary bandwidth or reliability to acquire the data via direct transfer over FTP or other similar protocol. To overcome this problem in the short term, it is necessary for us to carry the data into the country on physical media and to have it accompanied by a data management system that can facilitate interaction with the large quantity of data. Thus, efficiency and portability are significant concerns.

2. DEVELOPMENT OF A SPATIAL DATABASE SYSTEM

Our solution for a spatial DBMS involves bridging a variety of software packages following the basic framework as described by Câmara et al (1996) for the development of the TerraLib GIS Library and the integration considerations posed for the MurMur project (Parent, Spaccapietra, and Zimányi 2006). First, we outline the conceptual framework, and second, we implement the design. Third, we describe the development of routines, batch, or other

TABLE 2 A Sample of the Subset of Kenya Census Data we Hold from the 1990 National Census

	cntry	year	sample	serial	persons	wthh	subsamp	gq	unrel	ubran	provke	distke	ownrshpd	electrc
1	404	1989	4041	1000	4	20.0000	26	10	0	2	1	1010	216	2
2	404	1989	4041	1000	4	20.0000	26	10	0	2	1	1010	216	2
3	404	1989	4041	1000	4	20.0000	26	10	0	2	1	1010	216	2
4	404	1989	4041	1000	4	20.0000	26	10	0	2	1	1010	216	2
5	404	1989	4041	2000	1	20.0000	76	10	0	2	1	1010	216	1
6	404	1989	4041	3000	4	20.0000	2	10	0	2	1	1010	216	1
7	404	1989	4041	3000	4	20.0000	2	10	0	2	1	1010	216	1
8	404	1989	4041	3000	4	20.0000	2	10	0	2	1	1010	216	1
9	404	1989	4041	3000	4	20.0000	2	10	0	2	1	1010	216	1
10	404	1989	4041	4000	1	20.0000	92	10	0	2	1	1010	140	2
11	404	1989	4041	5000	1	20.0000	81	10	0	2	1	1010	216	1
12	404	1989	4041	6000	12	20.0000	5	10	0	2	1	1010	216	1
13	404	1989	4041	6000	12	20.0000	5	10	0	2	1	1010	216	1
14	404	1989	4041	6000	12	20.0000	5	10	0	2	1	1010	216	1

preconfigured shell scripts that can be selected to run either from the command line or through an interactive GUI prompt whereby a user can add and recall raw data files or query the database to return a mash-up of spatial data files or metadata. Finally, we develop a set of SQL triggers (code set to run when activated by a defined action) to enforce data integrity.

2.1. Conceptual Model

Figure 2 demonstrates our conceptual model for a spatial DBMS. In contrast to previous implementations of MySQL, Postgres, and other common spatial databases, modern DMBS models facilitate raw data and metadata to be stored together, embedded in the database (Elmasri and Navathe 2004; Watson 2004). The proposed spatial computing environment uses open-source, community-supported software and standards, providing a solution to the data-management problem that is temporally extensible. The database is portable in that we can copy the database and software binaries to a portable drive that can be carried to Kenya. Of critical concern to us in selecting software components was the interoperability of the system, and the ability of components to interface and work together. Our selected DBMS is PostgreSQL[5] (Postgres), an advanced, readily available, open-source, object-relational database management system. Using standard SQL syntax, Postgres allows for complex query capabilities, including spatial queries, and facilitates strict rule and primary key enforcement. Postgres is also extensible, allowing for the addition of new functionality (Stonebraker and Rowe 1986; Stonebraker and Kemnitz 1991).

PostGIS[6] is an extension to the Postgres language that adds functionality for the storage and retrieval of spatial data files. PostGIS is, at its core, a suite of tools that serves as the back end for spatial functionality in Postgres (Ramsey 2005). Of particular interest is the WKTRaster[7] (Beta 0.1.6) project, which extends the ability of a Postgres database to store and index raster data, a first of its kind. The project mirrors the inherent vector-based functions (of Geometry type) for raster data. The result is a single set of SQL functions that handle both spatial data types. This extension has the potential to greatly enhance and facilitate the utilization of raster data by end users. Figure 3 presents the conceptual model for the user interface to the Postgres DBMS. We incorporate a variety of software packages, explained later, each of which provides the user with statistical, visual, and geoprocessing capabilities; the user can interact with these packages through a GUI or through a command line interface.

GRASS (geographic resources analysis support system)[8] is one of the few open-source options for handling raster GIS data. Developed by the Open Source Geospatial Foundation, GRASS is an increasingly popular solution for the use and analysis of spatial data in academic research. Like the many other

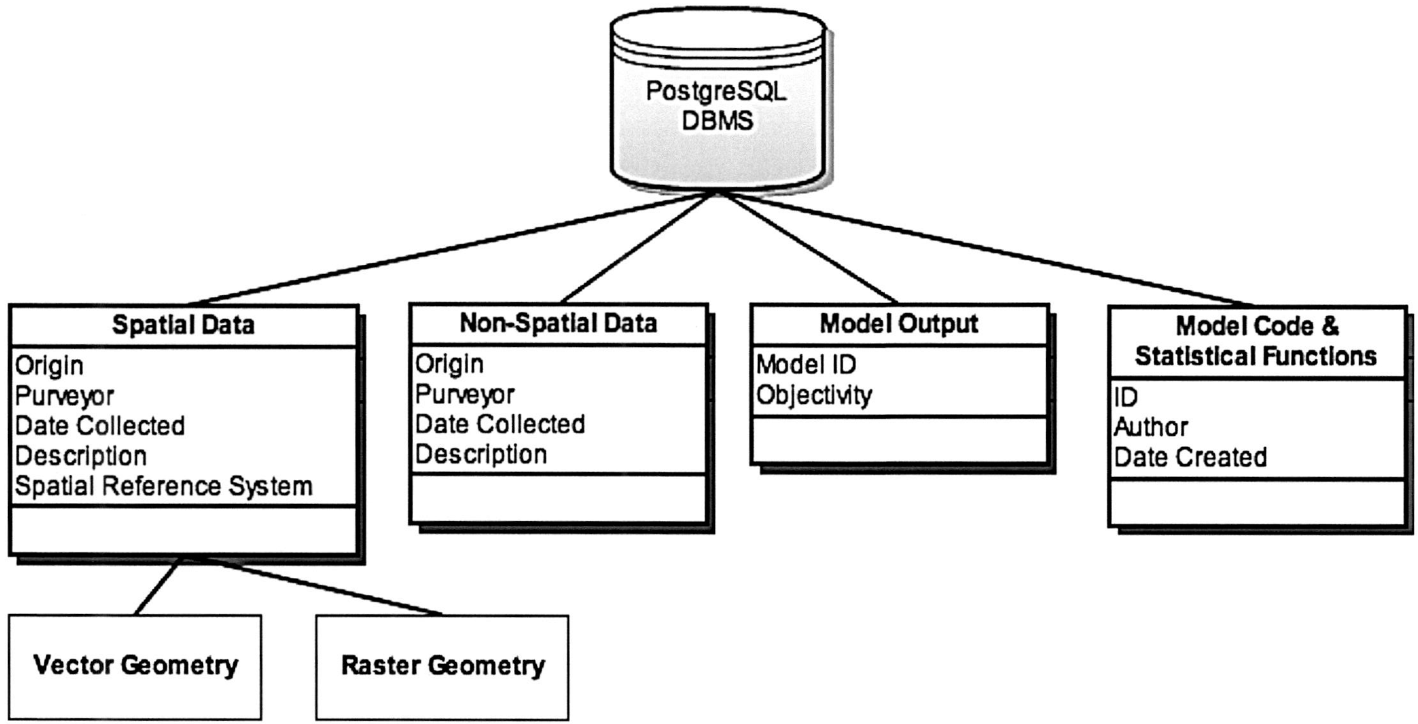

FIGURE 2 A conceptual model framework for the spatial DBMS.

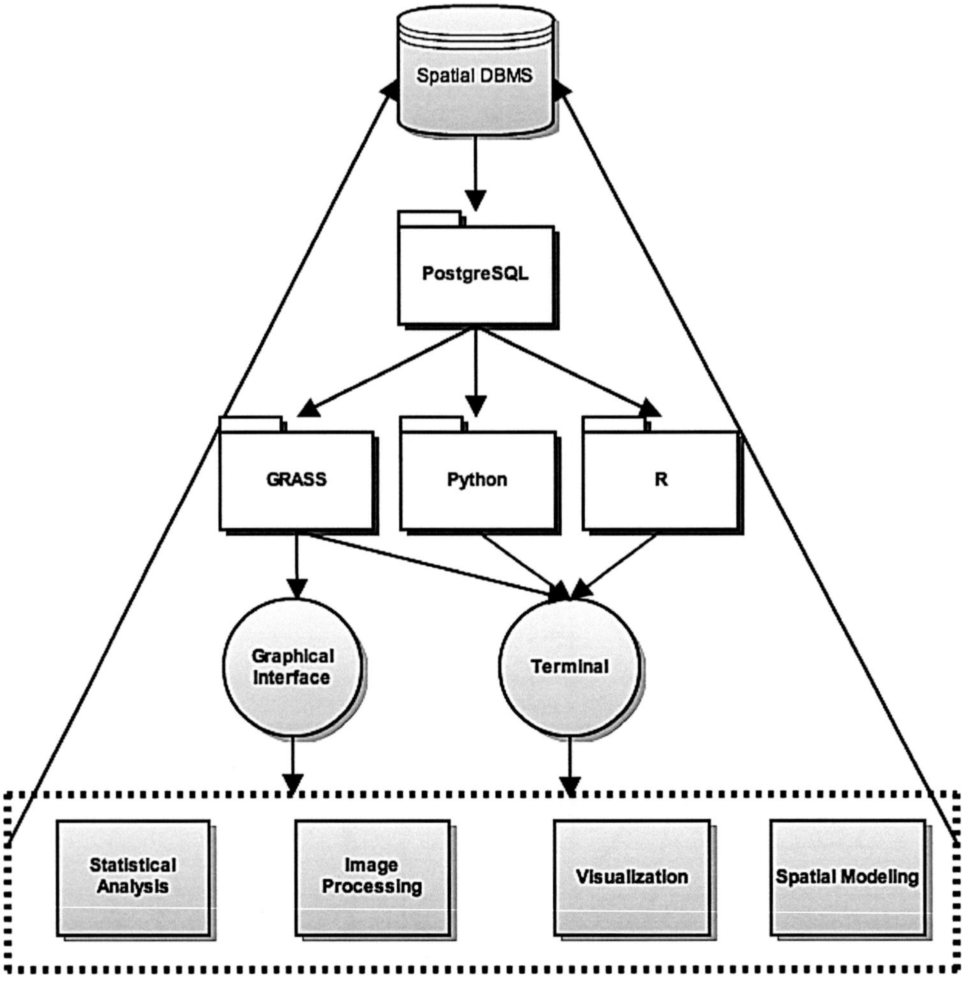

FIGURE 3 Flow of data through the model implementation as users interact with the system. It should be noted that flows are one-directional, meaning that although users can interact with the data to generate analysis, the results must be stored as a separate entity in the database. This ensures that the underlying data cannot be changed.

components selected for the system presented here, GRASS is interoperable with Python and Postgres, and is extensible, allowing users to create and add new functionality.

Although there is a plethora of statistical packages available, R is our preferred statistical package,[9] in large part because it interfaces easily with GRASS and Postgres. We can do so without needing to install any additional software components. R is an open-source solution, developed by an international community of users, to create an alternative to the often expensive and restrictive programs offered by statistical companies. Although R lacks a graphical interface, it uses far less computer memory than most other comparable statistical packages. This allows us to perform complex analyses with fewer hardware demands, an important consideration for maintaining portability of the project.

Finally, Python is an object-oriented programming language developed by Guido van Rossum in 1991 and maintained, in large part, by the open-source community (Python Software Foundation 2010). Python is an efficient scripting language that facilitates interoperability between our database (Postgres), statistical analysis software (R), and GIS (GRASS) (Neteler and Mitasova 2008). Python is a highly intuitive, object-oriented programming language, easy enough to learn and use that it makes for a good solution to bridge our project components. Furthermore, the open-source nature of the language fits well with the other components, enabling us to incorporate additional extensions written by the community.

The most critical considerations for long-term data storage are persistence and security (Elmasri and Navathe 2004; Watson 2004). Digital data are inherently ephemeral in that over time physical storage media will fail or degrade, thus requiring continuous rewriting on digital media to ensure persistence. Though drive technology has progressed significantly in the past decade, drive failure is not uncommon; the volume of data and frequency with which the data are accessed puts immense stress on the physical mechanisms. Therefore, it is necessary to employ a strategy that ensures the long-term viability of the data. To this extent, we employ a redundant array of independent disks (RAID) as our secondary storage medium, mirroring data between groups of drives. This enables corrupted data resulting from disk failure to be recovered in real time, without the need to create tertiary backup regimes. Furthermore, we enforce constraints to access of the data in making the data read-only, reducing the chance a write error will occur or values will be inadvertently changed. Finally, all files will have MD5 checksums (a cryptographic hash code generated from a file's binary data) included as an attribute of the file allowing us to verify the integrity of any data file (Rivest 1992). The strategies employed here will also enable us to protect against accidental user error, which may result in inadvertent modification or deletion of data. Security restrictions, though a good first line of defense, are frequently circumventable. The ability to roll back changes within Postgres, as well as being able to restore data from the RAID, will ensure the long-term integrity of the data library.

2.2. Database Standards

Generic frameworks for database development, such as the one we outline here, should use established ontologies in their component descriptions, which we satisfy by conforming to the formal ontology described by the Open Geospatial Consortium (OGC).[10] The OGC is an independent group tasked with the purpose of developing and maintaining a set of standards for the management of spatial data to promote both consistency and interoperability across GIS platforms. The Geographic Data Abstraction Library[11] (GDAL) stands as a single standard for interoperability of raster data within the GIS community. As a library, it facilitates the conversion between data products. However, as is the case when working with proprietary data, conversion between formats requires a commonly understood intermediate. The GDAL standards and abstraction libraries used in our project facilitate this conversion between data formats by providing a commonly understood intermediate.[12] Custom GDAL libraries are used largely in our implementation of GRASS as a mechanism to add support for a range of occasionally unsupported data formats.

There are an inordinate number of disparate standards for metadata generation and inclusion, none of which are remotely universal. Regardless, it is necessary for our own data management that we accept and enforce a single standard for metadata management. The fact that our DBMS facilitates the storage of raw data within the system precludes the need to store metadata separately as this information is included within the database as discrete variables (the raw data are technically also included as an attribute value). However, it is foreseeable that we may need, on occasion, to transfer data outside the realm of the database. Under this scenario, it is necessary to have a mechanism to recreate the metadata files discarded earlier. Thus, we incorporate custom scripts that can be called to assemble the necessary metadata precursor information from the data table. The resulting metadata report meets the formatting and content criteria specified by the OGC and ISO19115 specifications.[13]

2.3. SQL-Rule-Based Interactions and Scripting

In an effort to ensure the integrity of the raw data and prevent accidental deletion or modification, all users are restricted in the ways they can interact with the DBMS. In most cases, raw data are restricted to read-only access by users at the database level. One way we achieve this is by restricting Update and Delete privileges to the database administrator account only. This ensures that raw data cannot be changed or deleted through unverified scripting. It further facilitates the simultaneous access and use of raw data by multiple processes. Figure 3 symbolizes the flow of data from the DBMS to the user. Even though the raw data are read-only, it is useful to permit users to save the output of models to the database, with the option to link to the source data. Indexing these data sets together is useful when new users explore the data. We will discuss this functionality further in the section "A User Perspective: Interfacing with the DBMS." Metadata for these model outputs will vary, but will at a minimum include the user identity and model code, as well as a summary of the model objective. A set of predefined rules or triggers is loaded into the DBMS, providing enforcement of the desired constraints (e.g., spatial/temporal mismatch encountered during scripted analysis). These rules serve to provide a minimal standard of validity and consistency for model output and statistical analysis (Shi, Goodchild, and Fisher, 2002; Devillers and Jeansoulin 2006).

The storage of raw data within the DBMS precludes the need to regularly interact with different data formats. Nevertheless, it may be useful to incorporate a mechanism whereby we can convert data among data formats or export data into a range of formats. Although most of these tasks can be accomplished within the GRASS interface, we include in our library a set of Python scripts to extend our ability to move among data formats (particularly useful for the range of raster imagery available). For example, our "data bank" includes raster imagery (*.img, .tif, .hdf, among others), vector data (*.shp and others), text documents (*.doc, .docx, .txt, .pdf, and others), metadata files corresponding to acquired imagery (*.xml, .pdf, .txt, and others), as well as an assortment of other types not specifically mentioned here.

2.4. DBMS Interface—A Manager Perspective

Implicit in the design of our database are SQL rules (and triggers) that constrain the ways users can work with data in an effort to prevent common mistakes. Because the database holds data at varying resolutions and extents, we constructed rules to check for common errors committed by users in selecting data layers. In the event that data layers are deemed incompatible, the user is alerted to the mismatch and encouraged, though not required, to restate their request. These rule sets operate at the point of data retrieval and storage. When importing data, we check and request that the user define the relationship between spatial data and metadata. If metadata are not available, the user is prompted to input known characteristics of the data file in an attempt to force this paired relation. Common examples of prompted information include the time stamp of data acquisition or generation, solar or view angle (for satellite-derived imagery), or a definition of codes that may occur within the data table (often the case with census data). Some of these data can be retrieved from the raw data, such as extent, summary statistics, or file type. Enforcing these relationships at the time of storage will greatly reduce the number of unpaired spatial data files and corresponding descriptors.

These rule sets also operate on a variety of demographic or other similar data types stored in our database. In our specific implementation of the database, we have sample volumes of census data collected by the Kenyan government and acquired from IPUMS.[14] As data are input into the database, users are prompted as to the type of data being input and plain English definitions of the variables (a long form description of the purpose of the data) included in the data set. We developed a means to query the data file for variables and return this list in memory to the rule set. In the event the data file does not return the correct list of variables, the user is prompted to specify the range of variables or create them.

2.5. DBMS Interface—A User Perspective

Though many incantations of interfaces are possible, one means by which users can interact with data is through a Web browser, which connects to the database via an application developed for Mac OS. Through the application, users have access to all the tools needed to query, utilize, and analyze data from the DBMS. From a set of menus, users are prompted to select a subset of data. Next, they are given the opportunity of selecting from either a set of precompiled models or statistical scripts that can analyze the data, or the data can be brought forward and immediately visualized in the browser window. Finally, the users are provided with command line tools that can augment their interaction with the data. This approach to data interaction lowers the learning curve for new users and gets them instantly connected with the data.

2.6. Statistical and Analytical Analysis

We extend the functionality of our DBMS to assist users in browsing the library of data by using the R package to automatically calculate descriptive statistics. These summaries are potentially most valuable to users not involved with the production of the data, or who may not be familiar with a region of interest. Furthermore, providing a means to compute descriptive statistics automatically enforces consistency between files that is often a symptom of user error when files are independently managed.

Perhaps the most common challenge users face in interacting with databases is retrieving data both correctly formatted and appropriate for use in a particular analysis (Longley 2005). The scripted analysis tools help bridge the gap in understanding for users not familiar with the R statistical package. With a simple menu prompt, the user can specify which data files and statistical methods are to be employed by the program. Though not a comprehensive selection, it provides a means to conduct a range of simple statistical comparisons. Further analyses can be performed though the R package directly linked to the database.

3. IMPLEMENTATION

To enable the reader to implement our DBMS model, we provide a general outline of the steps needed to install and configure the software packages. We make no assumptions as to the hardware on which the model is implemented. Our solution requires a number of software components, including PostgreSQL, PostGIS (with GDAL and WKTRaster extensions), Python, GRASS, and the R statistical package. In this section we will detail the required steps for the implementation of each component within open-source Debian distributions of Linux.

3.1. Software Packages

Debian distributions of Linux take advantage of the aptitude system for software distribution, and therefore you can install all packages from the terminal. To install, type

```
sudo apt-get install python postgresql
sudo apt-get install gdal-bin postgresql -8.4 -postgis postgis grass r-base
```

You may also be interested in installing the Quantum GIS (QGIS) program, another convenient GUI that interfaces with GRASS, which can also be installed with aptitude:

```
sudo apt-get install qgis
```

To allow interaction between GRASS and the GDAL libraries, you need to build and configure the GRASS plugin for GDAL. Download and follow the installation instructions provided by

http : //trac.osgeo.org/gdal/wiki/GRASS

Finally, you need to install optional extensions to the R package. Start R from a terminal by typing R; then install packages with

```
install.packages ("ctv")
library (ctv)
install.views ("Spatial")
```

3.2. Initializing Postgres

You will need to log in to Postgres for the first time using the default "postgres" login. From the terminal window you will then be able to create user accounts, set access restrictions, and create the database for the project data. First start Postgres from a terminal by typing

```
psql -U postgres
```

You can now create your user accounts. In our implementation of the project, all users are granted limited permission by default. Additional rights can be given later depending on the needs of the user.

```
CREATE USER <username>;
CREATEDB <dbname>;
GRANT ALL to <username> ON <dbname>;
```

It is necessary to configure the database to enable spatial functionality with PostGIS. The instructions given are also available from the PostGIS documentation at

http : //postgis.refractions.net/documentation/

First, type

```
CREATELANG plpgsql <dbname>
```

Now, copy the PostGIS spatial definition files into your new database and navigate to the PostGIS installation directory specified during installation and type

```
psql – d <dbname> -f postgis.sql
\q #Quits the Postgres session
```

For additional security options available, you can refer to the Postgres documentation.[15] You can now log in to your new database from a terminal window by typing

```
psql -U <username><dbname>
```

Use caution when performing upgrades to PostGIS, as you will likely have to rebuild support for your database.

3.3. WKT Raster Extension for PostGIS

WKT Raster is not yet included in the PostGIS precompiled binary as it is (as of 09/15/2010) still in beta testing. Therefore, you will need to download and compile the extension. The following instructions are available from the WKT Raster project documentation.[16] Depending on your specific system configuration, it may be necessary to build the PostGIS libraries from source as well as the required dependencies. Download the source code from

http : //www.postgis.org/download/

Unpack the tar file and navigate to the wktraster directory. Generate a configuration profile by typing

./autogen.sh

Now run a configuration script. You will need to locate the installation directory for PostGIS:

./configure - -with-postgis-sources=/thesrc/postgis-version

If no errors were generated, you can install wktraster. Because you are already in the installation directory, simply type

make & make install

3.4. Configuring GRASS

The first time you start GRASS, you will have to specify a location and path for your data. Choose the data path that you set up earlier (it should already be the default entry). To create a new location, it is easiest to have a georeferenced data file that spans the region of interest. Although not necessarily required by the software, it greatly simplifies the process of adding a spatial reference system to the data library to specify it right away. Start GRASS by navigating to the icon or from a terminal:

grass64 - gui

Click on the Location Wizard icon on the right-hand side of the window. Follow the on-screen instructions, selecting your georeferenced data file when prompted. Alternatively, you can create a new location by entering GRASS with the default example "spearfish60." From the GRASS terminal navigate to the directory where your data are stored and type

r.in.gdal i=<yourimage> -o <mapname> location=<newlocation>

The function r.in.gdal will parse the image file and automatically define the region based on the extent of the selected image.

3.5. Loading Data and Interfacing GRASS with Postgres

There are a great many possibilities for importing data and interfacing with GRASS. Here we demonstrate several examples of importing data into Postgres and accessing those data within GRASS. Landsat7 data are downloadable from the USGS as georeferenced TIFF files for individual bands. To import them into a sample database Kenya, use a Python loader script:

```
gdal2wktraster.py -r * .tif -t Landsat -s 4326 -k 100 × 100 -I >
    Landsatloader.sql
```

The script does not directly load the data into the database; rather it creates the necessary SQL script to do so. In this example, the -r option enables multiple files (selected with the asterisk) to be imported simultaneously into a single table. The -t option specifies the table name the data will be imported to. With the -s option, we specify the spatial reference system using SRID numbers (spatial reference identifier, OGC specifications), WGS84 in this example (Herring 2006). The –k option splits each raster into tiles that are 100 × 100 pixels. Finally, the –I option requests that a spatial index file be created for each raster tile. Next, pass the SQL loader for processing with

```
psql -U <username> -f Landsatloader.sql <yourdatabase>
```

If you do not want to create a spatial index or you forgot to do so in the first step, you can easily create one at the Postgres prompt:

```
CREATE INDEX Landsat_SI ON Landsat USING GIST
    (ST_ConvexHull (rast));
```

In this example, the GIST (generalized search trees) index is used, which has a balanced tree index structure similar to a B-tree (Hellerstein 1999; Kornacker 1999). An example of a common format vector data type is the ESRI shape file and an example is a digitized map of fly belt regions FLY.shp. Postgres facilitates the importing of vector data from the terminal with

```
shp2pgsql -s 4326 -I -D FLY.shp <yourdatabase> .flybelts > flybelts.sql
```

Here the –s flag specifies the spatial reference system using SRID codes. The –I option requests the script initialize a GIST spatial index on the geometry column of the data. Finally, the –D option creates a dump file (sql loader) that can be imported into Postgres from the terminal, a faster means of adding data to the database. Now pass the sql loader to Postgres with

```
psql -U <username> -f flybelts.sql <yourdatabase>
```

Alternatively, import vector data using a graphical interface by loading

```
shp2pgsql -gui
```

To load the data into GRASS, initialize the Postgres driver from within the GRASS terminal. Start GRASS specifying a work location (see previous instructions for the generation of Location). Now, load the driver defining the connection between Postgres and GRASS:

```
db.connect driver=pg database="host=localhost,
dbname=<yourdatabase>"
db.login user=<username>
db.connect -p
db.tables -p
```

After initializing the connection, you can query the database, for example, retrieving the fly belts data described earlier:

```
v.in.ogr dsn="PG : host=localhost dbname=<yourdatabase>
user=<username>" layer=????? output=flybelts type=boundary,
centroid
v.db.select flybelts
v.info -t flybelts
d.vect flybelts
```

Data in HDF formats can be read only with additional GDAL libraries, which are not included with the standard distribution. However, the version of GDAL made available through the Ubuntu repositories appears to support some limited functionality. If further interaction with HDF is required, you will need to compile GDAL manually, inputting development files downloadable from the HDF Group.[17] HDF formats are containers, and thus may hold multiple data sets. Header data are accessed with

```
gdalinfo sample.hdf
```

Subdata set names are formatted as

HDF4_SDS:subdataset_type:file_name:subdataset_index

A portion of the output reads:

SUBDATASET_8_NAME=HDF4_SDS:MODIS_L1B:GSUB1.A2001124.0855.003.200219309451.hdf:7 SUBDATASET _8_DESC=[408×271] Range (16-bit unsigned integer)

Detailed headers for this subdata set can be viewed with

```
gdalinfo\SUBDATASET
  _8_NAME=HDF4_SDS: MODIS_L1B: GSUB1.A2001124.0855.003.
  200219309451.hdf : 7
```

Inasmuch as the GRASS plugin was compiled with HDF support, image data, by individual band, are directly imported into GRASS with r.in.gdal.

r.in.gdal HDF4_SDS:MODIS_L1B:GSUB1.A2001124.0855.003.200219309451.hdf:7 out=hdfexample

Once the data are loaded into the GRASS interface, they can be imported into Postgres either directly with db.connect or by exporting the image as .TIF and importing with the gdal2wktraster.py script.

4. LIMITATIONS AND FUTURE EXPANSION

The initial phase of our project is limited to the objectives addressing the misuse, misrepresentation, and effective archiving of our data library. As advances and improvements are made to the telecommunications infrastructure in Kenya, we will be able to share a common, easily-accessible repository for data with our colleagues outside the United States. The DBMS framework, including necessary software packages and data, can be packaged together and distributed via portable hard drive. Future updates to our software model will include a Web-based interface that will allow users to interact with the DBMS, including the suite of analysis and visualization tools (R and GRASS), without the need to install and configure these programs locally. This reduces the hardware requirements for working with the data, allowing a potentially broader base of users to share in data access. This approach has been extensively applied in many of the institutional projects commonly referenced in the literature (Câmara et al. 1996; Parent et al. 2006).

5. SUMMARY

Disease ecology is a transdisciplinary field, exploring the complex interactions between diseases and the environment. Computational and collaborative barriers inhibit meaningful advances in the field. Major problems include data management schemas to facilitate the scalability (data are resampled dynamically to avoid redundant storage), reliability (concurrent access to data permitted while ensuring that the raw data cannot be changed), and data security (the database allows for a dynamic security access policy while meeting HIPAA and Institutional Review Board [IRB] requirements). As data become aggregated with decreasing spatial resolution, many of the privacy concerns disappear but tracking and management problems proliferate. The DBMS must dynamically alter the restriction rule-set to account for aggregation and application challenges. Previous implementation of data management systems required that multiple instances of the data be stored, creating a problem of exponentially increasing data storage demands. Currently, no framework for data management that addresses this set of integrated concerns exists.

Over the course of our research on AT, we have accumulated a large library of data. Our database model utilizes open-source software to allow for flexibility and extendibility in model implementation. We take advantage of the new PostGIS extension, WKTRaster, to allow for the storage of raster imagery within the database. This allows us to enforce a single standard in the way all data formats, irrespective of the contents, are managed. With this development, we are finally able to store our entire data library, spatial and nonspatial, explicitly within a single database implementation, and the restrictions and rule sets coded into the DBMS should ensure the long-term integrity and security of the data.

The overarching goal of this project is to create a multiscale predictive model for the tsetse and AT to provide a means whereby governments, communities, and Nongovernmental Organizations (NGOs) can make informed decisions for disease control or suppression that are spatially and temporally aware. Given the variable background and technical expertise of the different groups, our solution should be simple enough for the most basic user, yet powerful enough to be useful for complex analyses by the most skilled. To maximize the utility of this system, we will use a participatory design framework to develop Mac, iPhone, and Web applications for interfacing with the models and data.

Open-source software is uniquely capable of rapid adoption of new technologies and functionality due to the base of community developers working on modular extensions to the software base. Spatial databases are increasingly common. Mobile data applications are becoming increasingly location aware (e.g., Facebook, Twitter, Loopt, Turn-by-turn Navigation [Waze]), with the purpose of providing users with context-specific information and opportunities. These GIS technologies increasingly promote Web-based interfaces to a spatial database. Perhaps the most exciting vision for geographic information systems (GIS) is the adoption of mobile technologies, now incorporating global positioning systems (GPS) technology, to provide for context-aware interaction with spatial database systems. The next step in our project is to implement an efficient, two-way Web portal for the spatial DBMS that will allow us to interact with data and model results from mobile devices in the field. Combined with automated scripting and model execution, this would have the potential to dramatically increase the amount of information shareable with local communities. Although not yet possible due to barriers in Kenya, we work toward the vision of achieving synchrony between science and practice.

NOTES

1. Data are publicly available.
2. Not all maps are publicly available.
3. International Livestock Research Institute (Nairobi, Kenya).
4. https://international.ipums.org/international/
5. http://www.postgresql.org
6. http://postgis.refractions.net
7. http://trac.osgeo.org/postgis/wiki/WKTRaster
8. http://grass.itc.it
9. http://cran.r-project.org
10. http://www.opengeospatial.org
11. http://www.gdal.org
12. http://www.opengeospatial.org/standards/is
13. http://www.iso.org/iso/iso_catalogue/catalogue_tc/catalogue_detail.htm?csnumber=26020
14. http://international.ipums.org/international/
15. http://www.postgresql.org/docs/
16. http://trac.osgeo.org/postgis/wiki/WKTRaster/Documentation01
17. http://www.hdfgroup.org

REFERENCES

Adam, N. R., and A. Gangopadhyay. 1997. *Database Issues in Geographic Information Systems: The Kluwer International Series on Advances in Database Systems.* Boston: Kluwer Academic Publishers.

Batchelor, N. A., P. M. Atkinson, P. W. Gething, K. Picozzi, E. M. Fevre, A. S. L. Kakembo, and S. C. Welburn. 2009. Spatial predictions of Rhodesian human African trypanosomiasis (sleeping sickness) prevalence in Kaberamaido and Dokolo, two newly affected districts of Uganda. *Plos Neglect Trop D* 3(12):e563.

Bauer, B., I. Kabore, A. Liebish, F. Meyer, and J. Petrich-Bauer. 1992. Simultaneous control of ticks and tsetse flies in Satiri, Burkina Faso, by the use of flumethrin pour on cattle. *Tropical Medicine and Parasitology* 1(43):1–74.

Brun, R., J. Blum, F. Chappuis, and C. Burri. 2010. Human African trypanosomiasis. *The Lancet* 375(9709):148–159.

Câmara, G., R. C. M. Souza, U. M. Freitas, and J. Garrido. 1996. SPRING: Integrating remote sensing and GIS by object-oriented data modelling. *Comput & Graphics* 20(3):395–403.

Campbell, D., H. Gichohi, A. Mwangi, and L. Chege. 2000. Land use conflict in Kajiado District, Kenya. *Land Use Policy* 17(4):337–348.

Campbell, D., D. P. Lusch, T. A. Smucker, and E. E. Wangui. 2004. Root causes of land use change in the Loitokitok Area, Kajiado District, Kenya. *Land Use Change Impacts and Dynamics (LUCID) Project Working Paper* 19.

Cecchi, G., R. C. Mattioli, J. Slingenbergh, and S. De La Rocque. 2008. Land cover and tsetse fly distributions in sub-Saharan Africa. *Medical and Veterinary Entomology* 22(4):364–373.

Cohen, M. L. 2000. Changing patterns of infectious disease. *Nature* 406(6797): 762–767.

Cox, F. E. G. 2004. History of sleeping sickness (African trypanosomiasis). *Infectious Disease Clinics of North America* 18(2):231–245.

Devillers, R., and R. Jeansoulin. 2006. *Fundamentals of Spatial Data Quality*. Newport Beach, CA: ISTE.

DeVisser, M., and J. Messina. 2009. Optimum land cover products for use in a *Glossina morsitans* habitat model of Kenya. *International Journal of Health Geographics* 8:39–39.

DeVisser, M. H., J. P. Messina, N. J. Moore, D. P. Lusch, and J. Maitima. 2010. A dynamic species distribution model of *Glossina* subgenus *morsitans*: The identification of tsetse reservoirs and refugia. *Ecosphere* 1(1):1–21.

Drew, P., and J. Ying. 1996. GeoChange: An Experiment in Wide-Area Database Services for Geographic Information Exchange. In *Proceedings of the 3rd International Forum on Research and Technology Advances in Digital Libraries*: IEEE Computer Society.

Egenhofer, M. 1994. Spatial SQL: A query and presentation language. *IEEE Transactions on Knowledge and Data Enineering* 6(1):86–95.

Elmasri, R. M., and S. Navathe. 2004. *Fundamentals of Database Systems*. 4th ed. Boston: Pearson/Addison Wesley.

FAO. 1979. *The African Trypanosomiases: Report of a Joint WHO Expert Committee and FAO Expert Consultation*. Rome: FAO.

Gyapong, J. O, M. Gyapong, N. Yellu, K. Anakwah, G. Amofah, M. Bockarie, and S. Adjei. 2010. Integration of control of neglected tropical diseases into health-care systems: challenges and opportunities. *The Lancet* 375(9709):160–165.

Hellerstein, J. 1999. *The GiST Indexing Project*. Available at http://gist.cs.berkeley.edu

Herring, J. R. 2006. OpenGIS Implementation Specification for Geographic Information—Simple Feature Access. Part 2: SQL option. Open Geospatial Consortium Inc.

Johnson, P. T. J., and D.W. Thieltges. 2010. Diversity, decoys and the dilution effect: How ecological communities affect disease risk. *J Exp Biol* 213(6):961–70.

Keesing, F., R. D. Holt, and R. S. Ostfeld. 2006. Effects of species diversity on disease risk. *Ecology Letters* 9(4):485–498.

Kennedy, P. 2005. Sleeping sickness—human African trypanosomiasis. *British Medical Journal* 5 (5):260–267.

KETRI. 1996. *Tsetse Distribution in Kenya Showing Tsetse Belts and Conservation Areas.*

Kornacker, M.. 1999. High-Performance Extensible Indexing. Paper read at 25th VLDB Conference, at Edinburgh, Scotland.

Longley, P. 2005. *Geographical Information Systems and Science.* 2nd ed. Hoboken, NJ: Wiley.

Messina, J., E. Walker, N. Moore, S. Grady, J. Maitima, J. Olson, and J. Kaneene. 2007. *A Dynamic Ecological Simulation Model of Tsetse Transmitted Trypanosomosis in Kenya.* Kenya: Research Sponsored by the National Institutes of Health, Office of the Director, Roadmap Initiative, and NIGMS: Award No. RGM084704A.

Moore, N., and J. P. Messina. 2010. A landscape and climate data logistic model of tsetse distribution in Kenya. *PloS One* 5(7):1–10.

Muriuki, G. W, T. J. Njoka, R. S. Reid, and D. M. Nyariki. 2005. Tsetse control and land–use change in Lambwe Valley, south-western Kenya. *Agriculture, Ecosystems and Environment* 106(1):99–107.

Neteler, M., and H. Mitasova. 2008. *Open Source GIS: A GRASS GIS Approach.* New York: Springer.

OGIS. 1999. Open GIS Consortium: Open GIS Simple Features Specification for SQL (Revision 1.1). www.opengeospatial.org (accessed November 28, 2010).

Olson, J. E. 2003. *Data Quality: The Accuracy Dimension.* San Francisco, CA: Morgan Kaufmann Publishers, Elsevier Science.

Ostfeld, R., F. Keesing, and V. T. Eviner. 2008. *Infectious disease ecology: The effects of ecosystems on disease and of disease on ecosystems.* Princeton, NJ: Princeton University Press.

Parent, C., S. Spaccapietra, and E. Zimányi. 2006. The MurMur project: Modeling and querying multi–representation spatio-temporal databases. *Information Systems* 31:733–769.

Python Software Foundation. 2010. *General Python FAQ—Python v2.6.5 Documentation.* Available at http://docs.python.org/faq

Ramsey, P. 2005. PostGIS manual. *Refractions Research Inc*, http://www.dcc.fc.up.pt/~michel/TABD/postgis.pdf

Rivest, R. 1992. *The MD5 Message-Digest Algorithm.* MIT Laboratory for Computer Science and RSA Data Security.

Shekhar, S., and S. Chawla. 2003. *Spatial databases: A tour.* Upper Saddle River, N.J.: Prentice Hall.

Shi, W., M. F. Goodchild, and P. Fisher. 2002. *Spatial Data Quality.* New York: Taylor & Francis.

Siringi, S.. 2003. Kenya rejects drugs deal. *Lancet Infectious Diseases* 3(6):320–320.

Smith, T. R, and J. Frew. 1995. Alexandria digital library. *Communications of the ACM* 38(4):62.

Stonebraker, M., and G. Kemnitz. 1991. The Postgres next-generation database-management system. *Communications of the Acm* 34(10):78–92.

Stonebraker, M., and D. Moore. 1996. *Object–Relational DBMSs: The Next Great Wave: Object–Relational DBMSs: The Next Great Wave.* San Francisco: Morgan Kaufmann Publishers.

Stonebraker, M., and L. A. Rowe. 1986. The design of Postgres. In *Proceedings of the 1986 ACM SIGMOD International Conference on Management of Data.* Washington, DC: ACM.

Sutherst, R. W. 2004. Global change and human vulnerability to vector-borne diseases. *Clinical Microbiology Reviews* 17(1):136–173.

Tatem, A. J., S. I. Hay, and D. J. Rogers. 2006. Global traffic and disease vector dispersal. *PNAS* 103(16):6242–6247.

van der Lans, R. F. 2007. *Introduction to SQL: Mastering the Relational Database Language*. 4th ed. Upper Saddle River, NJ: Addison-Wesley.

Watson, R. T. 2004. *Data Management: Databases and Organizations*. 4th ed. Hoboken, NJ: Wiley.

Wint, W. 2001. Kilometre Resolution Tsetse Fly Distribution Maps for the Lake Victoria Basin and West Africa. Vienna: PATTEC.

World Health Organization. 2001. "Report on African Trypanosomiasis (sleeping sickness)." Paper read at Report of the Scientific Working Group meeting on African trypanosomiasis, Geneva, June 4–8, 2001.

———. 2005. Control of Human African Trypanosomiasis: A Strategy for the African Region. World Health Organization, Regional Committee for Africa.

———. 2006. *African Trypanosomiasis*. Available at http://www.who.int/mediacentre/factsheets/fs259/en/ (accessed February 10, 2007).

Analyzing Geographical Access to HIV Sentinel Clinics in Relation to Other Health Clinics in Zambia

IMELDA K. MOISE and EZEKIEL KALIPENI
University of Illinois at Urbana-Champaign, Urbana, IL, USA

LEO C. ZULU
Michigan State University, East Lansing, MI, USA

This paper illustrates that in countries such as Zambia where available sentinel clinic data lack patient use information while including location and clinic type, advanced geospatial modeling can be a good proxy for measuring access to health care facilities including HIV sentinel clinics. The analysis shows mapped patterns of potential accessibility to HIV sentinel clinics versus all other clinics, while taking into consideration the spatial distribution of the country's population. The results indicate that Zambia has developed a relatively impressive set of health facilities—so much so that 98% of the population is within 50 km of a health facility, a reasonable distance for a day's bike ride, and nearly three in four are within 20 km. However, when it comes to HIV sentinel or surveillance clinics, this target is far from being realized, with only 52% percent of the population being within 50 km of a sentinel clinic.

INTRODUCTION

During the past two decades, sentinel surveillance of HIV in Zambia has relied on women attending antenatal clinics. Data collected through anonymous testing of pregnant women attending designated HIV sentinel clinics have the potential to provide a wealth of information about current trends in the epidemic, changes in infection rates over time, and they help warn health officials of possible dynamics of future spread of HIV/AIDS (UNAIDS/WHO 2004). If the data taken from such clinics are to be reliable, then these clinics need to be accessible to the majority of pregnant women in terms of travel time and distance. This paper employs a geographic perspective using geographic information systems (GISs) to examine the physical locations of HIV sentinel clinics in relation to all other health clinics and population levels in Zambia.

Many studies have been conducted to highlight the deleterious impact that HIV and AIDS have brought on the peoples of Zambia. However, few of these studies have directly focused on the geographic accessibility to HIV sentinel clinics. This is in spite of the fact that numerous studies have shown that geographic location and distance to health care facilities are crucial factors to health service utilization (see, for example, Atting and Egwu 1991; Gething et al. 2004; Tanser, Gijsbertsen, and Herbst 2006; Wilkinson and Tanser 1999). Many of these studies show that the location of health facilities influences the level of prenatal care in an area (McLafferty and Grady 2004; Ngoma and Mbukwa 2008). For example, several studies in Kenya showed higher utilization of antenatal clinics in urban areas than in rural areas due to close proximity to users in urban areas (Noor et al. 2003). Indeed, Noor et al. observed that people in urban areas were more likely to have shorter travel time to health facilities than their counterparts in rural areas, mainly due to higher densities and quality of health facilities and transport infrastructure.

It is in this context that this paper highlights the importance of taking into consideration the spatial location of and access to health care clinics, and utilization of clinics by both women and men. More importantly, if government, donors and nongovernmental organizations responsible for the planning and location of such clinics took into consideration the geographic aspects of locating them equitably in relation to population (rural versus urban and distance or travel time to nearest clinic) more seriously and consistently, then HIV/AIDS data derived from such clinics would be more representative of the entire population, and reduce the analytical impact of sampling limitations associated with the rather narrow focus on pregnant women visiting sentinel centers. This paper argues that careful geographic location in relation to distance would increase the quality, accuracy, and reliability of HIV/AIDS incidence and prevalence estimates spatially, allowing for a more equitable geographic distribution of resources to combat this disease.

Jackman (1972) offers a study that examined the planning and location of health care clinics with reference to distance and population in Zambia. Jackman's prescription for the location of new health care clinic sites for the flying doctor program in Zambia was simple. She noted the following: "The Flying Doctor Service should so site its clinics as to ensure that every person in Zambia lives within thirty-five miles of medical services with a doctor."

She used a simple geographic technique to allocate the entire population of Zambia to the nearest clinic. First, she identified areas that were served at the 35-mile (approximately 56 km) maximum distance to eliminate them as sites for new clinics. Second, she entered the coordinates of underserved population centers or places in a computer (Figure 1a). The computer was then programmed to recommend the smallest number of new sites needed to cover all the population at a distance of up to 56 kilometers (about 290,000 people), and to print out the coordinates of the population locations that could be used as clinic sites (Figure 1b).[1] According to Jackman, this method, as well as ensuring the least possible overlap of service areas, meant that each computer-recommended site was an approximate "center of gravity" of population. This paper uses Jackman's 56-km recommended distance from a health facility as the benchmark against which to gauge the progress of development of health facilities, particularly their location relative to population in Zambia since her study.

In addition, several case studies have recently examined geographic access to and utilization of health services using GIS techniques in the African context. Using homestead-clinic distance to delineate catchment areas with GIS tools, Tsoka and Le Sueur (2004) demonstrated that geographical access to primary health care centers (PHCs) was inadequate (only one third of the targeted population lived within 5 km of a clinic), and accessibility based on the catchment areas (96% of the population used the nearest clinic) decreased with distance. The study was in rural northern KwaZulu-Natal, South Africa. This convinced health officials not only to increase the number of PHCs, but also to upgrade them and decentralize malaria control programs to PHC level. In a more sophisticated study for Hlabisa, KwaZulu-Natal, Tanser et al. (2006) used GIS and survey information from 23,000 homesteads regarding which health care facility they used regularly to estimate and map mean travel time from any location to the nearest PHC or hospital. They also found wide variance in time-based access levels according to the means and quality of transportation and infrastructure. In short, although these kinds of studies are rare in Africa, there is a growing body of literature that utilizes GIS techniques to assess travel-time or distance-based accessibility and inform planners how to redress chronic spatial inequalities in access to PHC and other health facilities. The present study contributes to this growing literature by examining the distribution of and access to HIV sentinel clinics compared with other facilities in Zambia, under developing-country conditions of relative data scarcity.

The primary aim of this paper is to demonstrate how information on HIV sentinel clinics can be linked to population data using a GIS and to assess accessibility to and potential utilization of HIV sentinel clinics compared with other health care clinics in Zambia. This aim is addressed by seeking answers to the following basic questions:

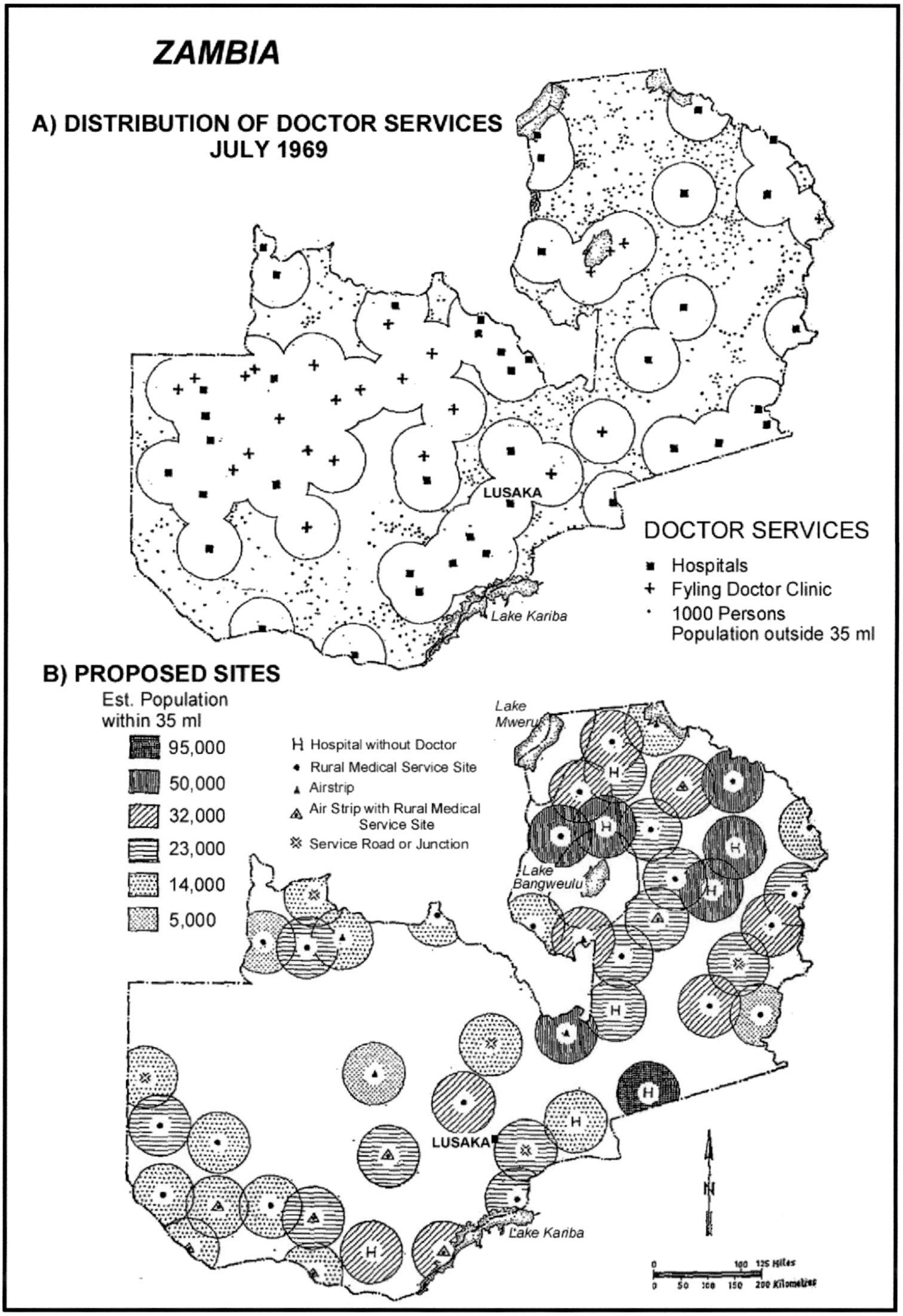

FIGURE 1 Distribution of doctor services and proposed sites for health care facilities in Zambia in 1969. Source: Jackman (1972:100), used with permission from Taylor and Francis Publishers.

a. What is the distribution of clinics in Zambia compared with population distribution, and does the distribution meet the benchmark set by Jackman in 1972 (see Jackman 1972)?
b. What is the average distance from any point in Zambia to any type of health care clinic? Does the average distance fall within acceptable accessibility norms for the respective population?
c. What is the average distance from any point in Zambia to an HIV sentinel clinic? Does the average distance fall within acceptable accessibility norms for the respective population?
d. What is the population potentially being served by the HIV sentinel clinics versus all other health care facilities, and what is the policy and analytical implications of the findings?

GIS AND SPATIAL STUDIES ON HEALTH CARE ACCESSIBILITY

The maturation of GIS technology and its functions of spatial and attribute data input, storage, manipulation, integration, display, and analysis; increasing computing power at declining cost; advanced locational technologies including the global positioning system (GPS), expanding availability of disaggregated spatial data including high resolution satellite imagery; and the inherently spatial nature of public health problems and solutions have promoted widespread use of GIS in geographic analysis of the relationship among disease, people, and place. GIS uniquely allows integration of spatial and nonspatial social, demographic, economic, political/institutional and ecological/environmental data in spatially explicit and sophisticated analysis. However, the GIS/health literature is too large to review here, and there are many useful reviews. Four categories emerged from GIS use in Nykiforuk and Flaman's (2011) review of issues, strengths, limitations, and future prospects in understanding public health outcomes and shaping decision making that covered 621 studies spanning 1990–2007: disease surveillance, risk analysis, access to health services and planning, and community health (utilization) profiling. The study at hand focuses on access and planning, itself a large area also adequately covered in recent reviews (e.g., Foody 2006; Higgs 2004, 2009). Selected recent GIS applications have ranged from identifying underserved locations where increased access could benefit a growing Hispanic population in Charlotte, South Carolina, using detailed health service use, socioeconomic and demographic data (Dulin et al. 2010) to assess health service utilization, and evidence of policy relevance of GIS findings (Higgs 2009; Nykiforuk and Flaman 2011), through implementing behavioral theoretical models of geographic access to health care (Graves 2009) to more sophisticated mathematical modeling and integration of temporal scale in space-time analysis (Foody 2006; Messina et al. 2006; Murray 2010).

Despite these advances and the proliferation of GIS use in public health problems, studies of urban environments and the urban-rural divide in developed countries have dominated work on health care access (Foody 2006). Less work has been done in developing countries where data availability and quality remain poor (Kalipeni and Zulu 2008; Tanser et al. 2006). Nevertheless, there has been notable progress from studies using partially manual delineation of catchment areas or production of Isocare maps of health-facility accessibility based using survey data, facility location, size, and level, and proportion of the population using them—see Jackman (1972) for Zambia, Iyun (1983) for Ibadan, and Atting and Egwu (1991) in Odukpani, Nigeria, and King (1966) in Mityama, Uganda. Some recent GIS studies in Africa have used automated techniques (e.g., Thiessen polygons) to spatially allocate locations and people to the nearest (Euclidean distance) health facility, for example, Gething et al. (2004) in Kenya and Tsoka and Le Sueur (2004) in South Africa. Even fewer studies (such as Tanser et al. 2006), have used GIS-derived travel times to assess accessibility, partly due to the wide variability in the means and quality of transportation and the scarcity of detailed digital data on transport networks. Integrating population data allows us to assess the equitability of access by comparing served populations with some desired standard based on targeted travel distance or time to the nearest health facility (e.g., Tsoka and Le Sueur 2004, described earlier). Access standards vary by case. Developing them is a major challenge in a data-scarce environment (see, for instance, Doherty, Rispel, and Webb 1996), but Bryant (1969) suggested a maximum target distance of 16 km, while Jackman (1972) thought 56 km—an average day's bicycle ride—would be right for Zambia in the 1970s. Findings can be useful regardless of target. Hlabisa, Kazulu-Natal, Wilkinson and Tanser (1999) showed that 36% of a target population was outside a 5-km catchment for PHCs, but that adding community-based health workers to the area reduced the excluded population to 3%. Tanser et al. (2006) showed later that median travel time based on survey data and GIS network analysis was 81 minutes to PHCs (65% traveled an hour or longer) and 170 minutes to the district hospital and that urban homesteads were 20 and 30 times less likely to use the PHCs than rural and peri-urban residents, respectively.

GIS use has limitations—much more pronounced in developing countries—including limited spatial data and quality, need for costly training and infrastructure, and more generic methodological issues including dependency of GIS outcomes on scale of analysis units (the modifiable areal unit problem [MAUP]), simplistic assumption of even distribution of population or measured phenomenon within the units, difficulty in integrating temporal dynamism, and concerns over privacy surrounding map-based results (Foody 2006; Gesler 1984; Higgs 2009; Nykiforuk and Flaman 2011). However, the spatial nature of public-health problems and solutions, some improvements in the availability and quality of some data, declining computer costs, and such advances as coupling GIS and location science and theory with modeling (see Murray 2010 for a comprehensive review) will broaden further the use of GIS in analyzing access-related and general public-health problems. The current study uses GIS and recently available high-resolution demographic data to assess distance-based accessibility to HIV/AIDS and general health centers in Zambia.

DATA AND METHODS

Sources of Data

In 2002, there were 568 health clinics in the Zambian health system, across a country that covers a contiguous geographical area of 290,586 square kilometers and has a population of about 13 million (Zambia Central Statistical Office 2010). Of the 568 health clinics, only 31 have been designated as HIV sentinel clinics for anonymous screening of pregnant women. The locations of these sentinel clinics were mapped using information obtained from a tabular (MS Excel) point dataset that was provided the authors by Centra Technology.[2] The Excel dataset had detailed information about HIV/AIDS seropositive rates from 31 sentinel surveillance centers in Zambia for women attending prenatal clinics. These data provided annual percentage HIV/AIDS rates dating back to 1985, as well as decadal rates for the past two decades. However, this study concentrated on the geographic patterns of the 31 centers in relation to population distribution using GIS analysis. The table included coordinate information (latitude and longitude) for each of the sentinel testing centers. The prevalence rates provided in the dataset were analyzed elsewhere (see Kalipeni and Zulu 2008; Moise and Kalipeni 2010), and are not dealt with in this paper.

Using the Excel dataset provided by Centra Technology, all the HIV sentinel points were converted into digital map points, and the data were loaded into ArcGIS 9.2 for further analysis. We also obtained the locations of all health care facilities in Zambia from the online GIS library at the Southern Africa Humanitarian and Disaster Management Network (SAHIM), which were available in Albers equal-area conic projection for Africa (Southern African Humanitarian and Disaster Management 2006). The spatial distribution of the 568 health facilities, including the 31 HIV sentinel surveillance clinics, is shown in Figure 2. The SAHIM Web site (no longer accessible) also provided other geographic data for Zambia, such as shapefiles for major roads, regions, provinces, districts, and other political boundaries, which this study used (Figure 3).

Zambia is divided into nine provinces, which are further divided into 72 districts, and then 150 constituencies, followed by wards. The number of districts in each province varies from three to twelve. Large parts of Zambia

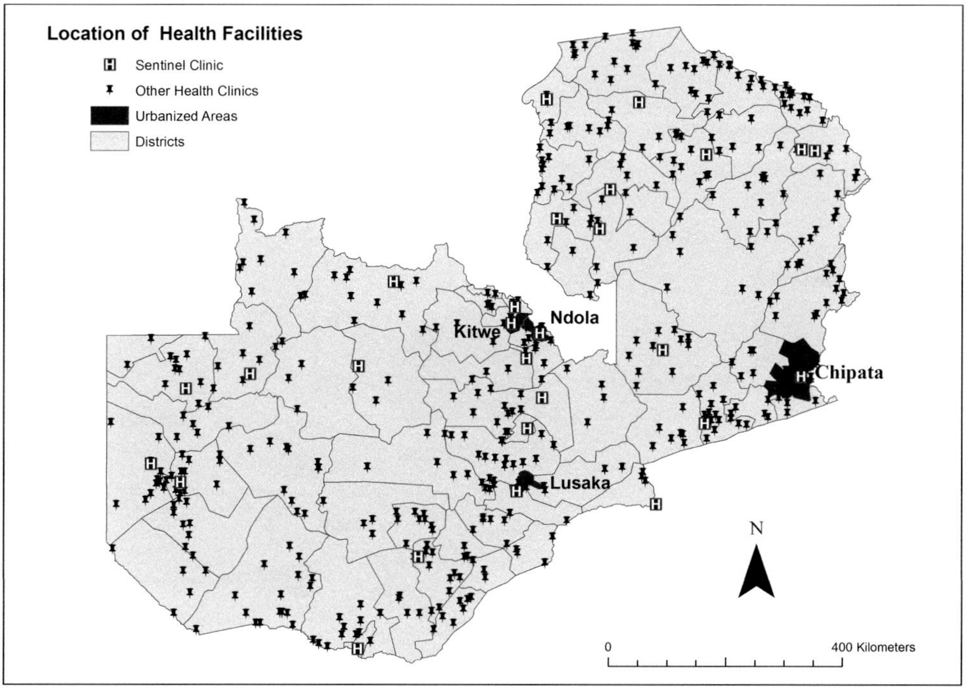

FIGURE 2 Spatial distribution of Zambia's health facilities and HIV sentinel clinics in 2002.

are predominantly rural with only about 40% of its population residing in urban areas and provincial headquarters (Figure 4).

Data Analysis

Recent research using *areal* (subpolygon or subzone) interpolation methods that seek to more accurately apportion and represent census-based population distributions spatially within commonly used mapping units or zones offer hope for dealing with the problems of coarse census units and even distribution of population or other variables across the units highlighted by Gesler (1984). Such mapping techniques are called *dasymetric mapping*; they have been used to improve census data distributions traditionally shown on choropleth maps (for the U.S., see Eicher and Brewer 2001; Holt, Lo, and Hodler 2004). The techniques depend primarily on remote sensing analysis–based land cover/use data and other ancillary data including maps of major roads and rail systems, elevation, slope, urban-area and administrative boundaries, town or village locations, and high-resolution imagery. They use these sets of data in a GIS to derive (dasymetric) weights by which to spatially allocate the population to most likely (dasymetric) subzones that "more accurately represent underlying data distributions" (Eicher and Brewer

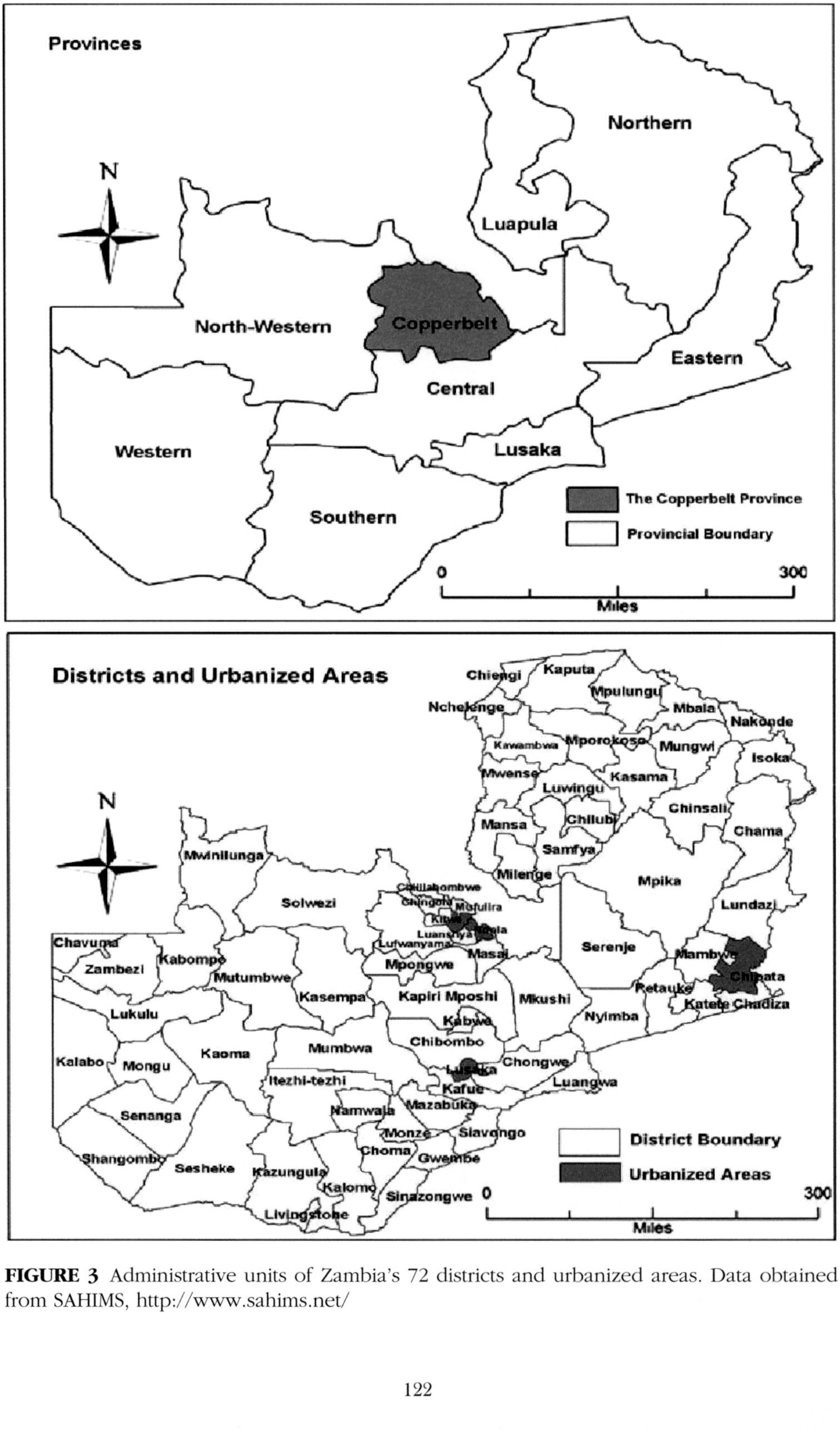

FIGURE 3 Administrative units of Zambia's 72 districts and urbanized areas. Data obtained from SAHIMS, http://www.sahims.net/

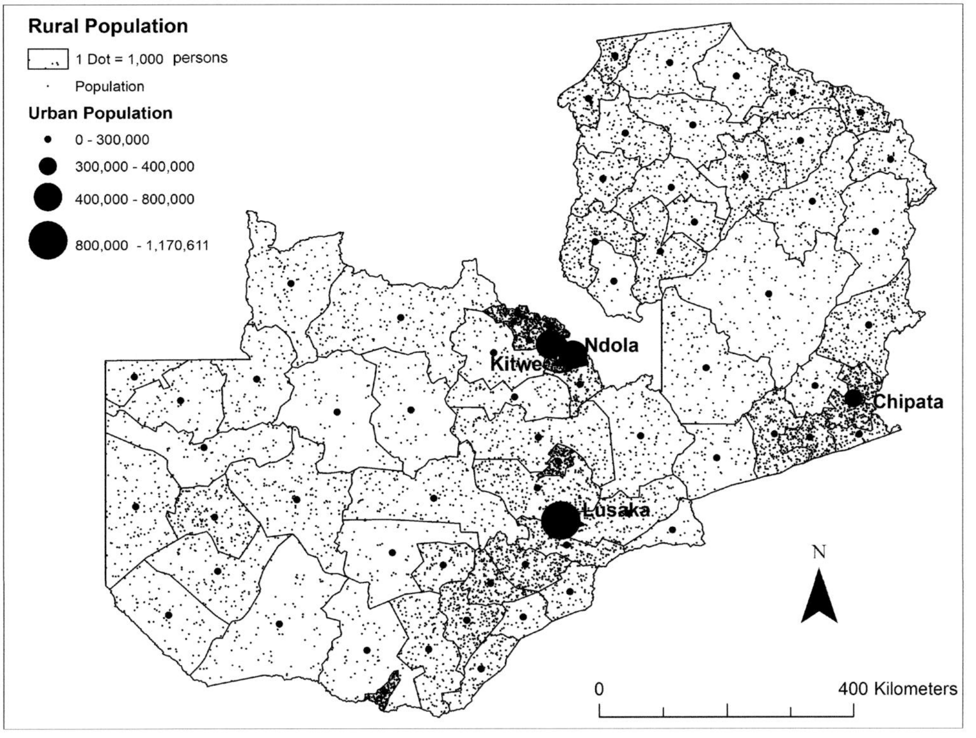

FIGURE 4 Spatial distribution of Zambia's rural and urban population, 2002.

2001). For instance, largely unpopulated water bodies, protected areas, and steep slopes are removed from population apportionment or given very low weights as necessary. Dasymetric mapping can considerably improve assessment of access to health care facilities and of optimum allocation of new ones, especially in developing countries where population data are often available only at district level or other coarse scale. In the case of Zambia, although the smallest administrative unit is the enumeration area, census data are reported only at the coarser ward level but are readily available mainly at district level. In the absence of readily available land cover or use data and other ancillary data at suitable resolution for Zambia, the Landscan 2008 Global Population Database produced using dasymetric techniques by the Oak Ridge National Laboratory were used. The spatially explicit population estimates are based on population projections from the latest census data for each country provided by the U.S. Bureau of the Census (Bhaduri et al. 2007).[3] In the case of Zambia, those projections were based on 2000 census data at constituency level. The data are provided at a resolution of 1 kilometer and show the ambient population count (average over 24 hours) within each 1-kilometer cell as of July 2008. This dataset was the basis for population-catchment estimates at various distances from health facilities suggested by

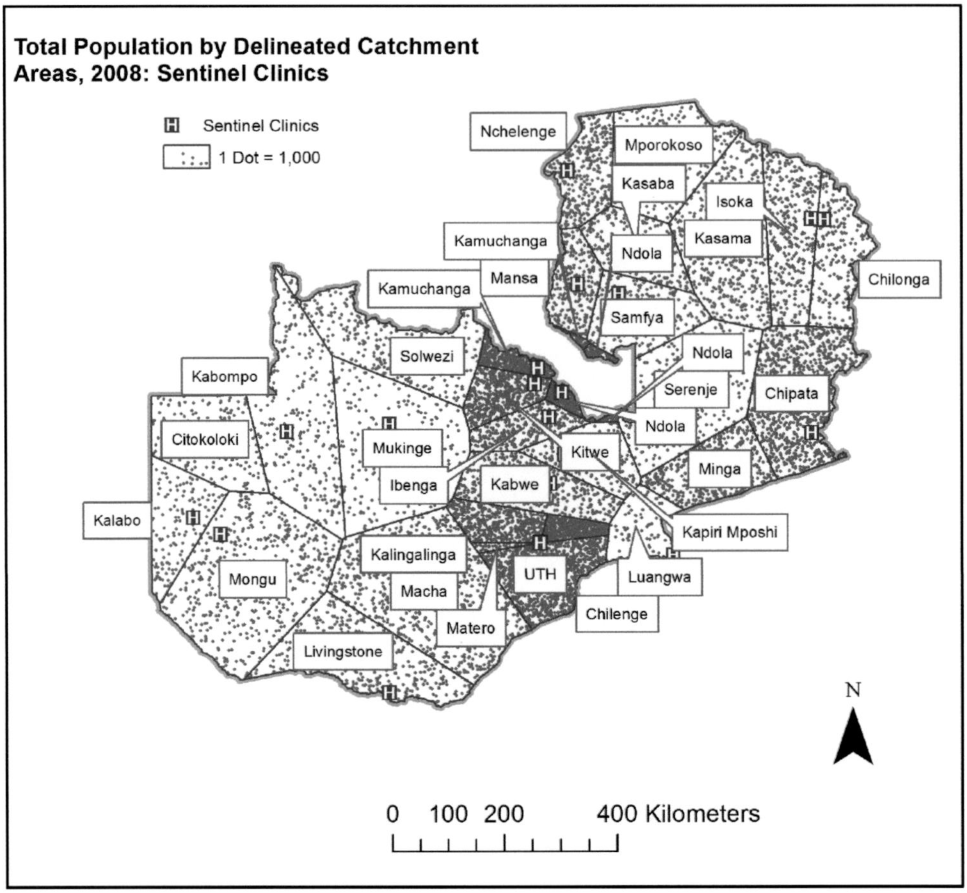

FIGURE 5 Thiessen polygon map with estimates of population in each HIV sentinel clinic service or catchment area.

the various researchers discussed earlier (see Bryant 1969; Jackman 1972, for example), using standard GIS extraction techniques in the Spatial Analyst module of ArcGIS.

The spatial pattern of HIV sentinel clinics in relation to other health facilities in the country and in relation to the population they could serve was analyzed using the Spatial Analyst module in ArcGIS (Esri 2006), which provides powerful tools for comprehensive raster-based spatial modeling and analysis. These tools were employed to generate the maps forming the basis of discussion for this paper. Kohli et al. (1995) used similar procedures in their GIS study of the distance of users to primary health centers. Travel time (represented by physical distance) to the closest existing sentinel clinic or health care facility was quantified using proximity analysis in the ArcGIS Spatial Analyst module. Proximity analysis included Thiessen polygon generation and calculation of straight-line distances from any geographic location

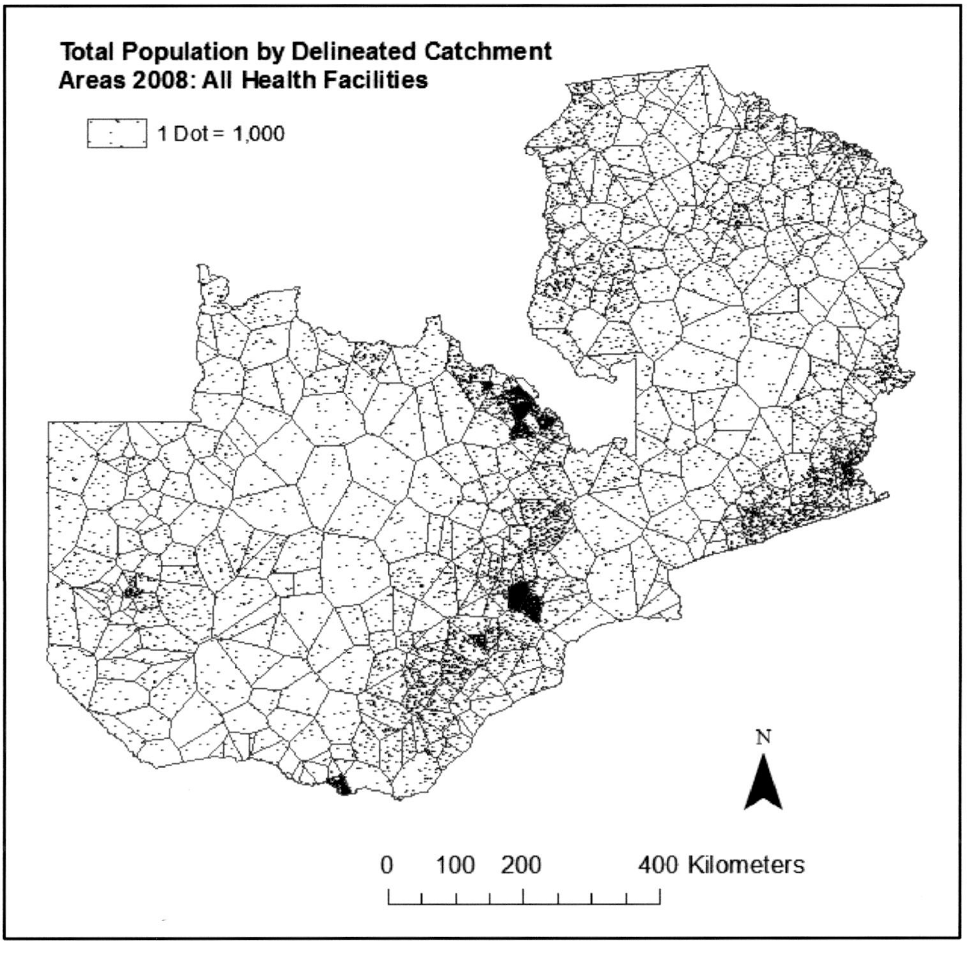

FIGURE 6 Thiessen polygon map with estimates of population in each health facility service or catchment area.

to health facilities for development of service areas and subsequent allocation of population to the nearest clinic. At a large spatial scale, straight-line distances have been found to be a good proxy for measuring access (Wood and Gatrell 2002). The analysis using this tool in ArcGIS resulted in a raster isoline/isoarea map[4] of average distances from any point on the map to the nearest sentinel clinic or health facility. GIS allowed automatic extraction of population tables along with basic information for all the health facilities, and sentinel clinics in dBase format. GIS analysis enabled the mapping of mean average distance to a health facility or sentinel clinic for that district interpolated within the Zambian boundary mask map. The assumption was that all else being equal, the closer the clinic, the better access people will have. Population density maps were also generated to show the projected location of people in the country and population statistics extracted and

TABLE 1 Population Served by Sentinel Clinics, 2008

Province	District	Sentinel Clinic	Population
Southern	Choma	Macha	1,115,040
Lusaka	Lusaka	Matero	941,437
Lusaka	Lusaka	Chilenge	848,027
Northern	Kasama	Kasama	572,715
Copperbelt	Luanshya	Ibenga	552,276
Copperbelt	Mufulira	Kamuchanga	542,499
Central	Kabwe	Kabwe	527,131
Eastern	Chipata	Chipata	519,145
Western	Mongu	Mongu	497,459
Eastern	Luangwa	Luangwa	485,143
Lusaka	Lusaka	Kalingalinga	458,931
Lusaka	Lusaka	Chelstone	417,444
N/W	Kasempa	Mukinge	380,796
N/W	Solwezi	Solwezi	361,254
Central	Kapiri Mposhi	Kapiri Mposhi	331,349
Northern	Mporokoso	Mporokoso	312,143
Luapula	Samfya	Samfya	306,946
Lusaka	Lusaka	UTH	288,852
Western	Kalabo	Kalabo	259,035
Northern	Mpika	Chilonga	258,243
Luapula	Samfya	Kasaba	242,448
N/W	Kabompo	Kabompo	235,401
Luapula	Mansa	Mansa	207,685
Luapula	Nchelenge	Nchelenge	204,104
Central	Serenje	Serenje	195,939
Eastern	Petauke	Minga	190,869
Copperbelt	Ndola	Ndola	171,401
Copperbelt	Kitwe	Kitwe	135,606
Northern	Isoka	Isoka	64,993
Southern	Livingstone	Livingstone	35,631

Note: These figures were extracted from the Thiessen polygon map (Figure 5) using estimates of population in each HIV sentinel clinic service or catchment area.

summarized at the catchment area level for each health facility and sentinel clinic.

Because the extent of the catchment area for each of the 31 HIV sentinel clinics was unknown, the Thiessen polygon module in ArcGIS was used to delineate the potential catchment areas for the sentinel clinics. In delineating catchment areas for given points, Thiessen polygons use the concept of *service area* in business analysis, and allocate locations to the nearest *service center*. In this case the HIV testing center is the service center, and locations are assigned to the nearest service center, regardless of national or subnational boundaries. The result is a layer consisting of a polygon for each data point (i.e., location of HIV sentinel clinic or health center in this case). Thiessen or Voronoi polygons have the unique property to apportion space to polygons such that each polygon contains only one input point (in this case, a health facility), and any location within a polygon is

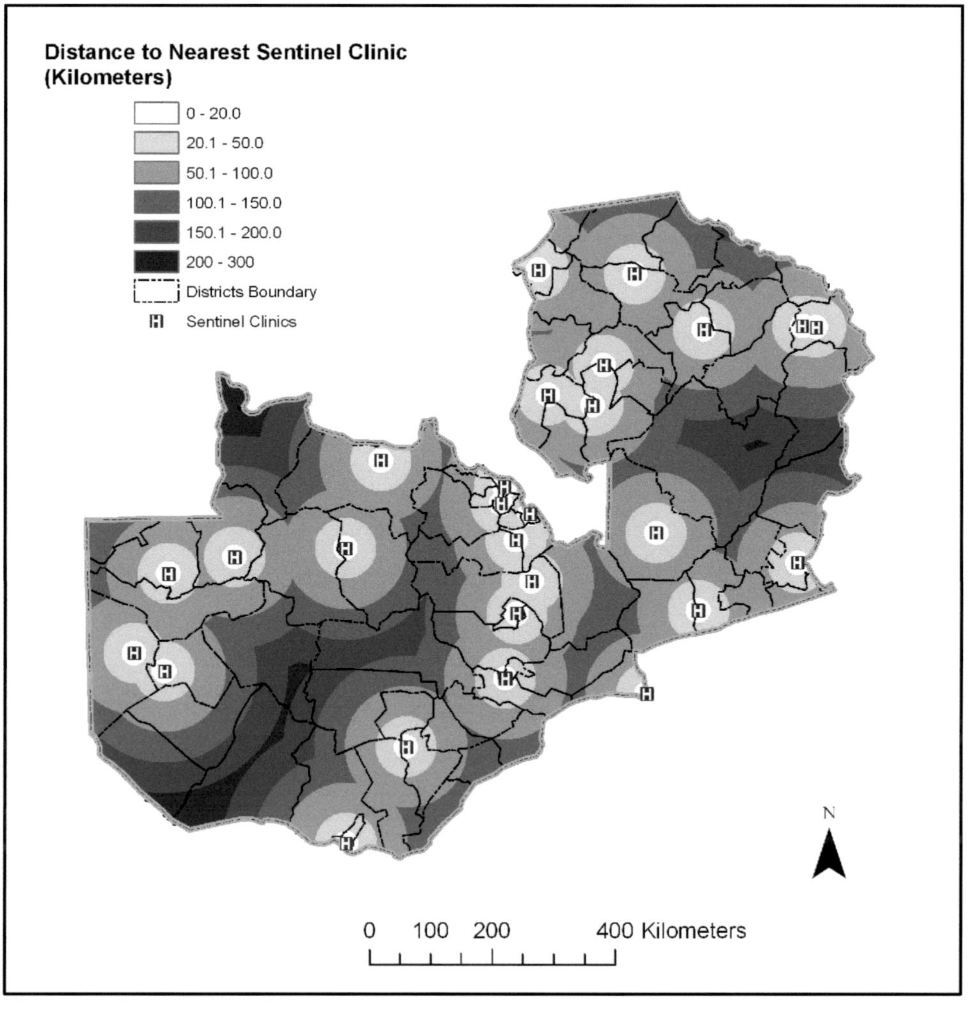

FIGURE 7 Distance to nearest HIV sentinel clinic in kilometers.

closer to its associated point than to points of any other polygon (Esri 2006; Tatalovich, Wilson, and Cockburn 2006; see also Figure 5). The Thiessen polygon algorithm in ArcGIS geometrically generates a polygon by drawing a perpendicular line through the midpoint of the distance between each data point and its immediate neighbors, and then joining the lines to form a closed polygon with the service point within it. Service-area allocation with Thiessen polygons is important in a country like Zambia where available sentinel clinic data contain basic information only including location and clinic type, lacking patient-use information and other capacity-related information. The use of Thiessen polygons in this context has been well established in related studies (Black et al. 2004; Gething et al. 2004). In addition to extraction of the 2008 dasymetrically, spatially interpolated population data by Thiessen polygon, thereby also bypassing limitations of traditional and coarse

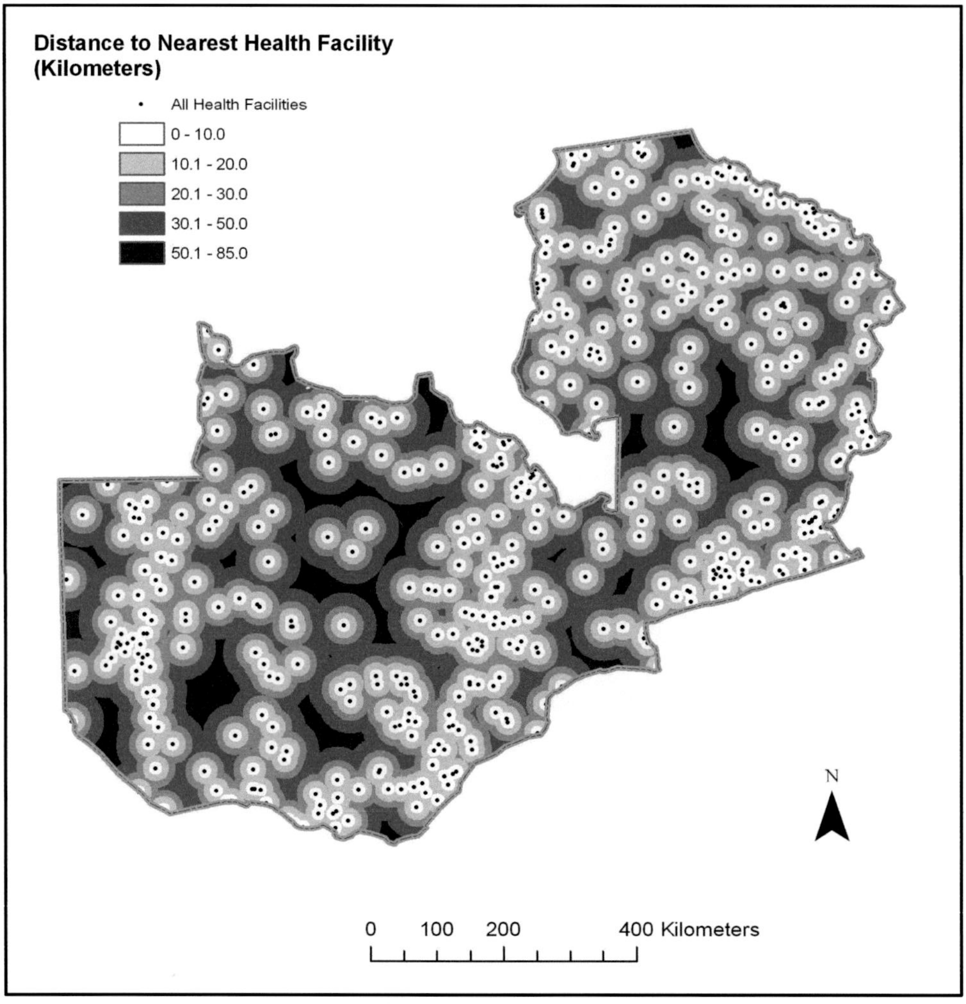

FIGURE 8 Distance to nearest health facility in kilometers.

census zones, access to health facilities based on average straight-line distances were also reported at district level (N = 72). The district level has been used as the geographic unit of data aggregation (N = 72) for some of the analysis and discussion in this paper. The discussion of the spatial patterns from the analysis also refers to some districts and provincial names (see Figure 2 for names of districts and provinces).

RESULTS AND DISCUSSION

Health Facility and Population Distribution

Results of this study indicate that there is generally equitable spatial distribution of health clinics in Zambia. This is in keeping with the implementation

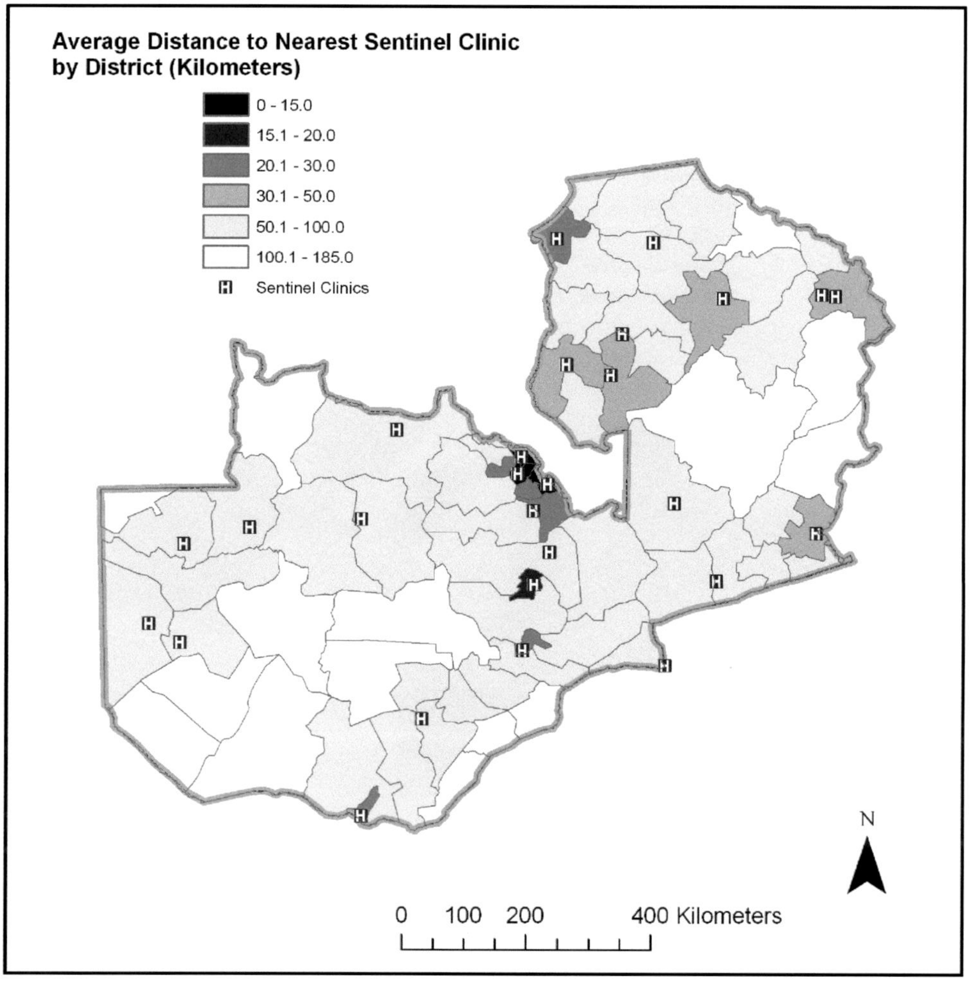

FIGURE 9 Average distance to nearest sentinel clinic by district in kilometers.

of plans that were drawn during the 1960s and 1970s (Figure 1; Jackman 1972). Access to health care in Zambia has also apparently increased considerably since then. Figure 2 depicts the 2002 locations of Zambia's 568 health facilities including HIV sentinel clinics. Clinic density is highest in the northeastern and eastern parts of the country, with a high concentration along major roads. The spatial patterns observed in the eastern and northeastern parts of the country could be due to the influence of early missionaries in these regions. Most clinics in these regions are mission hospitals. In contrast, few HIV sentinel clinics exist across the country. This is a glaring spatial inequality that requires to be redressed for the majority of Zambia's population.

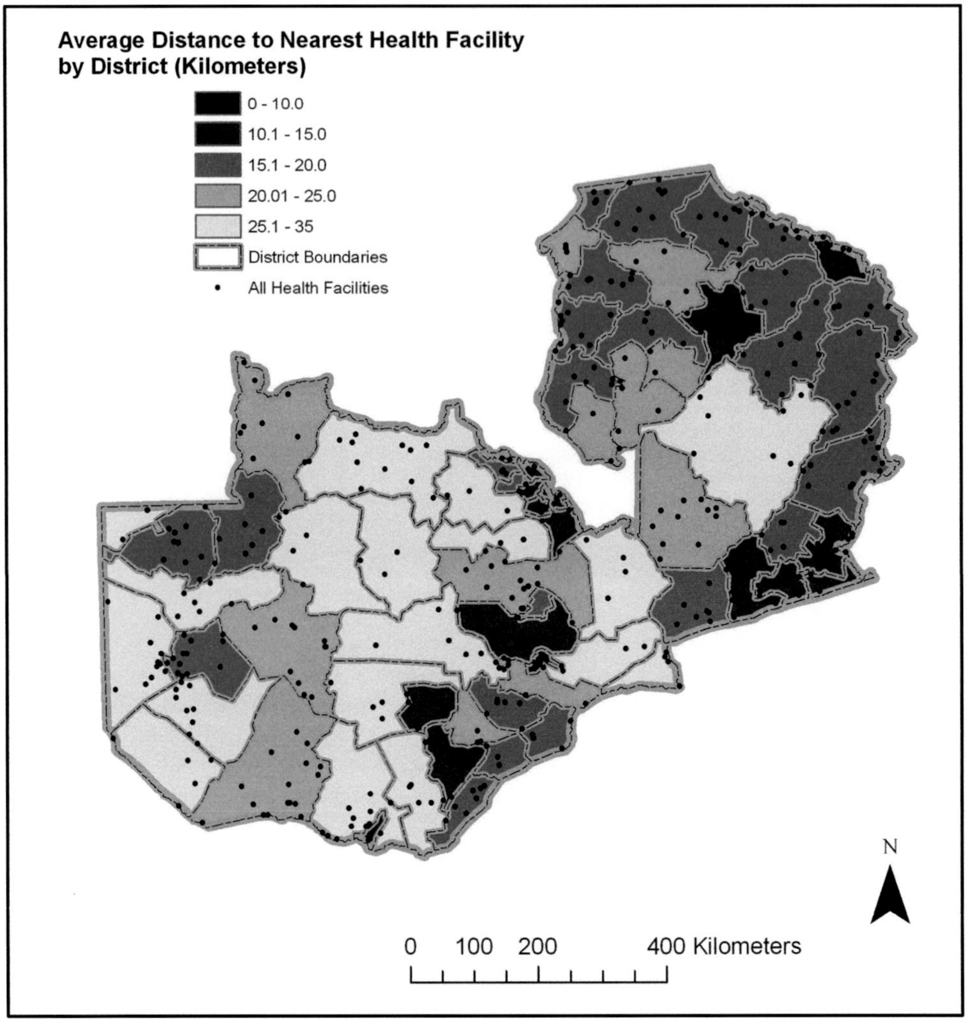

FIGURE 10 Average distance to nearest health facility by district in kilometers.

Figure 4 depicts the spatial distribution of Zambia's population by district and urbanized areas. As expected, most of Zambia's population is found in the two mining cities of Kitwe and Ndola in the Copperbelt Province, in the capital city of Lusaka, and in the Chipata District of the Eastern Province. The northern and northwest parts of the country have the lowest population densities. Approximately 10% of Zambia's population is concentrated in Lusaka. Apart from that, most of the population is sparsely distributed across the country, with provincial headquarters having more people than areas surrounding them. This concentration of people in the few cities is testament to the fact that Zambia is the most urbanized country in Africa south of the Sahara (excluding South Africa), with 40% of the population living in urban areas (Krabacher, Kalipeni, and Layachi 2009, 194). Although urban areas are few in the country, rural population tends to thin dramatically away from the cities. To the north and northwest parts of the country, population declines to some of the lowest in the country. In general, there are more people in bigger cities than there are in rural areas. Southern cities such as Livingstone, Kafue, and Siavonga do not appear visually prominent on the map in Figure 4 but are important districts in the distribution. Studies of urbanization in Zambia have shown that since independence in 1964, the country has witnessed a high rate of rural-to-urban drift, which has been caused by two factors: the relative stagnation of rural areas and an unprecedented and unanticipated rise in both real and money incomes in the few cities (Mutale 2004).

Accessibility to HIV Sentinel Clinics

As found in many other studies on primary health care utilization or uptake, access to sentinel clinics should increase with reduced distance (see, for example, Stock 1983; Atting and Egwu 1991; Gething et al. 2004). Thus, HIV sentinel clinics for pregnant women will be needed most in areas where there is a large population. Figure 4 depicts the number of people in each polygon living within each sentinel clinic service catchment area, as described in the Data and Methods section, with the population in each polygon denoted as a dot density map. Similarly, Figure 6) shows a map of Thiessen polygons or catchment areas for all the other health clinics in Zambia. As expected, higher concentrations of population are found around the Lusaka Province through Central Province and Copperbelt Kitwe and Ndola. The same information is given in Table 1, which clearly shows that though urban areas have fewer HIV sentinel clinics, they do, however, have a higher number of people who could utilize services at these clinics. Conversely, it might be argued that the few HIV sentinel clinics located in the major urban areas of Zambia are well equipped to handle large populations. However, it would be more equitable to establish more HIV sentinel clinics in the major urban areas inasmuch as these are also where most Zambians live. This would certainly ease congestion and improve access by most of the people residing in urban areas.

Figures 7 and 8 highlight the distances to the sentinel or other health clinic, respectively. Figure 7 clearly shows that the sentinel clinics are inaccessible to the majority of places and people in the country. Many patients must travel distances of 50 to 300 kilometers to access the nearest HIV sentinel clinic. Under the assumption that pregnant women can walk for only 30 to 60 minutes, it is very unlikely that most women would be able to access these clinics. On the other hand, the results shown in Figure 8 for all other health facilities indicate that most of the country is well covered. Most of

TABLE 2 Estimated Population (2008) Within Straight-Line Distance Based on Catchments of Health Facilities

	HIV/AIDS Sentinel Clinics Only (2002)				All Health Facilities (2002)			
Distance from Clinic (km)	Population (Number)	Population (%)	Area (km^2)	Area (%)	Population (Number)	Population (%)	Area (km^2)	Area (%)
5	2,405,970	21.10	2,176	0.30	2,815,590	24.69	37,044	4.92
10	3,112,630	27.31	8,124	1.08	4,742,060	41.58	126,591	16.82
15	3,356,460	29.45	18,238	2.42	7,086,100	62.13	240,299	31.93
20	3,603,860	31.62	31,623	4.21	8,372,430	73.4	357,564	47.51
30	4,401,670	38.62	67,731	9.01	10,194,000	89.37	546,721	72.64
50	5,948,450	52.19	163,685	21.77	11,201,500	98.21	714,403	94.92
100	9,434,650	82.78	473,245	62.93	11,405,900	100.00	752,611	100.00
150	10,788,300	94.66	652,772	86.80				
300	11,396,800	100.00	752,020	100.00				

Note: There are minor variations in total area and population size because of some resampling and minor differences in boundaries and extraction of data from the 1-km scale source. The 2008 population data were derived from the LandScan (2008) High Resolution Global Population Data Set copyrighted by UT-Battelle, LLC, operator of Oak Ridge National Laboratory under Contract No. DE-AC05-00OR22725 with the U.S. Department of Energy.

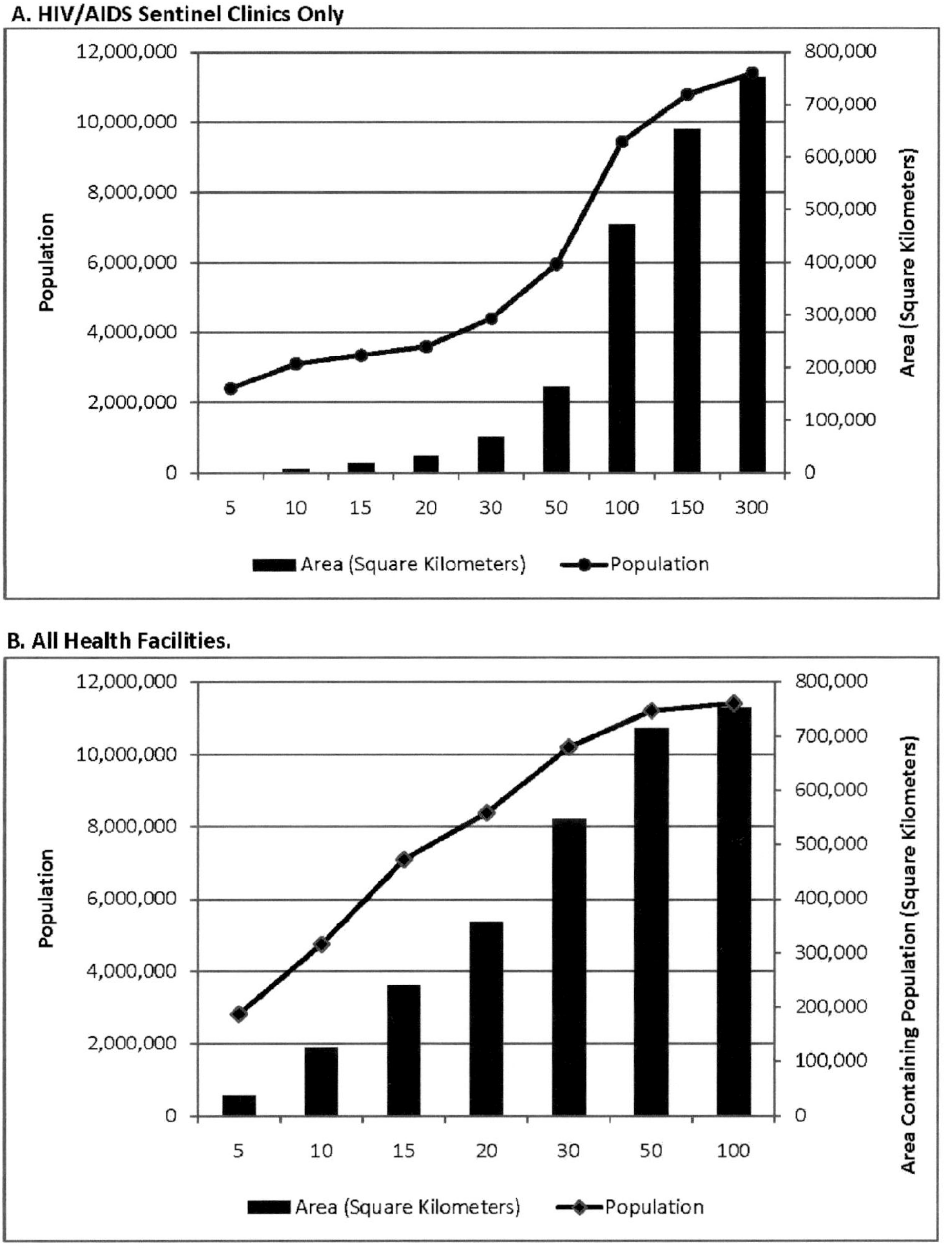

FIGURE 11 Population served by health facilities by catchment size in Euclidean distance.

the places in Zambia are within 50 kilometers of a health clinic, within Jackman's (1972) recommended distance. Within highly populated areas such as Lusaka, Copperbelt, Luapula, and districts in the central, northwestern, western, and eastern provinces, these distances are short, indicating that health clinics in general are very accessible to the Zambian population. These results are not overly surprising given the existing high population density and number of HIV–education program services in these areas. However, in reality, in any geographical area several other variables would affect health care accessibility and utilization (Chansa et al. 2008; Biritwum and Jackson 1997; Gage and Guirlène Calixte 2006; le Bacq and Rietsema 1997). As confirmed by Figure 9, which shows average distances at the district level, a significant number of people must travel mean distances of 50 to 185 kilometers to access the nearest HIV sentinel clinic. At the same time, because of the multiplicity of health clinics widely distributed throughout the country, the average distance an individual has to travel to a health clinic is below 35 kilometers (Figure 10).

In essence, these findings show continuing low levels of access to health facilities based on Euclidean distance, especially for the HIV/AIDS sentinel centers whose numbers have not changed much since the start of the reconnaissance program in the early 1990s. About 21%, or one in five people, lived within five kilometers of a sentinel center compared with 24.69%, or one in four people, for all health centers (Table 2 and Figure 11), while some nine in ten people were within 30 kilometers of any health facility and virtually all (over 98%) were within Jackman's (1972) target, here represented by 50 kilometers. This recommended catchment-size capture of 50 kilometers has just over half (52%) the population for sentinel centers (see Table 2 and Figure 11). The slow gains in population served as we go from 5 to 30 kilometers illustrates the concentration of these sentinel centers in urban areas, so the largest gains in population served would come from improving access from 100 to 50 or—even better—to 30 kilometers (Figure 7). For all health clinics, any improvement from 30 down to 5 kilometers would pay significant dividends in gains in population covered at shorter travel times and lower cost.

CONCLUSION

With reference to sentinel and other clinics, these service estimates indicate lower access to health services than in Kwazulu Natal, for instance, where a third of the population lived within 5 kilometers of a PHC (Tanser et al. 2006). The number (568) and spatial arrangement of the health facilities in 2002 captured 42% to 62% of the population in the 10- to15-kilometer service-area targets, making Bryant's (1969) suggestion of a maximum of 16 kilometers still a long way away for all clinics. Improvements and current needs make Jackman's 50-kilometer policy adequate for all clinics but still a desirable target for sentinel centers. The health-facility data used for 2002 are rather dated, and indications are that the number has increased significantly since then. Even so, the Fifth National Development Plan 2006–2010 indicated broadly that less than half the population lived within 5 kilometers of a health facility in rural areas compared with 90% in urban areas (Zambia Government 2006). So the urban-rural divide is worth more exploration, and the relative benefits of improving urban versus rural health access should be evaluated. The findings clearly show the need for increasing sentinel centers, using some of the widespread existing health facilities.

In the Zambian health system, HIV prevalence has been monitored primarily through antenatal surveillance and population surveys. Women attending antenatal clinics for the first time undergo unlinked anonymous testing for HIV to monitor trends in the epidemic as well as to estimate prevalence rates in the adult population (WHO/UNAIDS 2003). Though there have been minimal differences between estimates obtained from antenatal HIV sentinel clinics and those from population-based surveys in selected areas (Glynn et al. 2001), studies from the central African region have raised debates about the reliability of HIV prevalence estimates derived from using antenatal sentinel clinic data (Grassly, Sandoy, and Fylkesnes 2004; Michelo et al. 2008). Grassly and colleagues report that HIV estimates obtained from using sentinel data either underestimate or overestimate the pandemic, although no reasons for this discrepancy are given. Other scholars have questioned the representativeness of these estimates to the general population given that not all pregnant women attend such clinics nor do the estimates include men (Boisson et al. 1996; Montana et al. 2005).

In concurrence with other studies (for example, Huang et al. 2005; Noor et al. 2003), our results indicate that that urban areas had higher population densities and more HIV sentinel clinics than did rural areas (Figure 2). However, the maps also demonstrate that urban areas have high population densities but a limited number of HIV sentinel clinics to serve the entire population effectively. Similarly, HIV sentinel clinics are also sparsely distributed across the country. More importantly, placement of HIV sentinel clinics is crucial if HIV sentinel clinics are to be accessible to the majority of the Zambia population. An earlier study from Ghana that used location-allocation models found that accessibility to primary health care facilities could be improved without adding additional health facilities (Oppong and Hodgson 1994) and that additional health facilities did not necessarily translate into access. At the moment, Zambia already has the necessary infrastructure in terms of health care clinics. All that needs to be done is to designate some of these existing health clinics as HIV sentinel or surveillance clinics. This would ensure that most of the population in Zambia has access to this very important service. Of course, there are other factors that need to be considered, such as the availability of trained staff, infrastructure, and health care funding.

Accessibility patterns to HIV sentinel clinics were based on Thiessen polygons and the straight line tool or Euclidean distance analysis as seen in Figures 4 and 5. It is important to acknowledge that there are some weaknesses with using this technique to measure accessibility. Use of straight line distance measurement to determine the actual travel distance to service areas fails to take into account geographical barriers to movement such as rivers, mountains, lakes, or railroads, or transportation routes in general (Wood and Gatrell 2002). Failure to take these aspects into consideration is a weakness that affects the results of this study, as neither the road network nor other modes of travel that could have shown a cost-path analysis, best route, or shortest distance to HIV sentinel clinics were used. The network analyst tool could have been the best option for this analysis. However, this was not possible at the time of the study in the absence of a complete and reliable road network for the study area, as is the case in many developing countries.

Additionally, although maps were made that show the locations of HIV sentinel clinics and the proportion of populations that could use the clinics, these maps do not translate into sentinel clinic usage. An analysis based on population data from surveys on usage and more comprehensive information on individual pregnant women in the region would probably yield more accurate conclusions. Such an analysis could take advantage of both the adjusted sentinel clinic distance and the distribution of pregnant women in the study area.

Despite advances in methods to assess access to health services and to plan better location of new facilities, especially with the use of geospatial technologies (GIS, GPS, and remote-sensing analysis), data limitations still make this study only an approximation of access to health facilities and HIV testing. Dasymetric population mapping is an improvement over regular choropleth mapping in terms of population distribution, and it has considerable potential for improving clinic access and allocation analysis, especially for developing countries such as Zambia because of the generally coarse scale of census units. Disaggregation of population data through dasymetric mapping is also an effective tool against the analytical scale problem, the MAUP. However, the same inadequacy of data also limits the degree to which dasymetric mapping can be improved. For instance, whereas a preliminary examination suggests that the Landscan global population dataset generally accounted for major land uses and cover (lakes, national parks, and towns), its weighting assumptions may have overemphasized proximity to roads in predominantly rural landscapes. Even though the Landsat dataset has the assurance of being at least as accurate in population numbers as regular population mapping—because numbers add up to the lowest census units made available—this product needs further accuracy assessment to give it a more empirical estimation of its accuracy as more data layers are available for Zambia. The census underway (2010) in Zambia will be useful in that regard. A reliable and recent land cover or land use map is also essential, as are finer-resolution digital elevation models and improved mapping of small-town boundaries.

In sum, this study has demonstrated the use of GIS and proximity (Euclidian distance) of populations to health centers based on recently available, high-resolution (spatially disaggregated) demographic data to assess the accessibility of health facilities offering HIV/AIDS services relative to general health-service accessibility. These data indicate considerable improvement in general accessibility since Jackman's (1972) study (98%; nearly three in four being within 50 and 20 km of a health facility, respectively; and average distance to a clinic being less than 35 km). However, based on 2008 population data, it also points to the need to further expand HIV/AIDS service facilities to more PHCs, given the gravity of the pandemic and condition of patients, beyond the 52% who are able to access services within 50 km of their homes (only 32% access it within 20 km while average distances by district range from 50 km to 185 km). The study also highlighted data quality and quantity limitations to exploit the full potential of GIS analysis and the importance of the Landscan global population data and dasymetric analysis to improve data quality and availability.

Beyond the current study, analysis of geographic accessibility to health care to ensure even, equitable, and effective access needs more detailed analysis beyond physical accessibility to other factors that also affect actual utilization of such services, as others have noted (e.g., Curris and Regan 1998; McLafferty and Grady 2004). Improvements in data availability and quality, including spatial disaggregation (also accuracy, consistency, reliability, and timeliness) and recording of utilization and other attributive data—health-facility name and locational coordinates (e.g., service level, numbers attending, main ailments, number of beds, lab-processing capacity), and detailed ancillary land use, terrain, and transport networks will open up more sophisticated use of existing and future GIS tools for health-service equity- and access- related problems. Messina et al. (2006) offer a recent application through spatial covering models such as the location set covering problems (LSCPs) which identify the minimum number and locations of facilities that serve demand points based on maximum travel time or distance using community hospitals in Michigan as a case in point. Other recent applications include demand-based models addressing the maximal coverage location problem by citing a given number of facilities so as to maximize demand met within given standards (e.g., Church and ReVelle 1974; Yang, Goerge, and Mullner 2006). Adapting such studies, including developing and evaluating measures of spatial accessibility to health as was done for Chicago (Luo and Wang 2003), to developing-country settings is a fruitful area of future research. Efforts by WHO under the Service Availability Mapping program for developing countries point in the right direction in building the capacity of developing countries for accessibility mapping facilities and building databases to aid in local planning.

NOTES

1. In location theory, such center models that seek a minimum set and locations of facilities to service demand points within a maximum distance are called the locational set covering problem (LSCP; Murray 2010, p. 340).

2. See the Web site http://www.centratechnology.com about Centra Technology, Inc.

3. This product was made utilizing the LandScan (2008) TM High Resolution global Population Data Set copyrighted by UT-Battelle, LLC, operator of Oak Ridge National Laboratory under Contract No. DE-AC05-00OR22725 with the U.S. Department of Energy. The U.S. Government has certain rights in this Data Set. Neither UT-Battelle, LLC, nor the U.S. Department of Energy, nor any of their employees, makes any warranty, express or implied, or assumes any legal liability or responsibility for the accuracy, completeness, or usefulness of the data set. <http://www.ornl.gov/sci/landscan/>.

4. An isoline map is a map that shows lines or areas that join places of equal value, much like a contour map.

REFERENCES

Atting, I. A., and I. N. Egwu. 1991. Indicators of accessibility to primary health care coverage in rural Odukpani, Nigeria. *Asia-Pacific Journal of Public Health 5*(3):211–216.

Bhaduri, B., E. Bright, P. Coleman, and M. Urban. 2007. LandScan USA: A high resolution geospatial and temporal modeling approach for population distribution and dynamics. *GeoJournal 69*:103–117.

Biritwum, R. B., and H. E. Jackson. 1997. Health care accessibility and utilization in sub-Saharan Africa: The case of Ghana. In *Issues and Perspectives on Health Care in Contemporary Sub-Saharan Africa*, ed. E. Kalipeni and P. Thiuri. Lewiston, N.Y.: Edwin Mellen Press, pp. 361–374.

Black, M., E. Steeve, A. P. Najera, M. Vidaurre, and Z. E. Morjani. 2004. Using GIS to measure physical accessibility to health care. World Health Organization. http://www.who.int/kms/initiatives/Ebener_et_al_2004a.pdf (accessed December 5, 2010).

Boisson, E., A. Nicoll, B. Zaba, and L. C. Rodrigues. 1996. Interpreting HIV seroprevalence data from pregnant women. *Journal of Acquired Immune Deficiency Syndromes 13*(5):434–439.

Bryant, J. 1969. *Health and the Developing World*. Ithaca, N.Y.: Cornell University Press.

Chansa, C., J. Sundewall, D. McIntyre, G. Tomson, and B. C. Forsberg. 2008. Exploring SWAP's contribution to the efficient allocation and use of resources in the health sector in Zambia. *Health Policy and Planning 23*(4):244–251.

Church, R. L., and C. ReVelle. 1974. The maximal covering location problem. *Papers of the Regional Science Association 32*:101–118.

Doherty, L., L. Rispel, and N. Webb. 1996. Developing a plan for primary health care facilities in Soweto, South Africa. Part II: Applying locational criteria. *Health Policy and Planning 11*(4):394–405.

Dulin, M. F., T. M. Ludden, H. Tapp, H. A. Smith, B. U. de Hernandez, J. Blackwell, and O. J. Furuseth. 2010. Geographic information systems (GIS): Demonstrating primary care needs for a transitioning Hispanic community. *Journal of the American Board of Family Medicine 23*(1):109–120.

Eicher, C. L., and C. A. Brewer. 2001. Dasymetric mapping and aerial interpolation: Implementation and evaluation. *Cartography and Geographic Information Science 28*(2):125–138.

Esri. 2006. *ArcGIS 9.2*. Redlands, CA: Environmental Systems Research Institute (ESRI).

Foody, G. M. 2006. GIS: Health applications. *Progress in Physical Geography 30*:691–695.

Gage, A. J., and M. Guirlène Calixte. 2006. Effects of the physical accessibility of maternal health services on their use in rural Haiti. *Population Studies 60*(3):271–288.

Gesler, W. M. 1984. *Health care in developing countries*. Washington, DC: Association of American Geographers.

Gething, P. W., A. M. Noor, D. Zurovac, M. P. Atkinson, I. S. Hay, S. M. Nixon, and W. R. Snow. 2004. Empirical modelling of government health service use by children with fevers in Kenya. *Acta Tropica 91*:227–237.

Glynn, J. R., A. Buve, M. Carael, R. M. Musonda, M. Kahindo, I. Macauley, F. Tembo, and L. Zekeng. 2001. Factors influencing the difference in HIV prevalence between antenatal clinic and general population in sub-Saharan Africa. *AIDS 15*(13):1717–1725.

Grassly, N. C., M. Morgan, N. Walker, G. Garnett, K. A. Stanecki, J. Stover, T. Brown, and P. D. Ghys. 2004. Uncertainty in estimates of HIV/AIDS: The estimation and application of plausibility bounds. *Sexually Transmitted Infections 80*:i31–i38.

Graves, A. 2009. A model for assessment of potential geographical accessibility: A case for GIS. *Online Journal of Rural Nursing and Health Care 9*(1):46–55.

Higgs, G. 2004. A literature review of the use of GIS-based measures of access to health care services. *Health Services and Outcomes Research Methodology 2004*(5):119–139.

Higgs, G. A. 2009. The role of GIS for health utilization studies: Literature review. *Health Services and Outcomes Research Methodology 2009*(9):84–99, doi: 10.1007/s10742–009-0046-2.

Holt, J. B., C. P. Lo, and T. W. Hodler. 2004. Dasymetric estimation of population density and areal interpolation of census data. *Cartography and Geographic Information Science 31*(2):103–121.

Huang, N., W. Yip, H. J. Chang, and Y. J. Chou. 2005. Rural/urban differences in access to health care: Does universal coverage reduce inequalities in health? Abstracts Academy Health Meetings 2005 22: Abstract No. 3339. http://gateway.nlm.nih.gov/MeetingAbstracts/ma?f=103622802.html (accessed August 23, 2010).

Iyun, F. 1983. Hospital service areas in Ibadan City. *Social Science and Medicine 17*(9):601–616.

Jackman, M. E. 1972. Flying doctor services in Zambia. In *Medical Geography: Techniques and Field Studies*, ed. N. D. McGlashan. London: Methuen, pp. 97–103.

Kalipeni, E., and L. Zulu. 2008. Using GIS to model and forecast HIV/AIDS rates in Africa, 1986–2010. *The Professional Geographer 60*(1):33–53.

King, M. H. 1966. *Medical Care in Developing Countries: A Primer on the Medicine of Poverty and a Symposium from Makerere, Based on a Conference Assisted by WHO/UNICEF, and an Experimental Edition Assisted by UNICEF*. Nairobi: Oxford University Press.

Kohli, S. K., K. Sahlen, A. Sivertun, O. Lofman, E. TreU, and O. Wigertz. 1995. Distance from the primary health center: A GIS method to study geographical access to health care. *Journal of Medical Systems 19*(6):425–446.

Krabacher, T., E. Kalipeni, and A. Layachi. 2009. *Global Issues: Africa*. Boston: McGraw-Hill Contemporary Learning Series.

le Bacq, F., and A. Rietsema. 1997. High maternal mortality levels and additional risk from poor accessibility in two districts of Northern Province, Zambia. *International Journal of Epidemiology 26*(2):357–363.

Luo, W., and F. Wang. 2003. Measures of spatial accessibility to health care in a GIS environment: Synthesis and a case study in the Chicago region. *Environment and Planning B: Planning and Design 30*(6):865–884.

McLafferty, S., and S. Grady. 2004. Prenatal care and access: A GIS analysis. *Journal of Medical Systems 28*(3):321–333.

Messina, J. P., A. M. Shortridge, R. E Groop, P. V. Varnakovida, and M. J. Finn. 2006. Evaluating Michigan's community hospital access: Spatial methods for decision support. *International Journal of Health Geographics*. doi:10.1186/1476-072x-5–42.

Michelo, C., I. Sandøy, and K. Fylkesnes. 2008. Antenatal clinic HIV data found to underestimate actual prevalence declines: Evidence from Zambia. *Tropical Medicine and International Health 13*(2):171–179.

Moise, I. K., and E. Kalipeni. 2010. Applications of geospatial analysis to surveillance data: A spatial examination of HIV/AIDS prevalence in Zambia. *GeoJournal*, doi: 10.1007/s10708-010-9349-7.

Montana, L., M. Neuman, V. Mishra, and R. Hong. 2005. Spatial modeling of HIV prevalence in Cameroon, Kenya, and Tanzania. http://paa2006.princeton.edu/download.aspx?submissionId=61479 (accessed June 22, 2009).

Murray, A. T. 2010. Advances in location modeling: GIS linkages and contributions. *Journal of Geographical Systems 2010*(12):335–354, doi: 10.1007/s10109-009-0105-9.

Mutale, E. 2004. *The management of urban development in Zambia*. Aldershot, UK: Ashgate.

Ngoma, M. C., and T. R. Mbukwa. 2008. Use of health institutions by pregnant women in Zambia. *African Journal of Midwifery and Women's Health 2*(2):14–17.

Noor, A. M., D. Zurovac, S. I. Hay, S. A. Ochola, and R. W. Snow. 2003. Defining equity in physical access to clinical services using geographical information systems as part of malaria planning and monitoring in Kenya. *Tropical Medicine and International Health 8*(10):917–926.

Nykiforuk, C. I. J., and L. M. Flaman. 2011. Geographic information systems (GIS) for health promotion and public health: A review. *Health Promotion Practice 12*(1):63–73.

Oppong, R. J. and M. J. Hodgson. 1994. Spatial accessibility to health care facilities in Suhum District, Ghana. *The Professional Geographer 46*(2):199–09.

Southern African Humanitarian and Disaster Management (2006). GIS library: Country datasets and geographical information. http://www.sahims.net/gis/GIS%20input/GIS_library_Zambia.asp?cmd=reset (accessed June 22, 2009).

Stock, R. 1983. Distance and the utilization of health facilities in rural Nigeria. *Social Science and Medicine 17*(9):563–570.

Tanser, F., B. Gijsbertsen, and K. Herbst. 2006. "Modelling and understanding primary health care accessibility and utilization in rural South Africa: An exploration using a geographical information system. *Social Science and Medicine 63*(3):691–705.

Tatalovich, Z., J. P. Wilson, and M. Cockburn. 2006. A comparison of thiessen polygon, kriging, and spline models of potential UV exposure. *Cartography and Geographic Information Science 33*(3):217–231.

Tsoka, J. M., and D. Le Sueur. 2004. Using GIS to measure geographical accessibility to primary health care in rural South Africa. *Science 100*(7–8):329–330.

UNAIDS/WHO. 2004. Guidelines for effective use of data from HIV surveillance systems. Geneva: World Health Organization. http://data.unaids.org/publications/irc-pub06/jc1010-usingdata_en.pdf (accessed June 22, 2009).

WHO/UNAIDS. 2003. Reconciling antenatal clinic-based surveillance and population-based survey estimates of HIV prevalence in sub-Saharan Africa. Geneva: World Health Organization and UNAIDS. http://data.unaids.org/UNA-docs/anc-population_surveys_report_en.pdf (accessed June 22, 2009).

Wilkinson, D., and F. Tanser. 1999. GIS/GPS to document increased access to community-based treatment for tuberculosis in Africa. *Lancet 354*(9176):394–395.

Wood, D. J., and A. C. Gatrell. 2002. Equity of geographical access to inpatient hospice care within North West England: A geographical information systems (GIS) approach. North West Public Health Observatory, Lancaster University. http://www.nwpho.org.uk/reports/inpatientgis.doc (accessed June 15, 2009).

Yang, D. H., R. Goerge, and R. Mullner. 2006. Comparing GIS-based methods of measuring spatial accessibility to health services. *Journal of Medical Systems 30*(1):23–32.

Zambia Central Statistical Office. 2003. *Zambia: 2000 Census of population and Housing*. Lusaka, Zambia: Central Statistical Office.

Zambia Central Statistical Office. 2010. *Zambia 2010 Census of Population and Housing Preliminary Report*. Lusaka, Zambia: Central Statistical Office. Accessed on May 22, 2011, at http://www.zamstats.gov.zm/

Zambia Government. (2006). *Fifth National Development Plan 2006–2010: Broad Based Wealth and Job Creation through Citizenry Participation and Technological Advancement*. Lusaka: Republic of Zambia.

Maternity Ward Closures in Philadelphia: Using GIS to Measure Disruptions in Essential Health Services

SARAH CORDIVANO
University of Pennsylvania, Philadelphia, PA, USA

GIS is a robust analysis tool capable of contributing to a more comprehensive study of public health issues than was possible using traditional methods. By analyzing the issue of maternity ward closures in Philadelphia, this paper explores the proper methods for utilizing, processing, and analyzing sensitive public health data. These analytical methods are underutilized in public health research due to widespread unfamiliarity with GIS technology as well as difficulty in accessing accurate data. Understanding and adopting GIS technology is valuable to the assessment, allocation, and delivery of health care services.

INTRODUCTION

The number of medical facilities providing obstetric care in Philadelphia has declined drastically in the past decade. In 1996 there were nineteen maternity ward facilities; today only six remain open. Some causes of these closures are the high cost of obstetric care, including malpractice costs and claims, threats of litigation, and insufficient revenue to support the facility (Kruse, Phillips, and Wesley 1989; Fondren and Ricketts 1991). The reduction of services provided in Philadelphia has led to a decrease in options for Philadelphia women and the danger of reaching capacity at the remaining facilities (Kolker 2007). There has been insufficient research done to predict the short- and long-term effects of these facility closures. Furthermore, research about the spatial implications is uncharted. This study seeks to address many questions regarding the effects of facility closures and the uncertain future of obstetric care in Philadelphia using geographic information system (GIS) tools.

The GIS is a powerful analytical tool for use in many fields. In health care, the GIS serves an important role in informing decisions and solving problems. Specifically, the GIS can be used for surveilling disease, measuring service allocation, and utilizing and assessing inequality of care access and need (McLafferty 2003). New advances in software development and awareness of the GIS as well as increased availability of spatial data have contributed to more widespread utilization and understanding of spatial analytical techniques. Using the maternity ward closures in Philadelphia as a sample study, this paper describes the most commonly used data, software, and tools, the process of database development, and the use of geospatial analytical methods in assessing the disruption of maternity ward closures in Philadelphia.

Literature Review

There is a long history of utilizing spatial data to approach problems in medicine. A common example of this is the mapping of the cholera outbreak in London during the 1850s by physician John Snow. Snow traced the outbreak to a tainted water pump by plotting the incidents of cholera to illustrate the clusters around the well. He disproved the popular theory of miasma or "bad air" (Hempel 2006). His contribution is considered a significant step in both the understanding of how diseases spread and the use of spatial methods to approach epidemiology.

However, there is a very brief history of the use of the GIS to chart access to care and the future of uncertain services. The issue of the decline of obstetrical services is not unique to Philadelphia, but is common in America and other countries (Bosanquet et al. 2005; Nesbitt, Scherger, and Tanji 2008). Access to care is of interest, especially in rural areas where closures have resulted in an increase in the rate of negative birth outcomes. Closures from 1990 to 2002 in Missouri have been determined to be the cause of an increase in the rate of low birth weight (Sontheimer et al. 2008). The Philadelphia obstetric care crisis has been tackled by researchers and local media. Jennifer Kolker of Drexel University has explored the implications of the closures in her report: *Obstetric Care for Philadelphia Residents* (Kolker 2007). She has addressed many important effects resulting from the closures including issues of capacity and impact on birth outcomes. However, the issue of obstetric care in Philadelphia has not yet been analyzed using geospatial analysis tools such as GIS software.

In other geographic areas, these methods have been used effectively to predict effects and inform decision making concerning the discontinuation of obstetric care. A study based in France used the GIS to determine the level of accessibility for women in rural areas after facility closures (Pilkington et al. 2008).

The GIS is an effective system for measuring access to services as well as predicting the future of care. Higgs explores these opportunities in his research and presents many suitable approaches for utilizing the methods (Higgs 2004, 2009).

This study uses geospatial methods to assess the impact of closing thirteen maternity wards in Philadelphia between 1996 and 2008. Specifically, this paper explores the facility shift preference of patients of the closed facilities, raising issues of facility capacity and an effective solution for future care. The software, tools, and data needed to conduct this analysis, as well as a step-by-step data processing procedure, are described.

A Primer on Spatial Data

Data that contain a spatial attribute such as an x-y coordinate or spatially identifying attribute are known as spatial data. There are two main forms of spatial data: vector and raster (Esri 2011). Vector data are used to represent geographic features; raster data represent cell grids or coverages. Vector data can be in the form of polygons, lines (or arcs), or points. Polygon vector data are used to represent areas such as bodies of water or counties. These can be symbolized in various colors or fills to show numeric graduation or qualitative attributes. Line or arc features can represent street centerlines, routes, or hydrology. These features can be symbolized with textured or weighted lines in various colors. Point features are used to represent discrete features such as cities, points of interest, and addresses. A centroid is known as the point located in the geographic center of a polygon feature.

Vector data can come in the form of administrative data, which are collected by government agencies and institutions. A few examples of this type of data are hospital records, unemployment data, and property valuation data. Perhaps the most well-known example of administrative data are U.S. Census data. These data are collected by the U.S. Census Bureau every decade at multiple geographic levels. From largest to smallest, these geographies are country, state, county, census tract, block group, and block. Data can also be collected at the metropolitan statistical area (MSA) or zip code level. The standard method for identifying a geography is known as the STFID code (Univ. of Texas 2004). This is a concatenation, or combined string, of numerical codes (Federal Information Processing Standards [FIPS]) signifying the geography. For example, STFID 4210100010001 indicates state (42 = Pennsylvania), county (101 = Philadelphia), census tract (0001 = tract 1), and block group (0001 = block group 1).

Raster features, on the other hand, are grid-based datasets that most often indicate a coverage or surface. In raster data, grid cells are of uniform size and each has one value associated with it. For example, elevation, slope, density, and land use classification are most often represented with raster features. These data values are often continuous and therefore are best represented by continuous grids as opposed to discreetly classified or quantified polygon features. Data can usually be converted from one form to the other; however, the precision of the data is dependent on the size of the grid cell.

Data used in a spatial analysis are often saved as feature classes stored in a file geodatabase, which is a relational database that can store, query, and manage both spatial and nonspatial data. This storage method is popular because it allows the user to organize and manage the entire data library as well as compress larger files.

GIS Software and Tools

There are several software products that can be used to analyze spatial data. Some products are open source while others require commercial licensing. A popular system is Esri's ArcGIS software package. ArcGIS Desktop suite is a set of software applications that is capable of storing, reading, and projecting spatial data. There are three licensing product levels with increasing functionality for ArcGIS Desktop: ArcView, ArcEditor, and ArcInfo (Esri 2011). For this analysis, ArcInfo, the product with the most complete functionality, was used. This product allows for advanced GIS data manipulation and cartography, as well as geodatabase development.

Some tools and software functions are especially useful in health analysis. ArcInfo includes a set of geocoding tools that allows the user to find the geographic coordinates associated with a table of addresses based on available spatial data, usually a complete street database. The user can convert a dataset of birth records including an address field, for example, to point spatial data. A *tabular join* is a function of the software that allows the user to join spatial data with a table based on a common field. When performing this join, the common field type must be identical, otherwise an error will occur. A *spatial join* is a function allowing the user to join two pieces of spatial data based on a shared spatial location. This is helpful when associating a broader geography with a more precise geography to eliminate identifying information.

Extensions, or add-on, software packages can increase the functionality of ArcInfo. Some extensions are especially helpful in analysis or interpretation of health data, specifically Spatial Analyst, Network Analyst, and Geostatistical Analyst. The Spatial Analyst extension is used for raster-based spatial modeling. For example, this extension can be used to create a density grid using point features, or service areas can be calculated by using the distance tool to measure the closest distance to each facility. The Network Analyst extension uses a network such as a road or rail transit network to calculate routes, closest facilities, and services areas. This can be especially helpful when allocating service areas based on shortest travel time or distance. This can be more precise than traditional methods of service area allocation that use Euclidian distance (as the crow flies) or administrative boundaries. The Geostatistical Analyst extension is helpful for visualizing and modeling spatial relationships or interpolating point data to create a continuous surface of values. For example, this could be helpful in predicting the amount of contaminate in soil based on several discrete measurements. It is also possible to utilize tools created by third party developers or independent users to increase the functionality of ArcInfo. For example, Geospatial Modeling Environment,[1] formerly known as Hawth's Analysis Tools, offers numerous tools created to conduct further analysis.

METHODS

Database Development

The first step in acquiring data is to identify the available data sources and select the most appropriate and accurate data for analysis. This can be difficult because there is no universally used database for storing and sharing health data in the United States, and the quality and availability of data vary drastically from region to region. For this analysis, the desired data were Philadelphia residential birth records from 1996 to 2008; maternity ward data for all facilities, open and closed, from 1996 to 2008; and last, demographic, socioeconomic, and birth outcome data for Philadelphia with the highest precision and accuracy available.

After identifying the desired data for analysis, the acquisition of accurate and current spatial data can be one of the biggest challenges. Birth record data is often maintained by state health departments, but it may be necessary to contact an intermediary who manages the data. Facility data, such as hospital and clinic data, may be available from a local health agency. In this study, the accuracy of the available facility data was insufficient, so it was necessary to create a new database of maternity wards by precisely geocoding the addresses of the facilities and joining this spatial data with a table of supporting information about the maternity wards including capacity, operation dates, and facility ID. The acquisition of demographic or socioeconomic data is slightly easier. The decennial U.S. Census collects much of the data that can be useful in analyzing health data. Demographic data such as race, age, sex, and educational attainment and socioeconomic data such as household income, rate of poverty, and median home value are also available at the census block level. These data types are 100% population data, meaning a complete survey of the population was used. Estimates or projections of current and future figures are also available from the U.S. Census. Available census data can be downloaded free from the U.S. Census Web site using the application American FactFinder.[2]

When accessing data containing sensitive patient information, such as name, home address, Social Security number, or telephone number, it is necessary to apply for institutional review board (IRB) approval. One way to bypass the application process is to request data that has already been de-identified, meaning the sensitive information has been removed from the dataset. In this analysis, the birth record data for Philadelphia County contained the home address of the birth mother and hospital ID of the birth facility. These are both extremely important to analysis, but because the home address is sensitive information, it is important to first de-identify the data. This process involves first geocoding, or assigning geographic coordinates to each address and then de-identifying the record by associating the data with the administrative polygon it falls within, most likely a census tract or block group, and removing the address field. By having the data managers conduct this process before receiving the dataset, it was possible to bypass the IRB application. In rural areas where there is low population density, caution must be used when de-identifying sensitive data. When associating a birth record with the containing administrative polygon, it must be first determined that there is significant population per polygon to make identifying an individual impossible.

Datasets may contain inaccuracies. As mentioned previously, the available hospital data were considered too inaccurate and out-of-date for use in this study, so it was necessary to re-create the data using current and factual information. Human input error can also cause data to be inaccurate. This can be specifically problematic when geocoding addresses included on birth records. The best method for troubleshooting this is to use a composite geocoder that utilizes more than one address locator to quickly find the most appropriate associated address. This method first tries to match the entire address. If this is unsuccessful, the locator tries to match the given zip code with one located in the city. If this returns a match, then the record is associated with the centroid of the zip code. If both locators return no matches, then the record is manually inspected for obvious mistakes such as a misspelling or the omission of a directional prefix. If this inspection is unsuccessful, then it is determined that the address cannot be geocoded properly. This is inevitable when geocoding large batches of addresses that have been subject to human input. Therefore, records with nongeocodable addresses were discarded for the purposes of this study.

Creating a geodatabase to store all datasets, spatial and nonspatial, is the best way to organize and maintain study data. Esri's file geodatabase system allows the user to organize files and identify relationships between datasets. The file geodatabases can store up to one terabyte of data, and they use about a third of the storage space required by other data storage methods. File geodatabases also allow multiple users to access the data simultaneously.

Keeping data accurately annotated and organized is imperative to proper spatial data maintenance. Providing notation about each dataset will make future access or sharing of the data much easier. Labeling the subject and date will help organize the data. Adding descriptive and accurate metadata is also imperative to data maintenance. Metadata can be easily added to spatial data or a geodatabase through the ArcGIS Desktop application, ArcCatalog. Information that should be cataloged includes keywords, description, status, date created and updated, source, owner, spatial reference, and attribute dictionary. Complete and accurate metadata will give future users all the necessary descriptive information about the dataset.

The data used in this study include the birth records of Philadelphia County residents from 1996 to 2008. The source of this dataset is the Pennsylvania Department of Health, which is managed by the department's Office of Maternal, Child, and Family Health Services. This dataset was geocoded according to the home address of the birth mother. This dataset was then de-identified by associating each record with the centroid of the block group the address falls within. A hospital ID number was included for each entry of the dataset that indicates the birth facility. Philadelphia residents who gave birth at facilities outside the city and those living outside Philadelphia County giving birth in hospitals within Philadelphia were excluded from this dataset. A database of open and closed maternity ward facilities in Philadelphia including capacity, operation dates, affiliation, for-profit/nonprofit status, and number of births per year was also used. Demographic, socioeconomic, and birth outcome data by census tract were also used.

Data Processing

The data procedures used in this study help illuminate the current obstetric care situation in Philadelphia after the numerous facility closures. The analysis began with data exploration and creation of catchment areas. In order to explore the impact of facility closures, it was necessary to determine a service area or catchment area per facility, the geographical area that a facility predominately serves. Once these areas are established, it is possible to see if any changes have occurred in the neighborhood after closure of the facility. There are many methods for designating the catchment area of each facility. Thiessen polygons are one option to determine unique catchment areas. These polygons are created by calculating the minimum distance between any two facilities and creating a border at that point. The result is that all points in the study area, Philadelphia County, will be assigned to the closest facility. An example of Thiessen polygons service areas is shown in Figure 1. However, this method has shortcomings that make it unsuitable for this study. This allocation of service areas assumes that clients will select a facility based on the sole criterion of proximity to the home address. And when two facilities are located close to each other, their service areas are much smaller compared with other facilities.

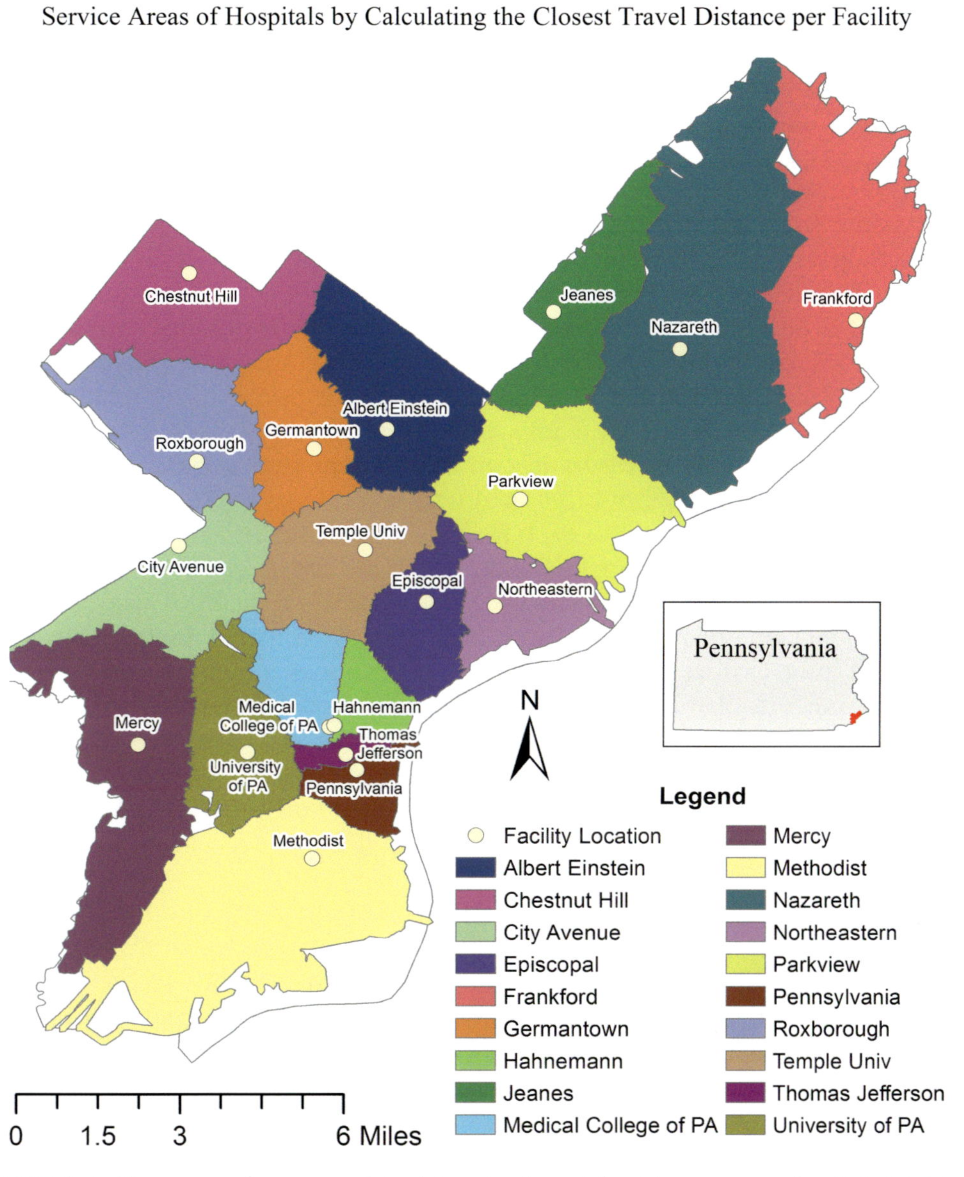

FIGURE 1 Thiessen polygons used to determine hospital catchment areas for Philadelphia facilities.

Facilities attract patients for many reasons such as reputation, type of insurance accepted, practices, and staff. It appears that, for Philadelphia residents, proximity is a very important factor when selecting a facility. Designing service areas that capture the geographic location of most of a facility's Philadelphia client base was the goal in determining the catchments of each hospital. In order to do this, a radial travel distance between 2.5 and 7 miles was selected per facility such that each service area would encompass 85%–90% of the facility's Philadelphia clients. An assessment of socioeconomic and demographic characteristics of each facility's catchment area follows. Administrative data by block group was aggregated for each facility catchment area.

Density indicates the frequency of an event (births) per unit of area (square mile), which can be useful in visualizing the distribution of births across the study area. Density mapping is also known as *hotspot mapping*. Density grids were created indicating the number of births per square mile, yearly, for all areas in Philadelphia. The result is a continuous surface of values at every point in the study area indicating the births per square mile at any location. Note that the locations of births are determined by the centroid of the block group in which the mother's home address falls. This method may create some artificial areas of high density because each block group's total number of births is concentrated in one geographical point instead of spread throughout the areal unit.

An assessment is made of each facility's catchment area facility shift preference, including change in Euclidian distance traveled to a facility before and after closure. To investigate how the closure of facilities has affected the residents of Philadelphia, the mean distance traveled by patients before and after closures is explored. These distances are measured using a point distance tool that calculates Euclidian distance between two sets of x-y coordinates. In this application, the first set of coordinates is the home address (aggregated to the block group centroid), and the second set is the location of the hospital of birth. Absorption rates and capacity issues for all Philadelphia facilities, as well as the effect of closures on staff and revenue, are explored.

An ordinary least squares regression analysis was conducted to determine whether there was a correlation between negative birth outcomes (preterm birth, low birth weight) and the Euclidian distance to the nearest obstetric care facility. The unit of analysis, the census tract, has the calculation of mean Euclidian distance from the nearest obstetric facility, as well as the 2005 rate of preterm birth and low birth weight recorded. This regression utilizes the GeoDa statistical software package.

A discussion follows, including an evaluation of the current situation of maternity care and an assessment of the results of the above data procedures. Lastly, a final recommendation is made for effective placement of new obstetric facilities.

RESULTS AND DISCUSSION

Study Area and Population

The age, race, and birth outcome characteristics of the dataset for two selected years was explored prior to any spatial analysis of the data (Kolker 2007).[3] This is displayed in Table 1. A few things of interest are the decrease

TABLE 1 Descriptive Details Of Birth Data Set for 1997 and 2004

Detailed Birth Data for Philadelphia Residents				
Year	1997	1997 Rate, %	2004	2004 Rate, %
Number of Live Births	22,038	100.00	21,585	100.00
White	9,139	41.47	6,045	28.01
Black	11,407	51.76	10,672	49.44
Asian	1,093	4.96	1,232	5.71
All other	399	1.81	2,804	12.99
Unknown/Refused	0	0.00	834	3.86
Age of Mother				
Under 19	4,053	18.39	3,384	15.68
20 to 24	5,590	25.37	5,980	27.70
25 to 29	5,565	25.25	5,419	25.11
30 to 34	4,341	19.70	4,185	19.39
35 to 39	2,012	9.13	2,046	9.48
40 and above	398	1.81	472	2.19
Birth Outcomes				
Low birth weight	2,490	11.30	2,612	12.10
Preterm birth	2,689	12.20	2,720	12.60
Infant mortality rate (per 1,000 births)	13	1.30	11	1.05

in births by mothers under the age of 19 between 1997 and 2004, and the rate of preterm birth and low birth weight,[4] which roughly held steady from 1996 to 2004 for all Philadelphia births. The rate of birth outcomes is important when assessing the impact of facility closures. High risk of birth complications often results in increased hospitalization time for mothers. This must be monitored closely because facility closures have decreased the amount of obstetric services in the city. Increased hospitalization time for Philadelphia mothers has the potential to exacerbate the current issues of facility capacity.

In establishing catchment areas, 1996 birth record data were used to determine the percentage of clients per facility catchment area because, in that year, all facilities in the study were operating with no restrictions and, with 19 facilities open across the city, residents were able to select their facility by considering all options. The facility catchment areas overlap because it is very likely that multiple facilities serve the same neighborhoods. Examples of two facility catchment areas, Frankford Hospital and Mercy Hospital, are shown in Figure 2. These catchment areas represent essentially the geographical area determined by travel distance, where most of the facility's Philadelphia clients live. Table 2 describes several characteristics of each catchment area. The figures indicate that percentage minority population, percentage vacancy, and percentage rental properties are higher for the catchment areas of open facilities. On the other hand, median income is higher for catchment areas of closed facilities. However, there is a larger population within the catchment areas of open facilities. The difference in characteristics of open and closed facility catchment areas may be due to the fact that the open facilities are located in Center City and lower north portion

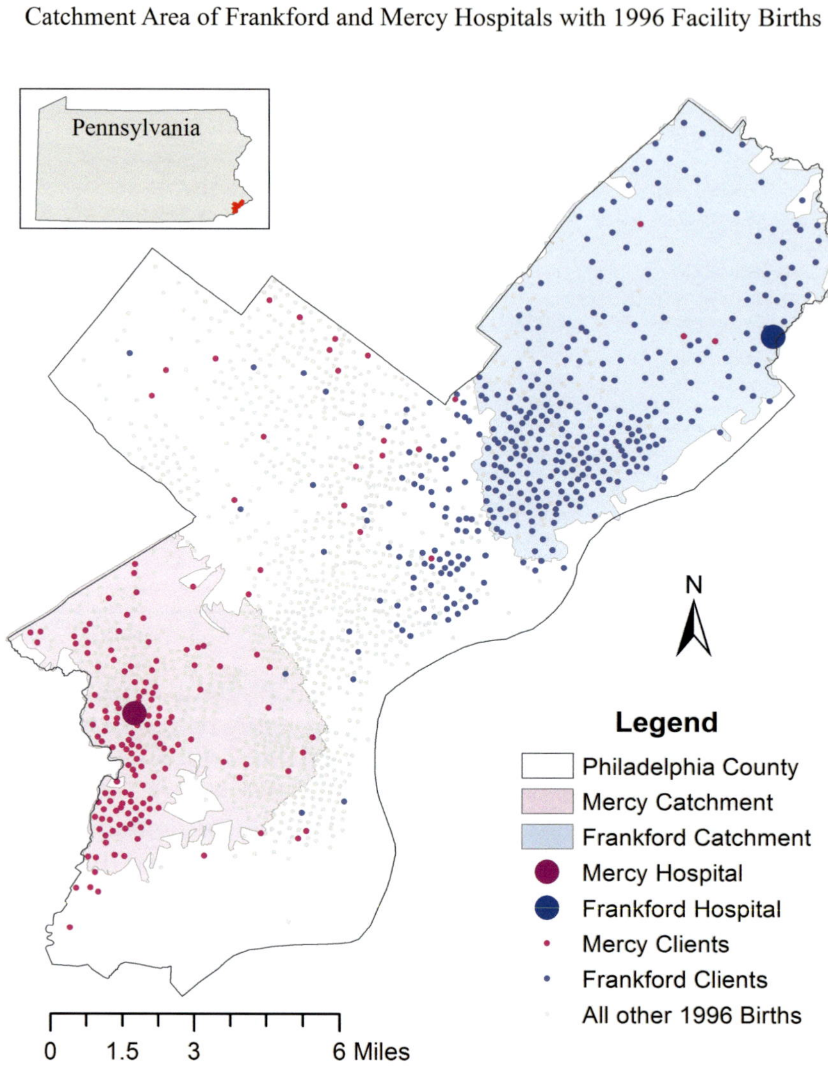

FIGURE 2 Sample catchment areas for two closed facilities including 1996 facility births and all other 1996 births.

of Philadelphia, neighborhoods that are struggling economically. However, many of the closed facilities were located near the edges of the city in the South, Southwest, Northeast, and Germantown neighborhoods. These areas have more diverse characteristics than Center City or North Philadelphia.

Birth Density in Philadelphia

It is evident that the demand for care has not declined in Philadelphia. During 1996–2008, births of Philadelphia residents have remained steady between 21,000 and 23,000 per year. Using the Spatial Analyst extension, a

TABLE 2 Demographic Data for Facility Catchment Areas

Hospital Catchment Area	2009 Est. Median Family Income	Percent Minority	Percent Black	Percent Hispanic	Percent Vacancy	Per. Renter Occupied Units	Median Age of Housing in Years	Operation Status
City Avenue	$46,029	80.87	67.57	8.75	14.19	41.71	55	Closed
Chestnut Hill	$70,278	76.29	66.07	5.04	9.24	35.44	55	Closed
Roxborough	$66,252	64.68	59.11	1.77	10.10	41.99	54	Closed
Parkview	$43,694	56.44	27.66	21.39	10.48	29.21	56	Closed
Nazareth	$58,733	24.61	9.70	8.27	5.33	29.82	46	Closed
Mercy	$46,474	72.54	62.84	2.32	12.78	44.12	55	Closed
Episcopal	$35,581	73.99	39.81	29.88	16.56	34.01	58	Closed
Northeastern	$38,321	66.37	34.69	26.57	15.18	33.96	57	Closed
Methodist	$41,867	68.99	51.89	10.36	14.90	41.32	54	Closed
Medical College of Pa	$44,337	69.38	52.13	10.26	13.35	39.06	54	Closed
Jeanes	$50,927	51.16	29.91	14.62	8.28	30.73	52	Closed
Germantown	$54,259	85.47	69.53	10.60	11.08	35.11	57	Closed
Frankford	$60,885	19.45	8.08	5.62	5.03	30.51	45	Closed
Univ. of Pennsylvania	$44,677	69.16	58.34	3.09	14.31	41.70	54	Open
Albert Einstein	$49,397	77.44	55.45	16.22	12.40	34.35	56	Open
Thomas Jefferson	$42,990	69.59	51.84	10.73	13.86	39.39	54	Open
Temple	$44,229	74.51	52.09	16.27	14.05	39.48	56	Open
Penn Hospital	$42,826	69.40	51.73	10.72	13.78	39.43	54	Open
Hahnemann	$42,219	70.23	53.29	10.40	14.70	40.69	55	Open
Average of all closed facilities	$50,587	62	45	12	11	36	54	Closed
Average of all open facilities	$44,390	72	54	11	14	39	55	Open

density grid of births was created for each year; this helps indicate any spatial changes in the birth patterns of Philadelphia residents. The evolution of birth density in Philadelphia between 1996 and 2008 is shown in Figure 3. The highest density areas, 500–900 births per square mile, have moved slightly over the years but remain in the same general areas, North, Southwest, and South Philadelphia. Areas with more than 900 births per square mile were evident only in 1996, 1997, 1998, 2005, and 2008. The geographical area of Philadelphia, by and large, has a birth density of approximately 1–500 births per square mile.

Facility Shift Preference

The Euclidian distance traveled was calculated for every birth of Philadelphia residents from 1996 through 2008. In 1996, the average Euclidian distance traveled by all Philadelphia residents giving birth at Philadelphia facilities was 2.80 miles. In 2008 this average increased to 3.24 miles. The difference in travel distance per client for each facility from 1996 to 2008 is included in Table 3. Mean Euclidian distance traveled increased more than 15% for patients of all facilities still open in Philadelphia, except for Pennsylvania Hospital, where travel distance decreased by 8.92%.

Density of Births:
1996-2008 Births per Square Mile in Philadelphia

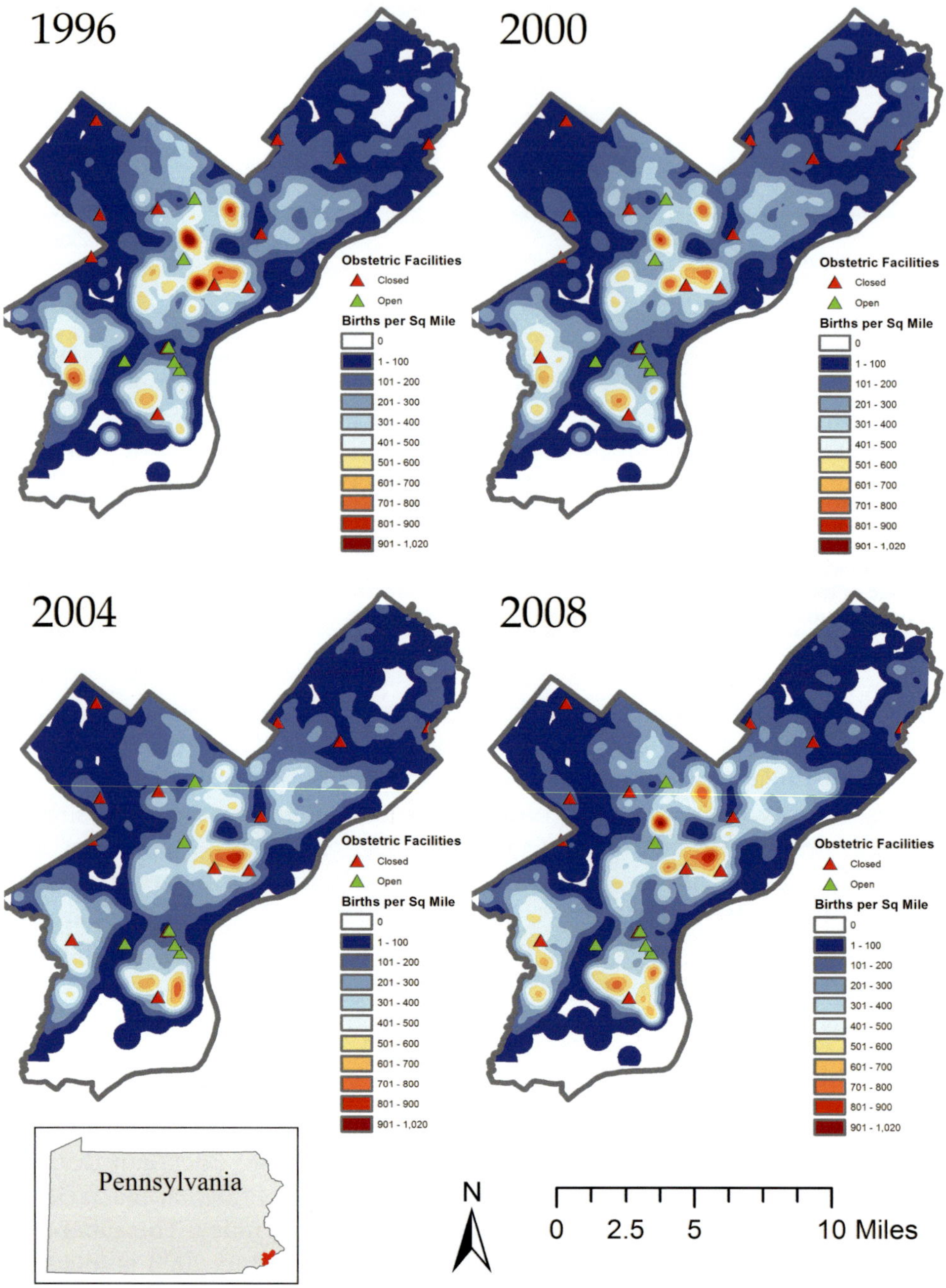

FIGURE 3 Evolution of density of Philadelphia residential births during the period of closures including open and closed facilities.

TABLE 3 Change in Euclidian Travel Distance per Hospital from 1996 to 2008

Hospital	1996 Births per Facility	1996 Average Miles Traveled per Facility	2008 Births per Facility	2008 Average Miles Traveled per Facility	Percent Change in Distance Traveled per Facility
Albert Einstein	1,390	2.19	2,720	2.87	31.23
Temple University	1,448	1.86	2,412	2.32	25.30
Hahnemann Hospital	1,343	2.99	1,754	3.63	21.78
Univ. of Pennsylvania	1,969	2.49	3,360	2.98	19.85
Chestnut Hill Hospital	576	3.44	602	4.10	19.27
Thomas Jefferson	1,514	3.59	1,785	4.21	17.53
Penn Hospital	2,635	3.85	3,906	3.51	−8.92
Germantown Hospital	428	1.70	0.00	0.000	Facility Closed
City Avenue Hospital	651	3.21	0.00	0.000	Facility Closed
Jeanes Hospital	463	3.16	0.00	0.000	Facility Closed
Medical College of PA	927	4.41	0.00	0.000	Facility Closed
Methodist Hospital	840	1.50	0.00	0.000	Facility Closed
Northeastern Hospital	803	1.68	0.00	0.000	Facility Closed
Episcopal Hospital	1,309	1.25	0.00	0.000	Facility Closed
Mercy Hospital	341	2.35	0.00	0.000	Facility Closed
Nazareth Hospital	354	2.74	0.00	0.000	Facility Closed
Parkview Hospital	874	2.09	0.00	0.000	Facility Closed
Roxborough Hospital	164	1.52	0.00	0.000	Facility Closed
Frankford Hospital	1,364	4.06	0.00	0.000	Facility Closed

Please note that travel distances in these estimates are calculated only for Philadelphia residents gaving birth in Philadelphia. By 2008, there was an increase in Philadelphia residents leaving the city for obstetric care. As previously mentioned, these patients are excluded from the dataset. Average travel distances of Philadelphia birth mothers would further increase with the inclusion of these figures. Another shortfall of this analysis is using Euclidian distance measurements. It is more realistic to calculate travel distance on route networks such as roads or transit lines. However, these datasets are too large, making calculating route travel distance too computationally intensive. For this study, it was necessary to assume that average travel distance was greater than average Euclidian distance.

It is also important to note that many of the facilities that closed accepted only private insurance. For low income or uninsured women, their obstetric care choices have remained generally the same despite closures. For Philadelphia uninsured women, the facility at which they must give birth is determined by the health center they visit for their prenatal care. Once they have visited a health center, they have no option in selecting an obstetric facility.

Absorption Rates and Capacity

As can be expected, the remaining facilities have had the task of absorbing excess births. This results in a substantial increase in patients to be served by other facilities in and outside the city. For example, in 1996, 9,094 of the 19,393 births of Philadelphia residents occurred in facilities that, by 2010, had closed. This is equal to 46.89% of Philadelphia births. Other facilities now have the task of accommodating the influx of patients. In 2008, every facility in Philadelphia still in operation accommodated a significant more number of patients than in 1996. For example, maternity patients at Albert Einstein Hospital increased by 95.7%, Hospital of the University of Pennsylvania by 70.6%, Temple University Hospital by 66.6%, and Pennsylvania Hospital by 48.2%. Table 4 shows the percent change from 1996 to 2009 for all hospitals. Figure 4 symbolizes the growth of facilities from 1996 to 2008. It is noteworthy that Chestnut Hill Hospital, which accommodated 602 births in 2008, closed their obstetric facility later that year. The gap of care left by this facility is not included in the previous calculations because 2009 birth records are not yet available. These figures account only for births of Philadelphia residents. Many women living outside the city rely on Philadelphia's hospitals as well. The area's remaining obstetric units have had the task of absorbing not only Philadelphia's excess births, but the region's.

The six facilities that remain open in Philadelphia are not able to completely absorb the excess births from the thirteen closed facilities. There was a 14.7% decrease in total births by Philadelphia residents at Philadelphia hospitals from 1996 to 2008 even though total births of residents increased by over 1,000.[5] This directly results in a decrease of revenue for Philadelphia hospitals as well as a decrease in jobs for obstetric staff (Kolker 2007).[6]

The remaining facilities in Philadelphia are operating very close to or beyond capacity. Using a dataset of resident and nonresident births as well as hospital data, Kolker was able to estimate the operating capacity of each facility (Kolker 2007).[7] This daily census calculation estimates the number of beds required for Philadelphia to maintain a 75% occupancy rate or below.[8] According to Kolker's estimates, as of 2004, five Philadelphia facilities were operating beyond the recommended capacity of 75% (Table 5). Furthermore, since 2004, three more Philadelphia facilities not included in these estimates have closed, so the current demand for Philadelphia obstetric care is expected to exceed 100% of capacity.

Correlation between Birth Outcomes and Facility Distance

The results of the regression analysis indicate that there is no significant correlation between negative birth outcomes and distance from an obstetric care facility. For example, the P value for the regression rate of low birth weight on mean Euclidian miles from an obstetric facility was 0.226, indicating insignificant correlation. Similarly, the P value for the regression rate of preterm birth on mean Euclidian miles from an obstetric facility was 0.142. It is unlikely that there is any relationship between distance from an obstetric

TABLE 4 Percent Change in Births per Hospital from 1996 to 2008 in Philadelphia

	Births per Year of Philadelphia Residents													
Philadelphia Hospital	1996	1997	1998	1999	2000	2001	2002	2003	2004	2005	2006	2007	2008	Percent Change from 1996 to 2008
Albert Einstein Hospital	1,390	1,464	1,909	1,834	1,960	1,992	1,903	2,280	2,229	2,115	2,405	2,671	2,720	95.68
Hospital of the University of PA	1,969	1,984	2,188	2,447	2,495	2,414	2,675	2,782	2,428	2,506	2,593	2,858	3,360	70.64
Temple University Hospital	1,448	1,731	1,934	2,093	2,156	2,604	2,482	2,540	2,556	2,492	2,506	2,728	2,412	66.57
Pennsylvania Hospital	2,635	2,566	2,414	2,697	2,766	2,886	2,911	3,031	3,366	3,265	3,664	3,911	3,906	48.24
Hahnemann Hospital	1,343	413	0	250	1,365	1,283	1,643	1,904	1,900	1,871	1,824	1,943	1,754	30.60
Thomas Jefferson Hospital	1,514	1,517	1,667	1,442	1,519	1,463	1,657	1,698	1,598	1,673	1,822	1,817	1,785	17.90
Chestnut Hill Hospital	576	585	612	595	836	813	794	770	728	795	784	844	602	4.51
Jeanes Hospital	463	413	462	499	474	445	571	646	697	887	1,177	498	0	−100.00
Frankford Hospital	1,364	1,395	1,579	1,647	1,626	1,466	1,346	1,173	1,183	1,112	321	0	0	−100.00
Parkview Hospital	874	887	856	820	839	1,046	1,123	552	0	0	0	0	0	−100.00
Mercy Hospital of Philadelphia	341	289	257	268	257	216	166	81	0	0	0	0	0	−100.00
Methodist Hospital	840	842	783	794	847	809	370	0	0	0	0	0	0	−100.00
Northeastern Hospital	803	716	669	637	639	707	760	0	0	0	0	0	0	−100.00
Episcopal Hospital	1,309	1,217	1,144	1,046	900	49	0	0	0	0	0	0	0	−100.00
Roxborough Hospital	164	177	144	95	0	0	0	0	0	0	0	0	0	−100.00
City Avenue Hospital	651	1,704	2,154	1,463	0	0	0	0	0	0	0	0	0	−100.00
Nazareth Hospital	354	101	52	0	0	0	0	0	0	0	0	0	0	−100.00
Germantown Hospital	428	271	0	0	0	0	0	0	0	0	0	0	0	−100.00
Medical College of Pa	927	532	0	0	0	0	0	0	0	0	0	0	0	−100.00
Total births at Philadelphia hospitals	19,393	18,804	18,824	18,627	18,679	18,193	18,401	17,457	16,685	16,716	17,096	17,270	16,539	−14.72

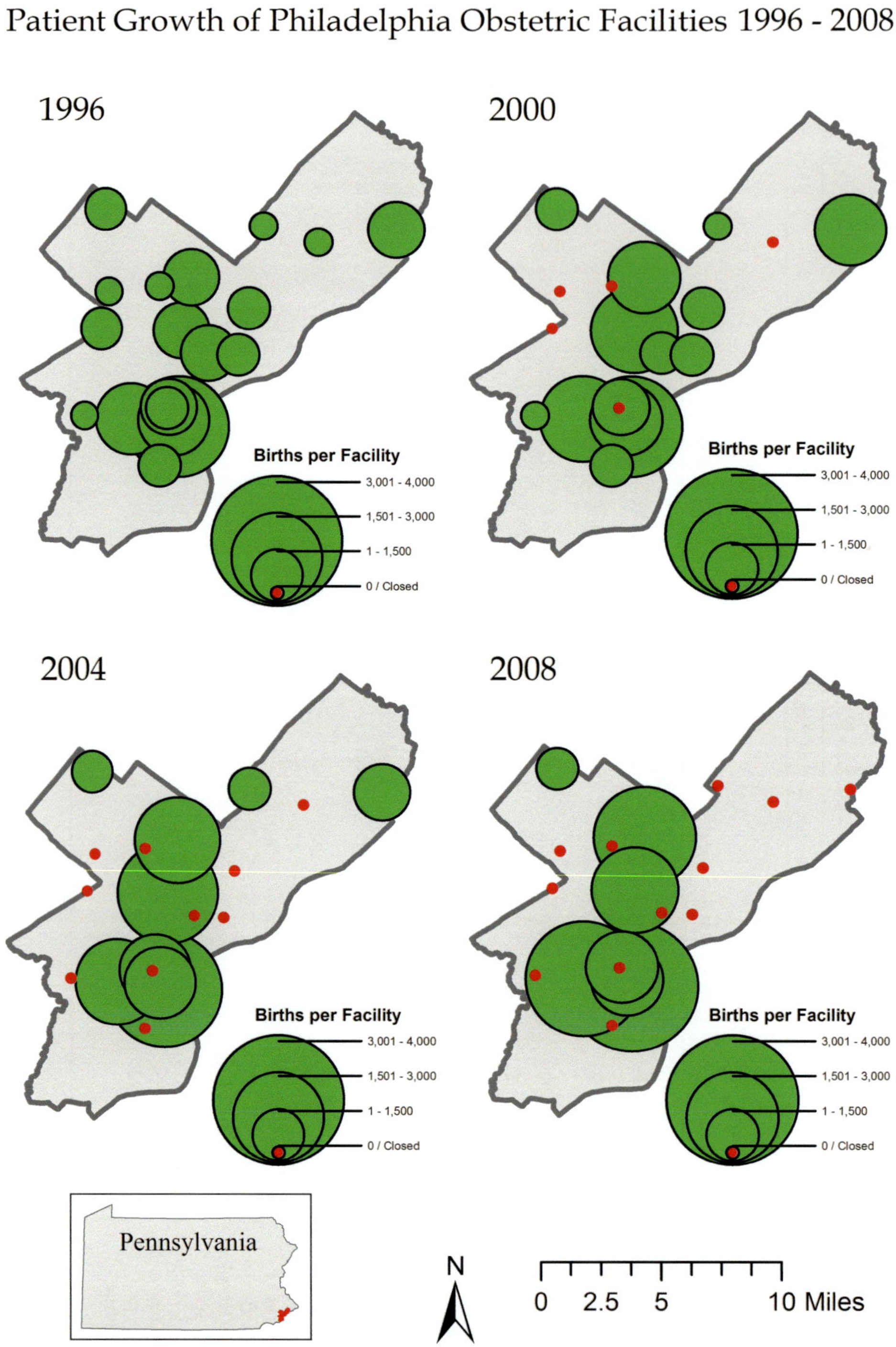

FIGURE 4 Philadelphia maternity ward facilities: patient growth displayed as graduated circles from 1996–2008.

TABLE 5 Occupancy Rate for Philadelphia Hospitals, 2004–2005

Philadelphia Hospital	2004–2005 Occupancy Rate for OB Care, %
Hospital of the University of Pa	107.3
Temple University Hospital	99.2
Albert Einstein Hospital	95.7
Hahnemann Hospital	86.2
Pennsylvania Hospital	85.3
Thomas Jefferson Hospital	66.2
Jeanes Hospital	56.6
Northeastern Hospital	54.9
Chestnut Hill Hospital	46.1
Parkview Hospital	Closed
Methodist Hospital	Closed
Episcopal Hospital	Closed
Germantown Hospital	Closed
Roxborough Hospital	Closed
City Avenue Hospital	Closed
Mercy Hospital of Philadelphia	Closed
Medical College of Pa	Closed
Frankford Hospital	Closed
Nazareth Hospital	Closed

facility and number of birth complications in Philadelphia because there is still a relatively short distance between facilities and all census tracts (the maximum mean Euclidian distance from any tract to a health facility is 4.62 miles). Travel distance is most likely not a discouraging factor in access to prenatal care services. However, if this study had been done in a rural area that was experiencing diminishing obstetric services and the distance to a facility increased drastically for residents, it would be possible that access and utilization of prenatal and preventive care services would decrease.

Recommendation

In consideration of the analysis and research conducted on obstetric facility closure in Philadelphia, it is imperative that a more effective method of care be instituted. The decentralization of prenatal, labor, and delivery care, support services, as well as approaching capacity issues make the future of obstetric care in Philadelphia uncertain. In order to encourage all Philadelphia women to obtain recommended prenatal services regardless of insurance status, changes in the system are needed. The establishment of three total obstetric care facilities in the city is recommended. These facilities would alleviate the burden on the large hospitals by serving all needs of insured and uninsured pregnant women, including prenatal checkups; complication screenings; women, infants, and children allocation; labor and delivery; and well-baby appointments. The establishment of these facilities would eliminate the need for pregnant women to visit several different facilities many times during and after their pregnancy. The location of these facilities was determined by the geographical areas containing the most underserved, demonstrating the most need for care, and being at the greatest risk for birth complications. Negative birth outcomes can often be correlated with social inequalities in neighborhoods that can lead to unusually high rates (Culhane and Elo 2005). It is vital to insure that these vulnerable areas are properly served. Figure 5 depicts fulfillment of these criteria. Each recommended location fulfills the following criteria: (1) more than 1.5 Euclidian miles from one of the six remaining obstetric facilities, (2) has a birth density (2008 totals) of more than 300 births per square mile, and (3) more than 15% of births are at high risk (either low birth weight or preterm). Figure 6 demonstrates areas that fulfill the above criteria and are suitable for the development of a total care facility. Adopting this recommendation for new total care facilities will help effectively serve the city, encourage better care practices, and alleviate the stress on current facilities. It is possible to alleviate the maternity care crisis as well as lower the high rates of negative birth outcomes for Philadelphia mothers. Informed decision making and new policies are desperately needed in the city. GIS methods can contribute to an informed and effective process of decision making for maternity care in Philadelphia.

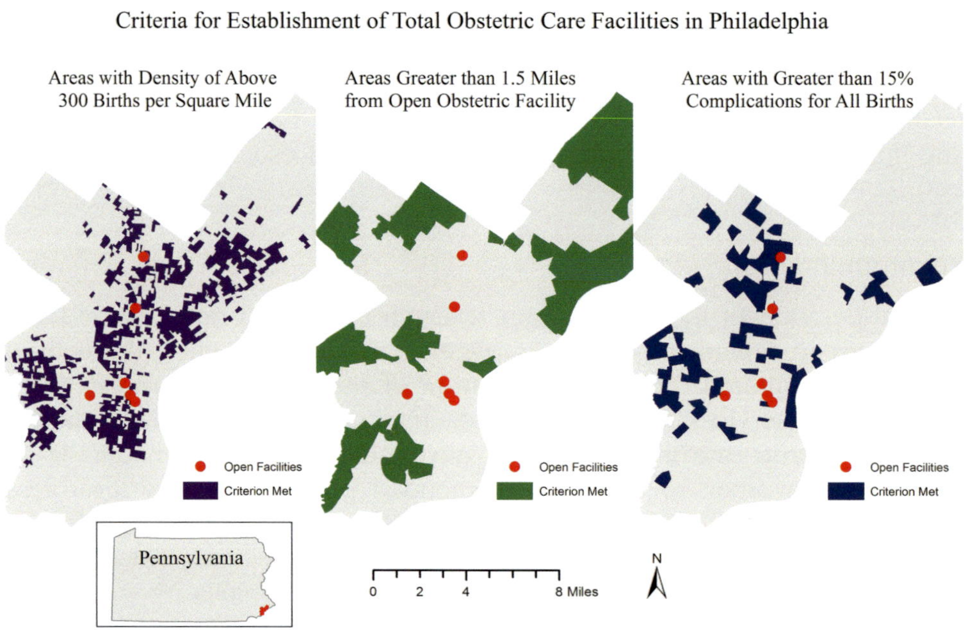

FIGURE 5 Geographical areas indicating fulfillment of each criteria for establishment of total obstetric care facilities in Philadelphia.

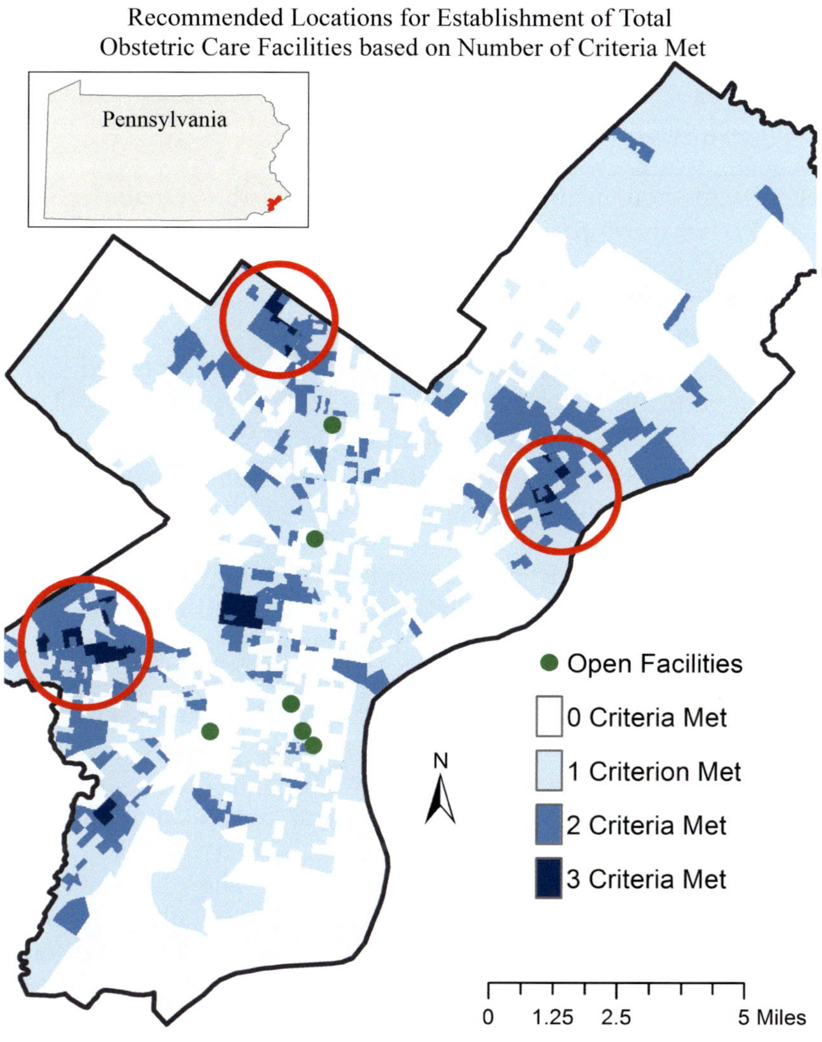

FIGURE 6 Geographical areas that fulfill all criteria and are suitable for development of total care facilities.

CONCLUSIONS

The results of this analysis indicate that access to care has diminished in the past decade due to numerous facility closures. The mean Euclidean distance traveled for Philadelphia residents visiting Philadelphia facilities has increased from 2.80 to 3.24 miles. This, however, is not a significant increase in distance—only .44 miles. The most pressing concern is the issue of approaching capacity facing Philadelphia hospitals. With five Philadelphia facilities estimated to be operating beyond recommended capacity, the potential for problems in the future is likely, especially if there is a large increase in the city's birth rate. If this system of care does not improve, it is possible that the rate of birth complications in the city will rise, which could exacerbate the capacity issue in Philadelphia. Lastly, the recent steep rise in unemployment[9] has caused a decrease in private insurance coverage for Philadelphia residents. The cost per patient of a normal vaginal delivery in the Philadelphia area is estimated at $8,728 and, for a cesarean, $12,175. Patients with private health insurance can expect to pay only 5%–7% out of pocket, with their insurance company paying the remainder (March of Dimes 2007). For those patients without insurance or with insufficient insurance, the out-of-pocket expense can be much higher. Facilities not receiving the total billed amounts for uninsured patients might result in their losing the revenue required to sustain their services.

There are certain limitations to this study which prevented a complete analysis. The geocoded dataset used did not have a complete set of attributes available, including age, race, birth outcome, and insurance or income status. It would be illuminating to repeat some procedures of this study with a detailed dataset. As mentioned previously, it would be beneficial to calculate travel distance using available routes as opposed to Euclidian distance. This would create more realistic estimates of travel time. Also in the future, it would be helpful to expand the dataset to include all regional births at all regional hospitals, facilitating accurately calculating the absorption rates of regional facilities. Also, this study would be enriched if the data included 2009 birth records to further illustrate the current situation. Finally, current information about negative birth outcomes would be helpful in elaborating on the postclosure situation in Philadelphia.

A comprehensive adoption of geospatial analytical methods among health professionals is not yet a reality in the industry. Barriers remain that prevent the more widespread utilization of GIS. The availability of easily accessible, accurate, and current data sources leaves much to be desired among health professionals. Data, subject to human error, are often incomplete or riddled with inaccuracies. Furthermore, software literacy and the prohibitive cost of software licensing further negatively affect the utilization of geospatial tools.

Two key initiatives would increase the adoption of these resources: encouraging the use of GIS methods for students in health care education and increasing the availability of easy-to-use, open-source or Internet-based software applications. This would help instill the importance and functionality of these methods early on in a health care career as well as make geospatial methods a ubiquitous tool among health professionals. The adoption of these tools can inform decision making and support the most effective and equitable allocation of care.

NOTES

1. http://www.spatialecology.com/gme/
2. http://factfinder.census.gov/home/saff/aff_transition.html
3. These data are not available in the geocoded birth dataset used for this study. The figures for this table are derived from the report by Jennifer Kolker, 2007.

4. Any birth with less than 37 weeks of gestation time is considered a preterm birth. Any birth weight measuring less than 2,500 grams is considered a low birth weight.

5. 1996 births of Philadelphia residents: 22,524. 2008 Births of Philadelphia residents: 23,559.

6. There was a loss of 214 medical professional jobs at Philadelphia hospitals between 1996 and 2005.

7. Number of hospital births multiplied by 2.9 projected maternity days. Projected maternity days/365 = average daily census.

8. 75% occupancy is recommended by American College of Obstetrics and Gynecology.

9. Current unemployment rate as recorded in February 2010 was 11.4%, up from 6.6% in February 2007, according to the U.S. Bureau of Labor Statistics.

REFERENCES

Bosanquet, N., J. Ferry, C. Lees, and J. Thornton. 2005. *Maternity Services in the NHS*. London: Reform.

Culhane, J. F., and I. T. Elo. 2005. Neighborhood context and reproductive health. *American Journal of Obstetrics and Gynecology* 192(5 Suppl): S22–S29.

Esri. 2011. *ArcGIS: A Complete Integrated System*. Available at http://www.esri.com/software/arcgis/

———. 2011. *Data Types and Models*. Available at http://www.gis.com/content/data-types-and-models.

Fondren, L. K., and T. C. Ricketts. 1991. *North Carolina Obstetrics Access and Professional Liability Study Research Summary*. Chapel Hill: University of North Carolina.

Hempel, S. 2006. *The Medical Detective: John Snow and the Mystery of Cholera*. London: Granta Books.

Higgs, G. 2004. A literature review of the use of GIS-based measures of access to health care services. *Health Services and Outcomes Research Methodology* 5(2): 119–139.

Higgs, G. 2009. The role of GIS for health utilization studies: literature review. *Health Services and Outcomes Research Methodology* 9(2): 84–99.

Kolker, J. 2007. *Obstetric Care for Philadelphia Residents*. Philadelphia: Drexel University.

Kruse, J., D. Phillips, and R. M. Wesley. 1989. Factors influencing changes in obstetric care provided by family physicians: A national study. *Journal of Family Practice* 28(5): 597–602.

March of Dimes. 2007. *March of Dimes Study Unveils New Data on Cost of Having a Baby*. Washington, DC: March of Dimes.

McLafferty, S. L. 2003. GIS and health care. *Annual Review of Public Health* 24:25–42.

Nesbitt, T. S., J. E. Scherger, and J. L. Tanji. 2008. The impact of obstetrical liability on access to perinatal care in the rural United States. *Journal of Rural Health* 5(4): 321–335.

Pilkington, H., B. Blondel, M. Carayol, G. Breart, and J. Zeitlin. 2008. Impact of maternity unit closures on access to obstetrical care: The French experience between 1998 and 2003. *Journal of Social Science and Medicine* 67(10): 1521–1529.

Sontheimer, D., L. W. Halverson, L. Bell, M. Ellis, and P. W. Bunting. 2008. Impact of discontinued obstetrical services in rural Missouri: 1990–2002. *Journal of Rural Health* 24(1): 96–98.

University of Texas. 2004. *Working with 2000 Census Data in ArcGIS*. Available at http://soa.utexas.edu/crp/gis/arcgis_tips/census2000/index.html

Role of Race and Ethnicity Predictive Modeling and Spatial Analysis in Addressing Health Disparities

ZACHARY D. VERNON
WellPoint, Inc., Roanoke, VA, USA

GRACE H. TING
WellPoint, Inc., Thousand Oaks, CA, USA

Health disparities are variations in quality or clinical outcomes of care, and they represent a major source of inefficiency within the U.S. health care system. Key strategies in addressing this challenge are developing data on the racial and ethnic demographics of patient populations and determining how best to allocate health plan resources to address disparities. This article examines the use of mapping tools and spatial analysis in the identification of health disparities among health insurance plan members (health plan members). The article also briefly explores the usage of indirect methodologies to determine a health plan member's race and ethnicity. In addition, case studies are examined to illustrate the role of mapping and spatial tools in the development of quality improvement interventions.

THE PREVALENCE OF HEALTH DISPARITIES

In 2002, the Institute of Medicine published *Unequal Treatment: Confronting Racial and Ethnic Disparities in Health Care*, a landmark report that concluded that racial and ethnic minorities receive lower-quality health care than whites, even when they have a similar age, a similar income level, and the same access to health coverage and care. Health services research has long revealed that race and ethnicity have been associated with variations in the quality of care (Smedley et al. 2003). These differences, called *health care disparities*, are pervasive and negatively affecting health care for minorities across many health-related domains: access to physicians and health care, receipt of evidence-based clinical treatment, health outcomes, mortality, and quality of life.

Extensive research has established that racial and ethnic minorities in the United States are in poorer health, suffer worse health outcomes, and have higher morbidity and mortality rates than their white counterparts (Institute of Medicine 2002).

Diabetes, growing at near-epidemic proportions, is a well-documented area of health disparities. According to recent estimates, the prevalence of diagnosed diabetes in the United States is projected to more than double from 2005 to 2050, from 5.62% of the population to 12.00%, to reach 48.3 million people with diagnosed diabetes by 2050 (Narayan et al. 2006). The same study forecasts that increases in the number of individuals with diabetes will be largest for minority groups; between 2005 and 2050, the number is projected to increase 481% among Hispanics, 208% among blacks, and 113% among whites. The age-race/ethnicity group with the largest increase, at 606%, will be for black seniors over 75 years of age (Narayan et al. 2006).

Studies have shown that African Americans are 1.4 to 2.2 times more likely to suffer from diabetes than whites. Overall, 10.8% of African Americans have diabetes compared with only 6.2% of whites (Mokdad 2000). Hispanics are 1.5 times as likely to have diabetes as whites. In addition, 2006 data showed that Hispanics had a 50% higher death rate from diabetes than whites (CDC 2009).

Cancer, the second leading cause of death in the United States, is another category of disease that has been closely linked to health disparities and health care disparities. The National Cancer Institute analyses of cancer incidence and death statistics reveal that certain groups in the United States suffer disproportionately from cancer and its associated effects, including premature death. African Americans/blacks, Asian Americans, Hispanic/Latinos, American Indians, Alaska Natives, and underserved whites are more likely than the general population to have higher incidence and death statistics for certain types of cancer (National Cancer Institute 2008).

For African-American women, even though they are diagnosed 10% less frequently for breast cancer than whites (CDC 2010), they are 36% more likely to die from the disease (NCI 2010). Disparities that may increase the risk of mortality in African American women include a later disease stage at diagnosis (Bach 2002) and a higher prevalence of comorbid conditions compared with white women (Tammemagi 2005). Similarly, Hispanics are more likely than whites to be diagnosed with breast and melanoma cancers at a later stage when the cancers are more difficult to treat and have spread to other organs (American Cancer Society 2009; Short et al. 2010).

Although the loss of lives due to health care disparities creates a moral imperative to address health equity policies, there are economic reasons for closing the health disparities gaps as well. Timothy Waldmann of the Urban Institute used data from the federal Medical Expenditure Panel Survey to project the financial impact of disparities. In 2009 alone, the study estimated that disparities cost the U.S. health care system $23.9 billion. Looking only at diabetes, hypertension, stroke and renal disease, and poor general health, disparities were responsible for costing private health insurers $5.1 billion in additional costs and $7.3 billion in additional health care costs for the Medicare program in 2009. Expectations are that these costs will more than double over the next 40 years as minorities become even larger segments of the overall population, and failure to reduce the incidence of these costly chronic diseases will result in higher excess costs to the public and private insurance sectors in the years to come (Waldmann 2009).

Another 2009 study out of Johns Hopkins School of Public Health found that more than 30.6% of direct medical expenditures by African Americans, Asians, and Hispanics in the United States were excess costs due to health inequalities, which cost the United States economy $229.4 billion over the four-year period between 2003 and 2006. Furthermore, the combined cost of these direct expenditures and the indirect cost of health disparities, such as lost productivity due to disability, illness, and absenteeism, was $1.24 trillion in 2008 inflation-adjusted dollars over the same time period (LaVeist et al. 2009).

The prevalence and persistence of health disparities have seen increased funding commitment and policy changes by the federal government to promote equitable health care and access to traditionally underserved minority populations. In April 2011, the U.S. Department of Health and Human Services (HHS) launched two strategic plans aimed at reducing health disparities: the HHS Action Plan to Reduce Racial and Ethnic Health Disparities outlines goals and actions HHS will take to reduce health disparities among racial and ethnic minorities, and the National Stakeholder Strategy for Achieving Health Equity, a common set of goals and objectives for public and private sector initiatives and partnerships to help racial and ethnic minorities and other underserved groups reach their full health potential. In addition, HHS's Healthy People 2020 has a renewed focus on identifying, measuring, tracking, and reducing health disparities through strategies that would address the social, environmental, and economic conditions that shape a population's health.

Reducing health care disparities and improving individual health for people of all ethnicities are key priorities for WellPoint, Inc. (WellPoint), the nation's leading health benefits company by membership, operating health insurance plans (health plans) in California, Colorado, Georgia, Virginia, Nevada, New York, Connecticut, New Hampshire, Maine, Indiana, Ohio,

Kentucky, Missouri, and Wisconsin. WellPoint health plans serve more than 33 million members; one in nine Americans carry some form of insurance products offered by a WellPoint affiliate company.

WellPoint has long recognized the negative health outcomes and increased medical interventions needed by patient populations that experience health disparities, and it proactively reviews administrative clinical health care quality measures to detect significant health care disparities trends among its affiliated health plan members and the communities served by those plans. Given limited resources, strategies to increase the access and quality of health care must be efficient and effective. When opportunities to address specific clinical health care disparities are identified, geospatial analyses are applied to geographic markets with the highest density of members and health care disparities to locate the most underserved micromarkets for member health education outreach or collaboration with local health authorities and community partners to promote mutual health care priorities.

DATA COLLECTION AND MODEL DEVELOPMENT

To effectively address racial and ethnic health disparities, a requisite first step is the collection of race and ethnicity data of the populations being studied. As reported by a number of studies and advisory groups, patient self-reported race, ethnicity, and language preference data represent the gold standard in building data sets to address health disparities (Fremont et al. 2005). Unfortunately, many health plans have been slow to collect patient self-reported data due to the high costs of technological system enhancements and data warehouse capabilities required to accommodate the collection and storage of these preferred or essential data attributes. Another major impediment is the hesitance among plans about potential legal and public relations issues related to asking members to provide their race and ethnicity data, even when such information is provided voluntarily. Currently, no state or federal laws prohibit the collection of this data after a person has become a health plan member, but a number of states, including California and Massachusetts, have laws limiting the amount of information that can be collected by a health plan at enrollment. In addition, internally, health plans often are concerned that asking for voluntary self-reported data will raise questions with potential stakeholders about the plans' intended use of the data (Bierman et al. 2002). Due to constant membership turnover and unwillingness of skeptical members to provide this data, health plans have not been able to collect this voluntary information on all members. In fact, it is probable that a large portion of members who choose not to voluntarily disclose their race or ethnicity are minority members who are the most underserved by traditional health care services and experience the greatest burdens imposed by health disparities. These problems bring focus to the need of health plans to overcome these barriers to better identify and prioritize patterns of disparities for strategic, targeted development of educational programs and interventions.

To overcome the gaps inherent with self-reported race and ethnicity data collection, health plans have turned to a number of indirect or predictive data models. Many of these methods rely heavily on data sets created by the U.S. Census. One of the most basic methods is the use of geocoding (Fremont et al. 2005), which relies on using residential addresses to determine spatial location. From this determination, the location can be linked to a census block group, of which the typical size is between 600 and 3,000 people with an optimal size of 1,500 (U.S. Census Bureau 2001). After determining an individual's census block, census data can be used to infer estimated demographic characteristics about an individual. For example, if a person lives in a census block group where 70% of the population is African American, then it can be inferred that a person has a 70% chance of being African American. Similar logic can be applied to a large spectrum of data including gender mix, age mix, and household size. Additional information can be gained by moving up a level to the census tract level data. Census tracts typically range in size from 1,500 to 8,000 people, with an optimal size of 4,000 (U.S. Census Bureau 2001), which remains small enough to give reasonable insight into community demographics. By examining census tract level data, additional fields become available including data on socioeconomic status, language preference, ancestry, and education. All these data can be very useful in examining the social determinants of health disparities. One very useful element of the application of geocoding and census data is that very little known data about a particular health plan member is required to derive estimated demographics about this member. In reality, the single necessary data element is residential address for this methodology. However, the application of geocoding and census data is not without limitations. In cases where populations are not fairly homogeneous, group mix can make demographic determinations difficult. Although more useful among locations with fairly homogeneous populations, for example, Chinatown or Little Italy in New York City, this methodology loses some of its usefulness in areas with a more diverse population. As found in previous research, the use of geocoding to infer race is most effective when used for African Americans as historically many members of this population have lived in more segregated neighborhoods. This type of inference is less effective for Hispanics and Asians, as neighborhoods where these populations tend to live often contain a more diverse racial and ethnic mix (Massey and Denton 1989). In rural areas, census block groups and tracts tend to be larger in order to reach the intended population sizes. As a result, whereas an urban block group might comprise a single city block, a rural block group may stretch over miles and across different communities. This can result in some loss of focus on particular groups. Finally, geocoding and census data alone rely on the assumption that a health plan's population is similar to the observed population of the community. This may not always be a valid assumption, as typical health plans' membership draws more from the white population and not as strongly from racially or ethnically diverse groups.

An alternative method of identifying a person's race and ethnicity is the use of surname data. Surnames can often provide valuable insight into a person's ancestry, hence race and ethnicity, provided a person's name can be successfully matched to a racial/ethnic surname list. Numerous surname lists have been developed (Falkenstein 2002; Lauderdale and Kestenbaum 2000; Word and Perkins 1996). Most of these lists focus on Hispanic or Asian surnames. The Asian lists in particular have provided useful, more detailed granularity for various ethnicities within the Asian race category. One major problem with these lists is in regard to African Americans who often have very similar or identical names as whites. An advancement in the use of surnames was a list released that provided demographics for all surnames appearing in the 2000 Decennial Census more than 100 times (Word et al. 2000). This new surname list consolidates into one master list the multiple races previously found in separate race and ethnicity lists, such as Perkins and Word or Falkenstein, that are lists specific to one race or ethnicity. This is most important in the case of names such as Lee that exist across several different races and ethnicities. In addition, this list did provide some insight into the surnames of African Americans. Though helpful in estimating race and ethnicity, surnames lists alone lack the additional demographic understandings provided by the census data linked to geocoding data. In addition, even with the improved Census 2000 lists, African-American surname analysis still yields limited success in estimating a person's race for the reasons stated above.

A number of hybrid methodologies have been developed to overcome the shortcomings of using geocoded data or surname data. One of the first hybrids used surname data to identify Hispanics and Asians, and then used geocoding to identify the persons not matched by surname as African American or white. This method proved to have had some success at identifying race and ethnicity (Fiscella and Fremont 2006). In order to increase accuracy rates, another methodology was proposed that employed Bayesian statistics to combine prior probabilities calculated from surname lists with geocoded probabilities. This methodology showed an increased level of accuracy by reducing the weighted average overall deviation from self-reported data from 6.2% for the previous hybrid method to 1.6% for the Bayesian hybrid (Elliott et al. 2008).

WellPoint has developed its own predictive methodology that combines the probabilities from surname lists with the probabilities from geocoded census data using logistical regressions. In the WellPoint model, the output for each individual is a probability of being white, a probability of being Asian, a probability of being Hispanic, and a probability of being African American;

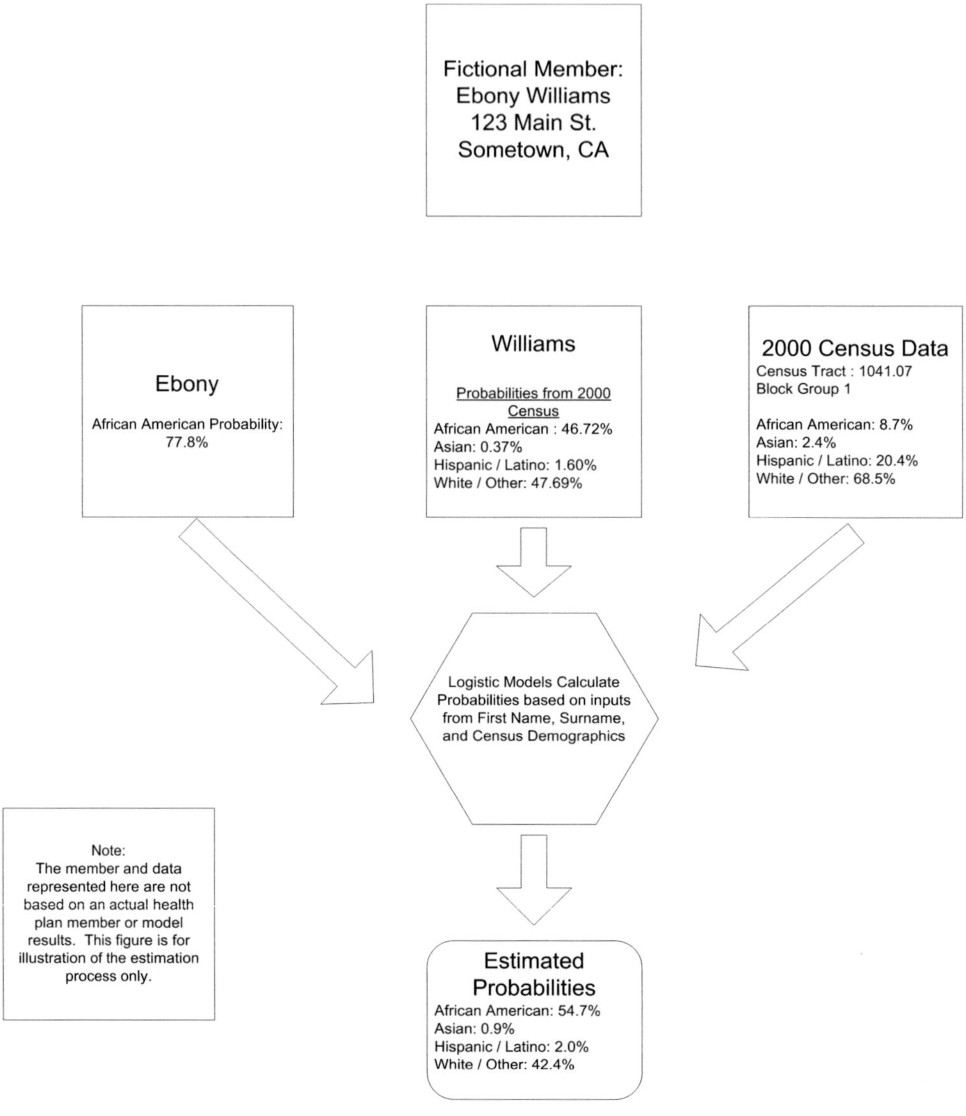

FIGURE 1 The WellPoint model uses logistic regressions to combine census data, surname data, and first name data into probabilities that a person is Asian, African American, Hispanic/Latino, or white/other. Probabilities are predicted at a member level and then combined to the appropriate 'aggregate level. *Source:* Internal WellPoint Analysis.

these probabilities sum to one (Figure 1). To examine the demographics of a particular geographic region, the probabilities for the individuals identified in that region are summed to yield aggregate demographics for that group. This methodology proved to be highly accurate, particularly when looking at aggregate groups such as state, region, county, zip code, or block group. Within test data, this methodology predicted the demographic mix within

Comparison of Aggregate Predictions

Approach N = 192,096	Hispanic (%)	Asian (%)	African American (%)	White / Other (%)
Surname	46.1	6.6	7.1	40.2
Geocoding	41.3	7.9	11.9	39.0
WellPoint Model	52.1	7.9	14.7	24.3
Self-Reported	52.0	8.0	14.8	25.2

FIGURE 2 Predictions from the WellPoint model are within 0.1% of the self-reported demographics. *Source:* Internal WellPoint Analysis 2008.

0.1% of the actual mix (Figure 2). By developing an internal proprietary model, WellPoint is able to more quickly implement updated and new data.

In addition, when used to determine the race and ethnicity at an individual level, overall imputed race and ethnicity were found to be correctly assigned for 86% of the test population and for members whose probability of being a particular race and ethnicity was greater than 80%, imputed individual race and ethnicity was found to be correctly assigned for more than 90% of the identified individuals (Figure 3).

As recommended in previous research by McCaffrey and Elliott, the most effective use of this data is not through determining one race for each individual, but rather in the usage of the probabilities. These probabilities can be effectively included in regressions, yielding a better overall result than using a single race, because the probabilities more effectively take into account the differences seen between members of the population who may have very different probabilities (McCaffrey and Elliott 2007). For example, the outcomes for persons with a 55% probability of belonging to a particular race and ethnicity may be different than the outcomes for persons with a 90% probability of belonging to the same group. Traditional binomial predictions would not account for this difference, as both sets of individuals would simply be shown as being in the same race and ethnic category.

The logical next step to effectively address racial and ethnic health disparities within a health plan setting is to determine how to apply imputed race/ethnicity data in the design of relevant services and products that will best serve the needs of its diverse membership.

In traditional programs designed to increase access to health care services, the standard approach has been to identify needs and then develop generic strategies that had not been culturally tailored to address them. There are certain implementation efficiencies with this practice, but given that health disparities continue to exist among racially and ethnically diverse members, new approaches were needed. Given limited resources, emphasis was placed on determining optimal capital and staff allocations to effectively address health disparities. Moreover, because members had already been

Comparison of Individual Predictions

Sensitivity

Approach N = 192,096	Hispanic	Asian	African American	White / Other
Surname	94.0	68.0	12.2	94.0
Geocoding	68.8	23.6	30.1	82.5
WellPoint Model	93.6	72.0	75.0	82.3

Specificity

Approach N = 192,096	Hispanic	Asian	African American	White / Other
Surname	81.2	99.4	99.5	79.3
Geocoding	77.0	98.1	96.3	71.7
WellPoint Model	92.6	99.3	96.3	91.4

Accuracy

Approach N = 192,096	All Members Accuracy Rate	Over 80% Accuracy Rate	Over 80% Member Count
Surname	74.5%	90.8%	130,150
Geocoding	62.9%	84.4%	54,092
WellPoint Model	86,2%	93.8%	145,009

FIGURE 3 The WellPoint model is much more accurate than Surname or Geocoding alone. By limiting imputed estimations to members with probabilities greater than 80%, overall accuracy is greater than 93.8%, and 145,009 out of 192,096 members are estimated. *Source:* Internal WellPoint Analysis 2008.

geocoded and linked to census data, the use of mapping and spatial tools represented a set of analysis tools worth exploring to identify populations and geographies in which quality improvement programs might have the most impact.

Initial attempts at disparities analysis focused on traditional analysis tools. Members were linked to states, regions, zip codes, and other segments. These groups were then tallied and compared across the population. Figure 4 illustrates how the screening rates of the four major race and ethnicity groups as derived by the indirect logistic model are compared across California for a single quality indicator measure, colorectal screening rate. Lower rates of screening received compared with whites were observed for diverse racial and ethnic groups across all regions of California, with Hispanics receiving the lowest rate of recommended colorectal screening. Rates with statistically significant differences from the white comparison group are indicated by black trend arrows (Figure 4).

One limitation in examining testing rates alone is the potential association of low rates and regions with low populations. In order to mitigate this

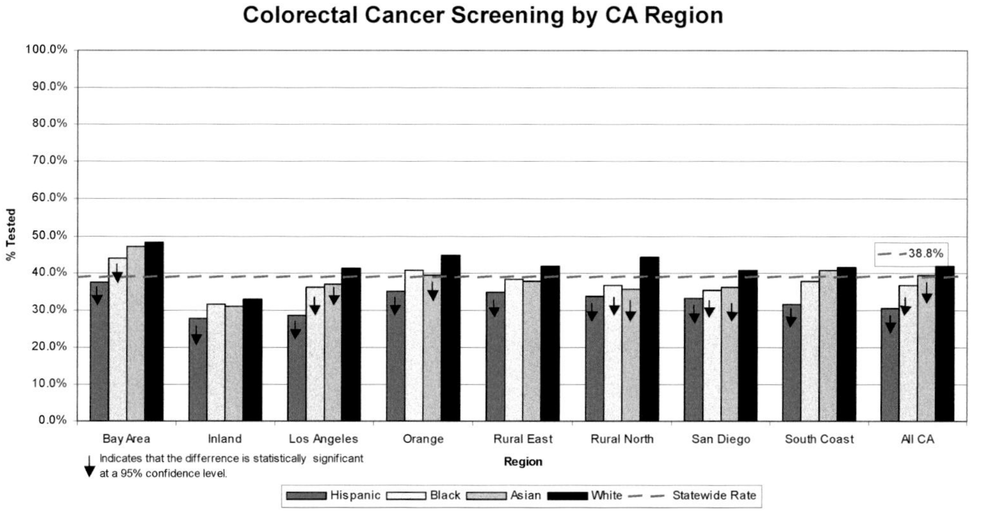

FIGURE 4 Nonwhite groups exhibit lower testing rates in all market regions. The Inland Empire has the lowest rates for all races, with a significant disparity between the Hispanic and white rate. *Source:* WellPoint data 10/07–9/08.

risk, a population-based chart was developed that related unscreened counts to the overall population (Figure 5).

Heath disparities analytic graphs like Figure 5 can provide a comprehensive view of the rate of interest for administrative region by race, as well as a distribution of the population across the state. Each stacked bar represents the total number of eligible members within a racial/ethnic group and a particular administrative region, of which the hashed portion of each bar represents members who have been screened within that group and region. The total screening rate appears above each bar. The obvious disparity is the higher screening rates among whites.

Figure 5 also presents data on population density and the absolute number of diverse members who had not received screening to support business planning decisions in allocation of budget for geographic or community-based quality interventions. For example, an area such as California Rural North has a significant disparity in colorectal screenings, but the overall minority population for that region is so small that it would probably not be the first choice for a planned intervention (Figure 6).

At the same time, the Inland Empire demonstrates not only low screening rates but large racially and ethnically diverse populations with significant disparities. Based on a population chart, the Inland Empire would therefore likely be a better candidate for community-based quality improvement interventions. At the same time, it was clear that a single number for a large region or county was not indicative of all of the communities based within that geographic area. For example, Los Angeles County has a large number

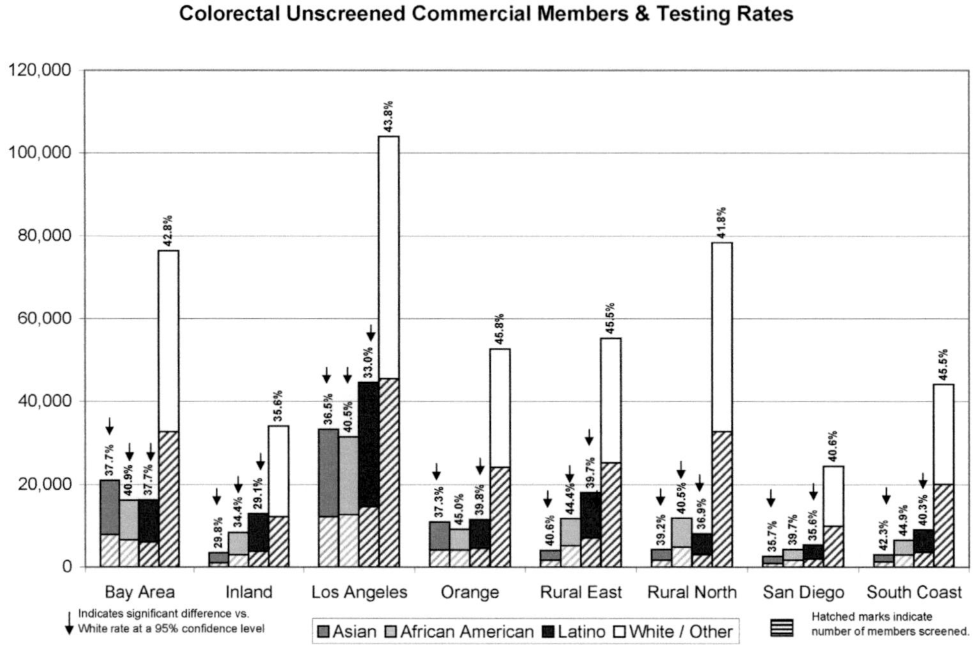

FIGURE 5 By looking at screened member counts instead of rates alone, interventions can be targeted to communities with the highest number of unscreened members or with the lowest proportion of screened members. This allows the development of interventions to target either the largest number of members or the populations with the most proportional need. *Source:* WellPoint data 10/07–9/08.

of members affiliated with the California-based WellPoint affiliate health plan. Los Angeles County has more than 10 million residents, covers 4,083 square miles, and contains 88 incorporated cities. More than half of these residents speak a language other than English at home and do not classify themselves as white. The county is home to traditionally very wealthy communities such as Malibu and Beverly Hills, as well as traditionally impoverished neighborhoods such as Compton and Crenshaw. With such vast diversity in one geographic region, a single measure could not capture the experience that reflects all its different residents. In a number of presentations and articles, Allen Fremont, MD, PhD, a natural scientist specializing in health care disparities at the RAND Corporation, and his colleagues at RAND had suggested using geographic information system (GIS) tools to map areas where measures fell below the expected performance (Lurie et al. 2008; Fremont 2007). In using this approach, key areas, (hot spots) could be identified. Once these hot spots were identified, targeted community-based approaches could be used to plan health plan interventions. Layering demographic information over the hot spot data, it became clear that many of these hot spots were also areas that contained demographically diverse populations. Health care quality improvement interventions could thus be tailored to meet the needs

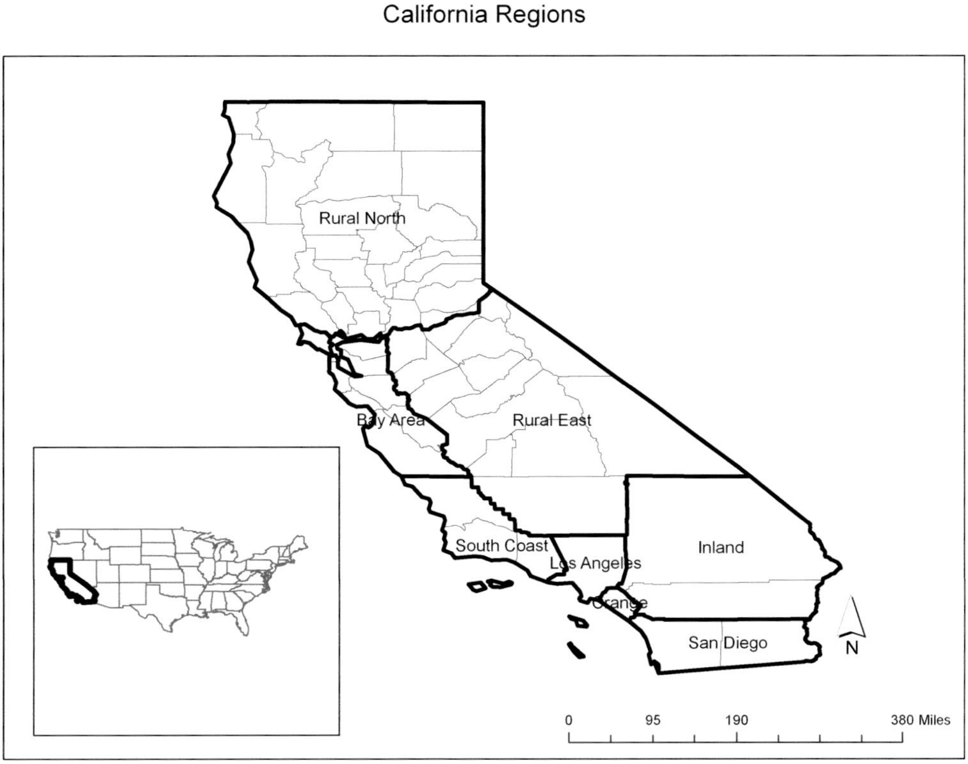

FIGURE 6 For business purposes, WellPoint focuses on eight different regions within the state of California. *Source:* Internal WellPoint data.

and culture of the target areas. If a particular neighborhood was identified as being predominantly Hispanic, programs could be tailored to match Hispanic cultural elements. For example, a diabetes health program might include recipe guides reflecting diverse Hispanic palates or communications tools such as *fotonovelas* might be distributed. If a community was identified as African American, then a separate set of culturally tailored tools might be deployed to better meet the needs of that group. The appropriate use of culturally tailored interventions can help health plans move beyond merely providing accurate information to members to focus on informing them in a manner better suited to their situation, lifestyle, and experience.

USE OF GEOSPATIAL ANALYSIS TO ADDRESS HEALTH DISPARITIES

The application of GIS in geospatial analytic methods is increasingly being used to aggregate and evaluate health-related data. Several definitions exist for the GIS (NBDPN 2004). The Healthy People 2010 guidelines from the

U.S. Department of Health and Human Services define it as "powerful tools combining geography, data and computer mapping" (U.S. Department of Health and Human Services 2000).

A number of factors have contributed to the increased adoption of GIS. Health care organizations are increasingly using electronic health information systems, thereby increasing the availability of geocoded health data that may be imported into GIS for analysis. There has also been a significant increase in the availability of digital geographic files that contain layers of geographical information, as well as data sources for environmental and medically related drivers that might affect the health of the population. Technological improvements in GIS technology (e.g., software with increased functionality that is easier to use and programs that run on a wider range of hardware including PCs) and increased compatibility with other software suites (e.g., statistical analytic packages) have also driven the implementation of GIS methodologies among a wider audience of users (University of Iowa 1997).

GIS software today offers powerful analytic functions, data integration and layering capabilities, and improved geographic visualization options. Both public and private sectors are rapidly developing methods for integrating health and environmental data to enable faster, better, and more robust understanding of factors leading to poor health. The resulting maps are becoming important business-decision support tools for allocating scarce resources to improve population health (Esri 2010).

The types of organizations adopting GIS within the health care sector are varied, and they are expanding. Initially, only public health departments and public health policy and research organizations were consistently using GIS techniques for epidemiological studies. Currently, hospitals, medical centers, laboratories, health insurance organizations, and many other health care service organizations are applying the data integration capabilities of GIS to create analytical, visually compelling, and descriptive tools for business planning and decision support. These organizations, including WellPoint, have found that GIS can play an important role in determining where and when to intervene to improve quality of care, increase accessibility of service, find more cost-effective delivery modes, and preserve patient confidentiality while satisfying the needs of the research community for data accessibility (Esri 2010).

GIS can support public health as well. Most importantly, GIS displays can improve understanding by health care executives, public health officials, and government policy makers to drive better decisions and support public health priorities. For example, elimination of health disparities is one of two primary goals of Healthy People 2010 and Healthy People 2020, the preeminent U.S. public health promotion and disease prevention plan in existence today. GIS can play a significant role in that effort, helping public health practitioners identify areas of disparities and ideally helping them identify and develop solutions to address these gaps.

CASE STUDIES

At WellPoint, GIS and geospatial analyses are applied to isolate trends and geographic areas of health disparities and to develop solutions for these disparities gaps. Using mapping tools at the small-area level and spatial analysis of health outcomes of racial, ethnic, and sociodemographic subgroups, analysts can illustrate health disparities patterns and highlight opportunities for intervention. The succeeding section illustrates a few initiatives at WellPoint from the past three years wherein GIS and geospatial analyses were used to detect health care disparity patterns in diabetes and cancer screening and to develop strategies to improve the quality of health care received by patients.

African-American Mammography Screenings in Brooklyn, New York

WellPoint was approached by a community group in the New York City area to collaborate on a public health initiative to address health disparities in mammography screenings among women in the major New York City boroughs. Both organizations agreed to collaborate, but they did not have a concrete population or geography identified, nor did they have a predefined intervention plan. WellPoint led the project ideation process with a preliminary analysis of the mammography screening rates for its Medicare health plan members in New York City. Geospatial applications of the members' mammography screening rates, layered with the members' estimated race and ethnicity composition, and the health plan's contracted mammography screening centers quickly revealed potential intervention targets and health outreach ideas. Inasmuch as the community cancer awareness group had a particular interest in educational outreach to African Americans, and as Brooklyn had a large African-American population and areas of low testing rates, the project team focused on Brooklyn for layered analyses of the region's demographics and health care resources. A density map was developed to identify areas with strong concentrations of members who had not received a recommended mammography screening; that base map was overlaid with pie charts that indicated the demographic proportions of members living within those zip codes (Figure 7). On the basis of that map, it was apparent that the zip codes within Brooklyn having the lowest rates of mammography screening rates were also communities with a high concentration of African Americans.

Next, density smoothing techniques were applied to highlight concentrated incidents of African-American women not receiving the recommended mammography screening (Figure 8). The resulting map analysis clearly demonstrated that the hot spots of unscreened African Americans were in the same zip codes with low mammography screening rates, indicating that there was indeed an African-American health disparity factor driving the low

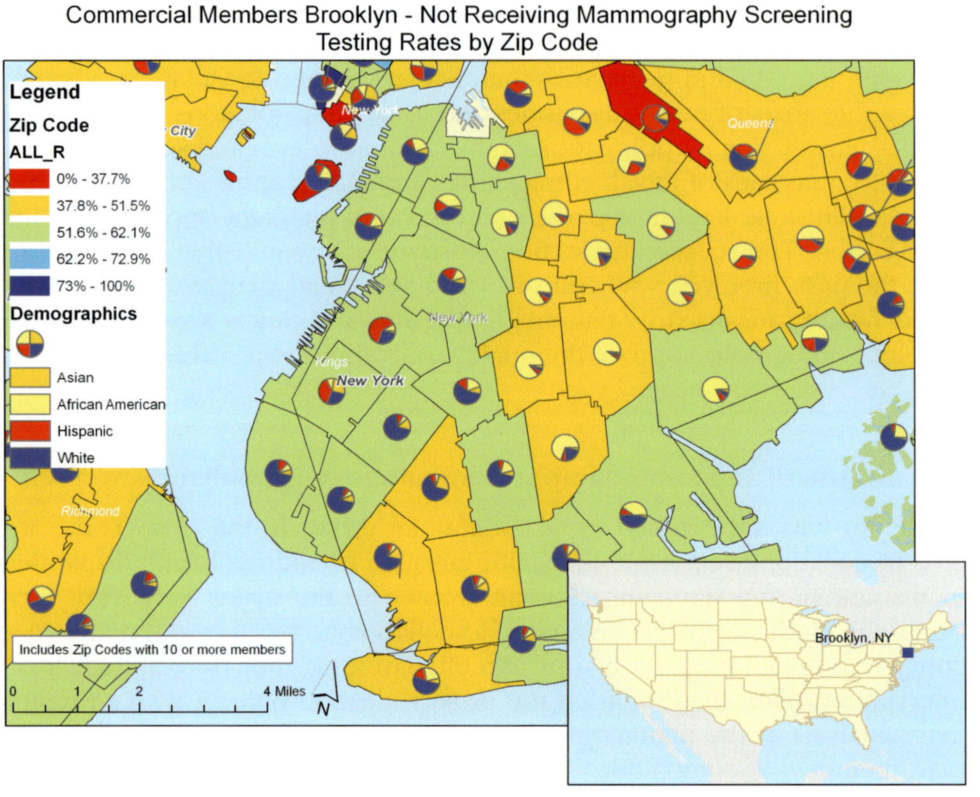

FIGURE 7 African Americans represent a higher proportion of the member population in neighborhoods with low testing rates. *Source:* WellPoint data 10/07–9/08.

mammography screening rates in the hot spot neighborhoods. The locations of contracted imaging facilities within Brooklyn hot spots were overlaid on the same map. Interestingly, this overlay revealed that the lack of screening was not due to access issues, such as insufficient provider network capacity or lengthy patient travel time, which might be alleviated with a resource-intensive intervention program such as a mobile mammography screening bus. Alternate hypotheses to the low screening rates were that African Americans have cultural barrier that influenced their lack of screenings or that a lack of culturally optimal communications meant that messaging around mammography screenings were not successfully reaching African-American members.

Based on the geospatial analyses, the collaborative organizations determined that a more effective solution would be an intervention that included outreach, education, and working with the local community hospitals and physicians serving the women in the hot spot communities.

Consequently, WellPoint and its community-based partner worked to jointly produce a continuing education symposium for primary care

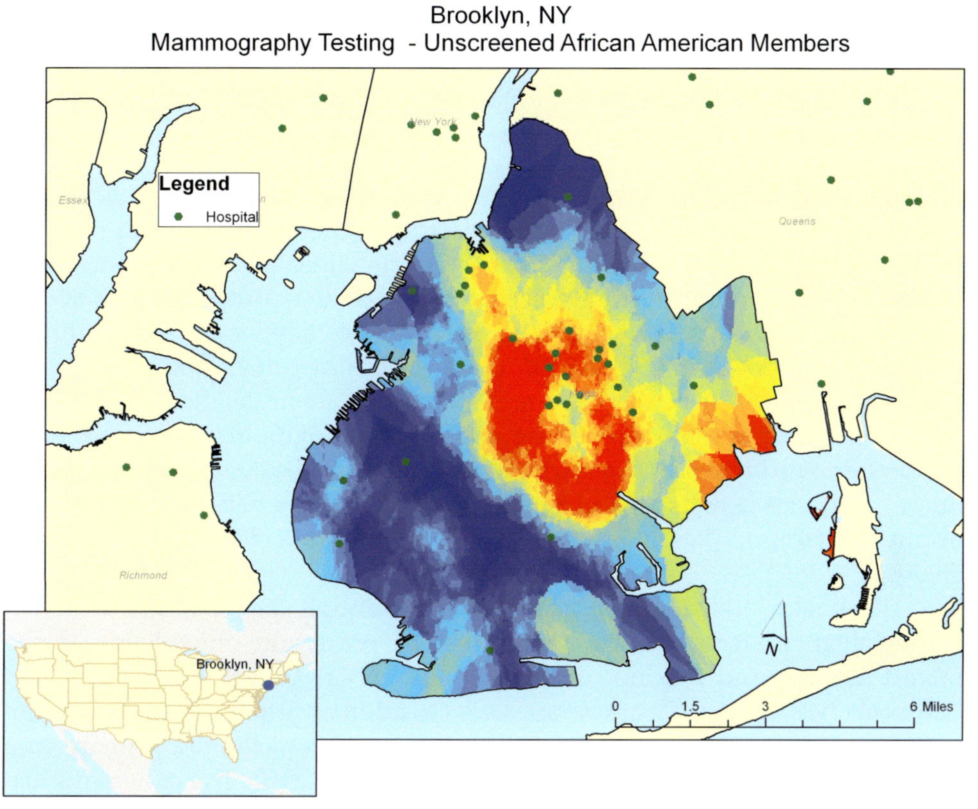

FIGURE 8 A density smoothed map shows a strong concentration of unscreened African-American members near hospitals. *Source:* WellPoint data 10/07–9/08.

physicians practicing within the Brooklyn zip codes having the highest rates of eligible women who had not received mammography screening. The symposium was conducted at a hospital located in the same neighborhood. A medical director from WellPoint's New York health plan and representatives from the community group provided detailed racial and ethnic health disparities statistics related to African-American women and highlighted the importance of early detection of breast cancer in these women. Mammography screening health care disparities data and maps were also presented to the physicians to increase the medical community's awareness of the particular needs of the patients within the impacted communities.

Taking Action Together Alliance—Southern California

Another successful application of geospatial analysis was in the design of a public health education program through a joint collaboration with a major pharmaceutical company. *Taking Action Together* is an alliance between

Merck, WellPoint, and WellPoint's affiliates, in collaboration with the American Diabetes Association (ADA) and other community partners. The purpose of the strategic alliance is to improve access to and quality of care for individuals and populations with diabetes and reduce the racial and ethnic disparities in successful self-management of Type II diabetes. The resulting education campaign was a set of community-based programs deployed within select service areas of WellPoint's affiliated California health plan.

Based on WellPoint's routine review of its clinical quality measures on recommended diabetes testing guidelines, the alliance project team selected Southern California as its intervention area. Specifically, two counties, Riverside and San Bernardino, located due east of Los Angeles County, are home to a large number of health plan members; these counties had traditionally struggled with low diabetes testing rates for hemoglobin A1c, low-density lipoprotein, and microalbuminuria. In addition, the Los Angeles and Inland Empire counties (Riverside and San Bernardino) have a very racially and ethnically diverse population, as confirmed by previous WellPoint demographic analyses.

The health education program offered through the Taking Action Together alliance targets all diabetic adults 18 years and older living in the Inland Empire, and it is not restricted to members of WellPoint's affiliated California health plan. The program seeks to address disparities in health care at the community level by removing access barriers to limited primary care physicians (PCPs) and certified diabetes educators (CDE). The program's diabetes health education ADA "conversation map" sessions provide a venue for enhanced in-person educational interaction and dialog between participants and CDEs. All activities and resources are provided at no cost to participants, and the program specifically addresses disparities due to cultural differences and language needs through provision of culturally-relevant resources and materials offered by bilingual, Spanish-speaking CDEs.

Given the size of the region, a primary question was how to best focus the intervention efforts. By mapping the location of members who have not received the recommended diabetes tests, identified hot spots allow prioritization of target communities with the greatest health care needs. Initially, unscreened members were mapped by zip codes, which were color coded to identify areas with the lowest testing rates and highest unscreened populations (Figure 9). To highlight hot spots more prominently, the data were converted to density maps (Figure 10). These density maps were raster rather than vector based, which provided smoothing and allowed distance between population concentrations to become more evident. One key area readily identified as a targeted intervention community within the Inland Empire was near Palm Springs, which has a large Hispanic population. The map analyses ensured that when the CDEs were scheduled for activities in the Palm Springs community, bilingual CDEs were on hand to facilitate the

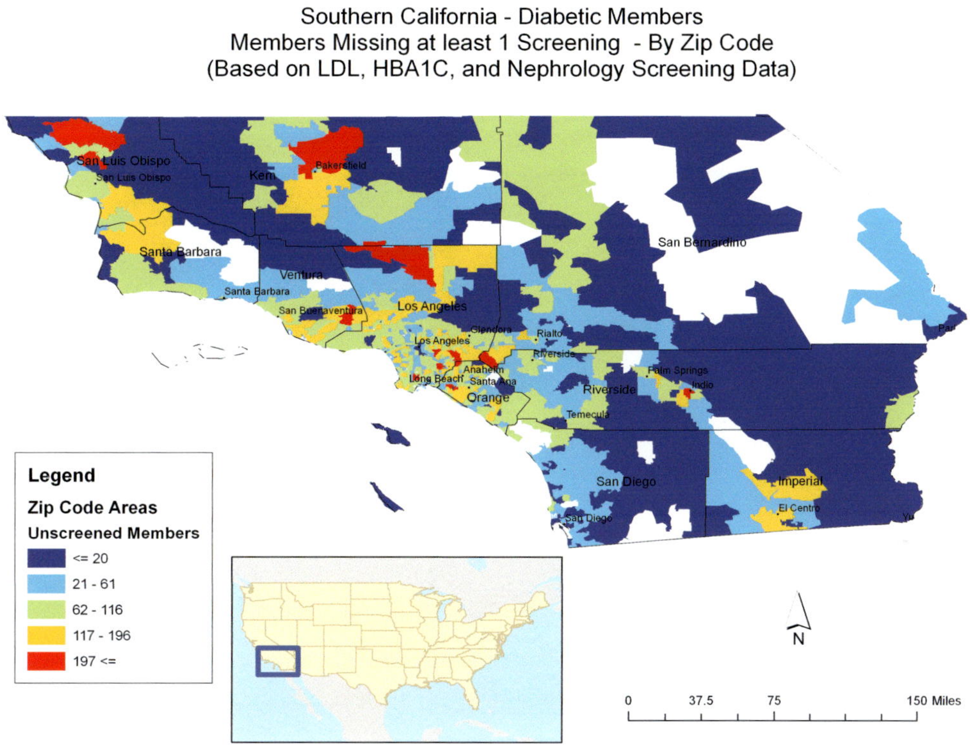

FIGURE 9 Analysis of unscreened members by zip code provides target areas. *Source:* WellPoint data 10/07–9/08.

health education sessions, and language and culturally appropriate program materials were available.

Another area of interest for the Taking Action Together alliance was near Bakersfield. Mapping became particularly important in this analysis because the hot spots were located clearly outside the more densely populated city. In addition, the question was raised as to which of the health plan's provider networks were servicing these members. By overlaying pie charts showing the ratio of unscreened members belonging to the plan's PPO to those belonging to the HMO networks, it became clear that members within the hot spots were more likely to be in the PPO network (Figure 11). This allowed for sufficient planning of the intervention and showed that interventions would not be as successful had they been coordinated through the HMO network of PCPs.

To meet the needs of these communities, the program tracked intermediate measures including number of conversation map sessions implemented, volume of participation, and participant satisfaction. The community-based nature of the program and concerns by participants about their privacy were

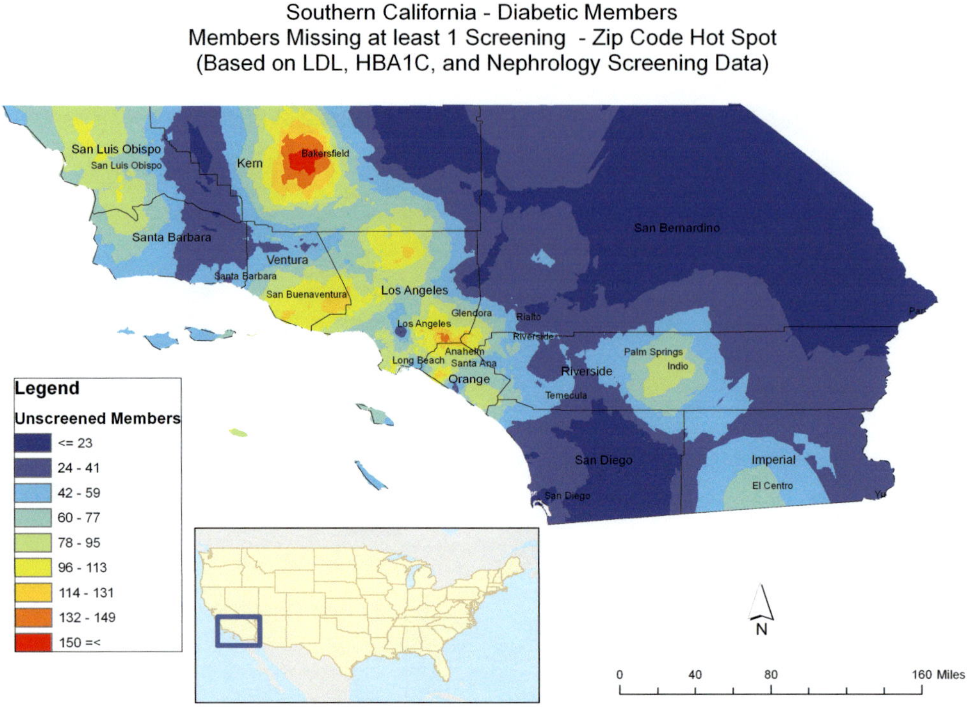

FIGURE 10 By creating a raster-based density map, hotspots become more apparent. *Source:* WellPoint data 10/07–9/08.

some of the challenges associated with tracking and measuring outcomes for this program.

Additionally, the hot spot maps allowed the Taking Action Together alliance to recruit additional stakeholders to support its outreach goals. Two local employers were identified and recruited within the hot spots to promote diabetes awareness in the workplace and help employees live healthier and more productive lives. The participating employer groups were offered free work site health screenings, and diabetes workshops utilized innovative teaching resources to educate participants about diabetes prevention and management. More than 200 employees and community members received diabetes-related health screenings at three mobile bus events hosted at the employers' work locations.

The alliance also focused on physician engagement and awareness within the identified geographic hot spots. In the Inland Empire, 2,353 physicians were contacted through two sequential rounds of notifications to encourage referral of diabetic patients to community diabetes workshops held in both English and Spanish. The second of such communications focused on the prevalence of diabetes among minorities in the Inland Empire and shared diabetes-related health disparities statistics to encourage

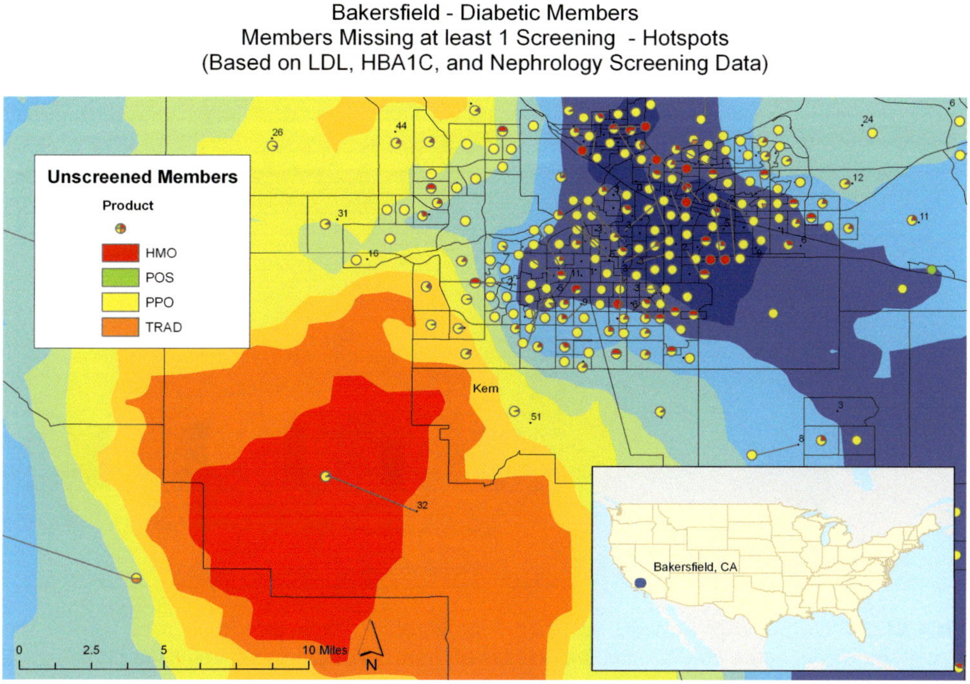

FIGURE 11 Overlaying pie charts showing network compositions shows that members in the area of greatest need are served by the PPO network. *Source:* WellPoint data 10/07–9/08.

physicians to refer their patients to the free diabetes health education workshops. As of January 2011, 172 individuals had attended 19 community workshops.

Physician Dashboard

As discussed in the previous case study, California's Inland Empire traditionally has exhibited lower adherence to evidence-based clinical guidelines, with statistically significant racial and ethnic health disparities among clinical quality indicators that are measured by the WellPoint-affiliated California health plan. Whereas the previous case study focused solely on community-based interventions, WellPoint and other health plans also address health disparities through provider-based interventions.

In 2008, WellPoint's affiliated California health plan launched a program to proactively engage physician practices in discussing observed racial and health care disparities in diabetes and colorectal screenings and to review resources the health plan could offer to support the physician practices in closing the disparity gap. First, medical groups with large patient populations were identified. Using imputed race and ethnicity, WellPoint's affiliated California health plan developed a medical group dashboard report that allowed

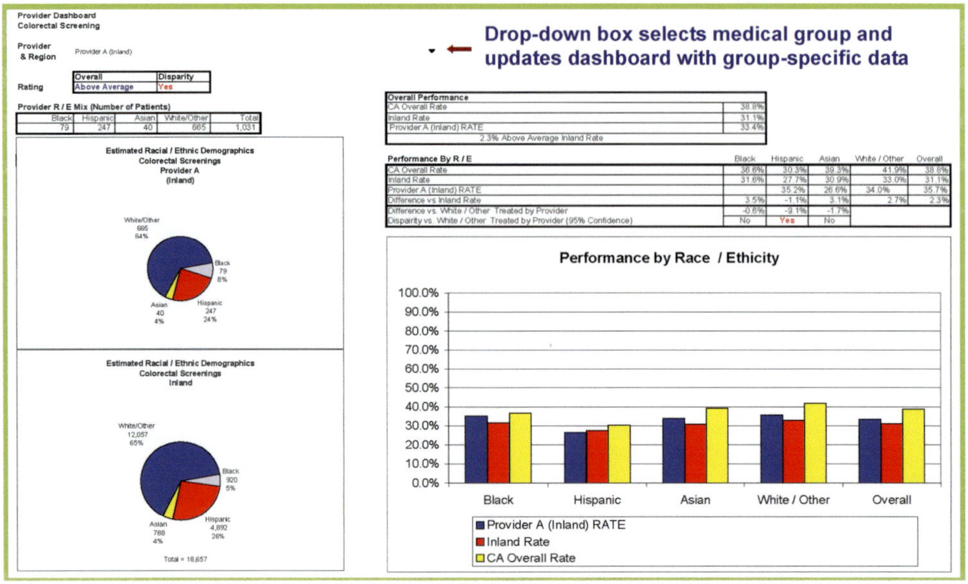

FIGURE 12 Dashboards provide member demographics for a provider group versus the overall members in the community. *Source:* De-identified sample from WellPoint HEDIS 2007 (2006 Data).

health plan staff to select individual medical groups to quickly review the overall demographics of the groups' patients, group performance by race and ethnicity for the clinical quality indicator being reviewed, and a comparison of the medical group's patient race and ethnicity demographics and performance on quality indicators with those respective overall rates for the region (Figure 12). In some instances, the dashboard report revealed that medical groups with high-quality indicator scores can sometimes have health care disparities. Conversely, these disparities may not necessarily be a factor in the clinical performance of groups with lower quality indicator scores. This differentiation allowed the health plan clinical quality team to tailor quality improvement discussions with individual medical groups to reflect whether the group needed additional support resources to health address their members' cultural and linguistic needs.

In addition, maps were created to show concentrations of health plan members served by the medical groups. These were overlaid on the screening rate maps in addition to shading showing areas with higher concentrations of minority members. The maps and dashboards enabled the medical groups to visualize whether they had higher concentrations of racial and ethnic minority patients in areas with low screening rates, which may indicate a need for improved culturally and linguistically appropriate medical services in those communities (Figure 13). Based on the dashboard reports and maps, health plan staff could initiate collaborative discussions to focus on

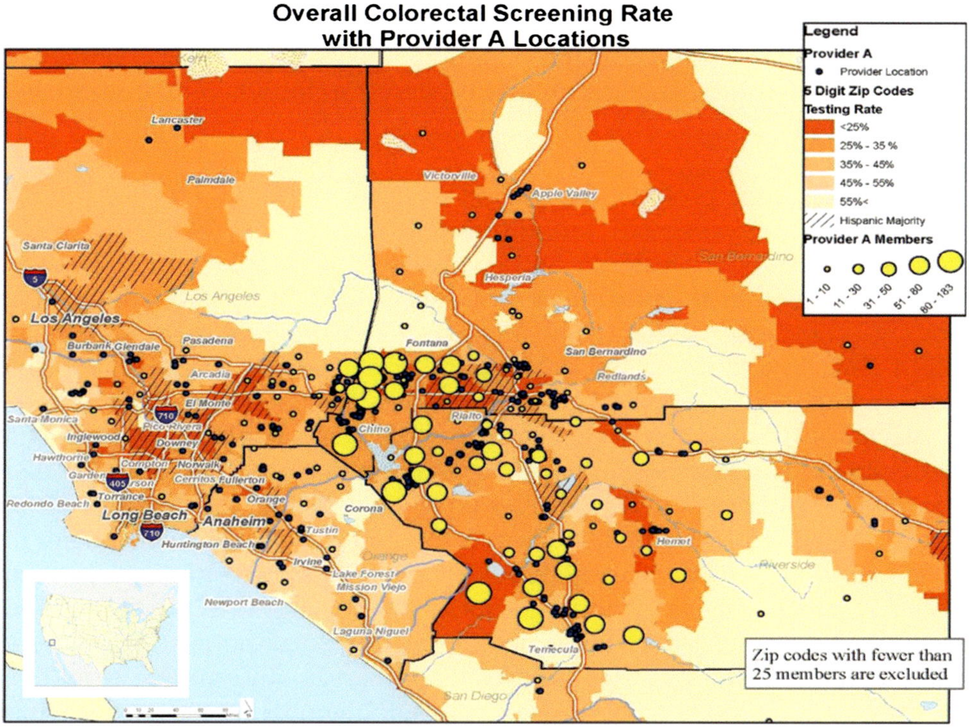

FIGURE 13 Overlaying patients and provider locations provides insight into the performance and demographics of facing the provider group. *Source:* De-identified sample from WellPoint HEDIS 2007 (2006 Data).

the health plan's and medical groups' joint priority to improve clinical quality performance for all the patients they serve. These open conversations helped raise awareness of health disparities and the need for culturally and linguistically appropriate services among doctors, and it helped the health plan and providers jointly address the issues of health disparities in the region.

Geospatial mapping and health disparities analyses may also be used to support provider network management activities, such as contracting and service access initiatives and physician cultural competency training initiatives. WellPoint's affiliated California health plan was able to couple the demographic overlay/screening density gradient map with additional specific provider network data to meet its regulatory mandated network management quality improvement and contract planning needs.

Cautions with Using Health GIS

GIS can be a powerful tool in analyzing and understanding the quality and appropriateness of health care received by patients and health plan members.

At the same time, this increased volume of information also opens the possibility of unintentional disclosure of an individual's private and confidential information. Mapping analysts should be very careful when choosing what level of granularity to display on maps. The most obvious case related to this issue is the plotting of an individual's exact location. Although this may be desirable for some projects, the analyst must be aware of where and how this data is being presented and ensure that security practices are in place to prevent inadvertent leaks of this data, because presentation of an individual's information in a public forum would likely be a violation of the patient privacy protections of the Health Insurance Portability and Accountability Act of 1996. In addition, when determining data summary levels, drill downs that result in very small populations may have the same effect. For example, displaying a block group with one or two diabetics could be viewed as a breach in these individuals' privacy. To overcome this problem, less granular geographic summaries may be preferred. By displaying data at zip code or tract levels, privacy may be better protected. Other possible solutions are to limit summary levels to those with 10 or more members or to use smoothed raster maps that blur individual locations. A positive side effect of these methods is the elimination of problems related to small populations that are particularly a problem in rural low population areas. An example would be the case of a zip code area with one diabetic member. A rate map of this individual would show a testing rate of 0% or 100% for this area and likely stand out on a map. Not only could this result in a privacy violation, but could also be misleading when planning intervention locations. Eliminating zip codes with fewer than 10 members or using a smoothed density map would amend this problem.

Although high-level summaries might be useful in protecting member's privacy, they may be an obstacle to developing accurate predictions about demographics. In most cases, zip code–level data do not contain enough granularities to effectively make predictions about individual demographics, and they might even result in misleading data. An example is probably the best method to illustrate this issue. Based on the 2000 U.S. Census, the population of zip code tabulation area 24017 in Roanoke, Virginia, is 26.9% white and 66.1% African American among its 23,000 residents. This same zip code's census tract 20 in Roanoke City is 93.7% white and 2.8% African American. The total population for this tract is approximately 4,500. Block Group 1 within Census Tract 20 is 96.3% white and 0.9% African American with a population of approximately 600. This clearly illustrates that using zip code as a proxy for someone within this block group would have produced a very strong estimation that this individual is African American. By looking more closely using tract or block group, models would likely show this person as white. The latter is likely to be a more accurate estimate, as modelers would probably expect the individual to have more in common with the 600 people in his block group than the 23,000 in his zip code.

As illustrated by this example, the most granular geography would likely produce the most accurate results.

CONCLUSIONS

A dominant focus in health care quality improvement—and perhaps the American health care system in general—is on addressing effectively racial and ethnic health disparities. This focus requires data analytic methodologies that help identify and prioritize geographic areas of disparities based on the regions given social, economic, and environment factors.

This article has focused on two critical concepts integral to addressing disparities. First, one must be able accurate identify populations experiencing health disparities through data mining and analyzing the health care experiences of an ethnically diverse pool of population, and, second, culturally and linguistically appropriate education through locally relevant channels for dissemination must be a priority in developing effective intervention programs to precisely target those populations that could benefit most from such services. Geospatial mapping has become an important component of WellPoint's analytic process for health plan operational support and for meeting its corporate public health priority in reducing health disparities for its members and the communities it serves. As described in the preceding case studies, the combination of traditional and spatial analysis can provide key insights when planning interventions to address health disparities.

Looking toward future areas for research, the development of models with a greater degree of granularity in regard to race, ethnicity, and language could unlock opportunities for further tailoring of interventions to meet the needs of individual communities most effectively. For example, current models do not drill down to ethnicities of members estimated as being Asian. Given the vast differences among the numerous cultures falling into this single race category, it is very difficult to tailor interventions to meet these groups' individual needs. It is the hope of the researchers that these further developments will do even more to eliminate the problem of health disparities.

REFERENCES

Altekruse, S. F., C. L. Kosary, M. Krapcho, N. Neyman, R. Aminou, W. Waldron, J. Ruhl, N. Howlader, Z. Tatalovich, H. Cho, A. Mariotto, M. P. Eisner, D. R. Lewis, K. Cronin, H. S. Chen, E. J. Feuer, D. G. Stinchcomb, and B. K. Edwards (eds.). 2010. SEER Cancer Statistics Review, 1975–2007. Bethesda, MD: National Cancer Institute.

American Cancer Society. 2009. *Cancer Facts and Figures for Hispanics/Latinos 2009–2011, September 15.*

Bach, P. B., D. Schrag, O. W. Brawley, et al. 2002. Survival of blacks and whites after a cancer diagnosis. *JAMA*. 287: 2106–2113.

Bierman, A. S., N. Lurie, K. S. Collins, and J. M. Eisenberg. 2002. Addressing racial and ethnic barriers to effective health care: The need for better data. *Health Affairs* 21(3): 91–102.

Elliott, M. N., A. M. Fremont, P. A. Morrison, P. Pantoja, and N. Lurie. 2008. A new method for estimating race/ethnicity and associated disparities where administrative records lack self-reported race/ethnicity. *Health Services Research* 43(5, pt 1): 1475–6773.

Esri. 2010. *GIS for Health Care Today and Tomorrow.* http://www.esri.com/news/arcuser/0499/umbrella.html. Accessed January 24, 2011.

Falkenstein, M. R. 2002. The Asian and Pacific Islander surname list: As developed from Census 2000. Paper read at Joint Statistical Meetings.

Fiscella, K., and A. M. Fremont. 2006. Use of geocoding and surname analysis to estimate race and ethnicity. *Health Services Research* 41(4, pt 1): 1482–1500.

Fremont, A. M. 2007. GIS tools for targeting disparities and interventions. CDC Assessment Initiative Conference. Atlanta, GA.

Fremont, A. M., A. Bierman, S. L. Wickstrom, C. E. Bird, M. Shah, J. J. Escarce, T. Horstman, and T. Rector. 2005. Use of geocoding in managed care settings to identify quality disparities. *Health Affairs* 24(2): 516–526.

Heron, M. P., D. L. Hoyert, S. L. Murphy, J. Q. Xu, K. D. Kochanek, and B. Tejada-Vera. 2009. *Deaths: Final data for 2006. National Vital Statistics Reports 57(14).* Hyattsville, MD: National Center for Health Statistics.

LaVeist, T. A., D. J. Gaskin, and P. Richard. 2009. *The economic burden of health inequalities in the United States*. Washington, DC: Joint Center for Political and Economic Studies.

Lauderdale, D., and B. B. Kestenbaum. 2000. Asian American ethnic identification by surname. *Population and Development Review* 19(3): 283–300.

Lurie, N., and A. M. Fremont, et al. 2008. The National Health Plan Collaborative to reduce disparities and improve quality. *The Joint Commission Journal on Quality and Safety* 34(5): 256 –265.

Massey, D. S., and N. A. Denton. 1989. Hypersegregation in U.S. metropolitan areas: Black and Hispanic segregation along five dimensions. *Demography* 26(3): 373–391.

Mathews, T. J., and M. F. MacDorman. 2008. Infant mortality from the 2005 period linked birth/infant death data set. *National Vital Statistics Reports* 57(3). Hyattsville, MD: National Center for Health Statistics.

McCaffrey, D. and M. N. Elliott. 2008. Power of tests for a dichotomous independent variable measured with error. *Health Services Research* 3(3): 1085–1101.

Mokdad, A. H., E. S. Ford, B. A. Bowman, et al. 2000. Diabetes trends in the U.S.: 1990–1998. *Diabetes Care* 23(9): 1278–1283.

Narayan, K. M. V., J. P. Boyle, L. S. Geiss, J. B. Saaddine, and T. J. Thompson. 2006. Impact of recent increase in incidence on future diabetes burden: U.S., 2005–2050. *Diabetes Care* 29(9): 2114–2116.

National Birth Defects Prevention Network (NBDPN). 2004. *Guidelines for Conducting Birth Defects Surveillance*. Sever, L. E., ed. Atlanta, GA.

National Cancer Institute. 2008. *Cancer Health Disparities Fact Sheet*. http://www.cancer.gov/cancertopics/factsheet/disparities/cancer-health-disparities#4. Last accessed January 25, 2011.

National Center for Health Statistics. 2007. *Health, United States, 2007 with Chartbook on Trends in the Health of Americans*. Hyattsville, MD: National Center for Health Statistics.

National Center for Health Statistics. 2010. *Health, United States, 2009: With Special Feature on Medical Technology*, Hyattsville, MD.

Short, L. J., M. D. Fisher, P. M. Wahl, M. B. Kelly, G. D. Lawless, S. White, N. A. Rodriguez, V. J. Willey, and O. W. Brawley. January 2010. Disparities in medical care among commercially insured patients with newly diagnosed breast cancer: Opportunities for intervention. *Cancer* 116(1): 193–202.

Smedley, B. D., A. Y. Stith, and A. R. Nelson, editors. 2003. *Unequal Treatment: Confronting Racial and Ethnic Disparities in Health Care*. Pp. 764. Washington, DC: National Academies Press.

Tammemagi, C. M., D. Nerenz, C. Neslund-Dudas, et al. 2005. Comorbidity and survival disparities among black and white patients with breast cancer. *JAMA*. 294: 1765–1772.

University of Iowa, Department of Geography, Department of Preventive Medicine and Program in Hospital and Health Administration. December 1997. *Improving Public Health Through Geographical Information Systems: An Instructional Guide to Major Concepts and Their Implementation*. Web Version 1.0. http://www.uiowa.edu/~geog/health/. Last accessed January 24, 2011.

U.S. Census Bureau, Geography Division Cartographic Products Management Branch. 2001. Census block groups: Cartographic boundary files descriptions and metadata. http://www.census.gov/geo/www/cob/bg_metadata.html#gad. Last accessed January 26, 2011.

U.S. Census Bureau, Geography Division Cartographic Products Management Branch. 2001. *Census Tracts: Cartographic Boundary Files Descriptions and Metadata*, http://www.census.gov/geo/www/cob/tr_metadata.html. Last accessed January 26, 2011.

U.S. Department of Health and Human Services. 2000. *Healthy People 2010* (conference edition, 2 volumes). Washington, DC: U.S. Government Printing Office.

Waldmann, T. 2009. *Estimating the cost of racial and ethnic disparities*. Washington, DC: Urban Institute.

Word, D. L., C. D. Coleman, R. Nunziata, and R. Kominski. 2000. *Demographic Aspects of Surnames from Census 2000*. http://www.census.gov/genealogy/www/surnames.pdf. Last accessed January 24, 2011.

Word, D. L., and R. C. Perkins Jr. 1996. *Building a Spanish surname list for the 1990s: A new approach to an old problem*. Washington, DC: US Census Bureau, Technical Working Paper 13.

Using Spatial Analysis to Improve Health Care Services and Delivery at Baystate Health

JANE L. GARB and RICHARD B. WAIT
Baystate Health, Springfield, MA, USA

Baystate Health has been recognized by the industry for its innovative and wide-ranging use of geographic information systems (GISs) to address problems in health. Spatial analysis is a key component in the effective use of GISs in health care for data exploration, hypothesis testing, and modeling. This paper describes GIS applications by the Health Geographics Program at Baystate Health. These applications include direct patient care, epidemiologic research, disease prevention and intervention, strategic planning, and marketing. We directed particular attention to the spatial analytic methods used in these applications. Finally, the challenges faced in obtaining and using health data for our analysis are discussed.

BACKGROUND

Baystate Health is an integrated health care delivery system serving a population of nearly 1 million people in four counties in western Massachusetts (Figure 1). It is one of the largest health systems in New England, with over 10,000 employees and an annual budget of over $1.4 billion. The major facilities and services consist of three hospitals, including a 653-bed, independent academic medical center and tertiary care hospital; multiple outpatient clinics throughout the region; a comprehensive cancer care center; a neurodiagnostics and sleep center; a visiting nurse association and hospice; multiple diagnostic laboratories and radiology facilities; respiratory and infusion facilities; a major private practice organization, and a for-profit health maintenance organization.

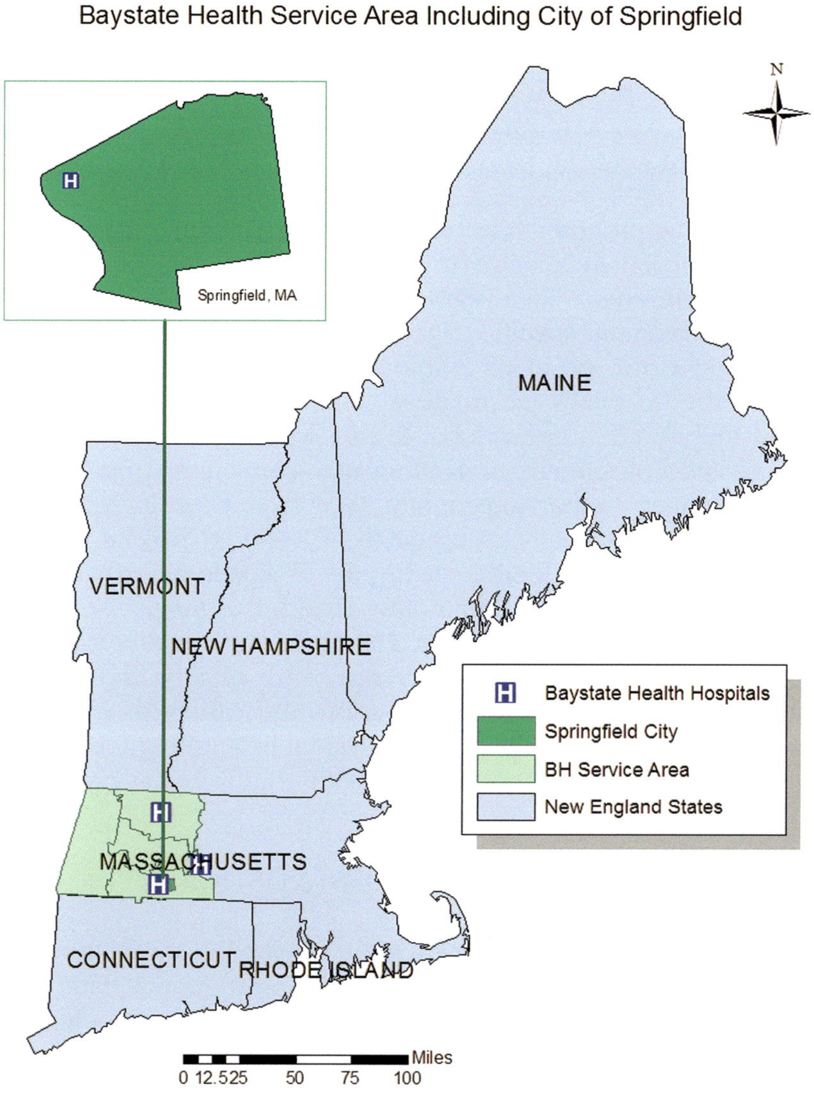

FIGURE 1 Location of Baystate Health service area and Springfield, MA.

In 1998, Dr. Richard Wait, chief of surgery, and Ms. Amy Pasini, injury prevention coordinator, instituted a GIS program at Baystate Health with three dedicated full-time staff. Initially the program was formed to support injury prevention initiatives. Recognizing these roots, the program joined forces with the city of Springfield's Injury Prevention Task Force to conduct several mapping projects. The program also developed strong ties with Esri, the industry leader in GIS software; as well as the American Community Survey of the US Census Bureau. The program received a contract from the Census Bureau in 2000 to conduct two demonstration projects using specially tabulated American Community Survey data in a GIS. These projects were on youth violence and late stage breast cancer, and they are detailed below.

Over time, the program initiators recognized the usefulness of GISs in many other areas outside of surgery, such as epidemiologic research, facilities management, and strategic planning, examples of which will be described in this article.

By 2002, the program had achieved international recognition in receiving Esri's Special Achievement in GIS award at the 22nd Esri International Users Conference.[1] Two years later the program received Esri's Vision award,[2] an achievement specific to the burgeoning health GIS field.

At its height, the program employed four full-time staff and worked closely with the hospital's information systems department to build a GIS server and mobile GIS applications. It also worked with another software vendor to design a proprietary emergency management mapping application. Although no longer a separate program, GISs have been integrated into the health care system, and they continue to be used by several departments, including Biostatistics/Epidemiology (a part of Academic Affairs), Strategic Planning and Marketing, and Community Health Planning.

The official mission of Baystate Health is "to improve the health of the people in our communities every day, with quality and compassion" (Baystate Health 2011). This paper describes the variety of ways in which GISs have been used by the health care system in fulfilling this mission.

GISs AND SPATIAL STATISTICS

A GIS is a set of hardware and software tools for the input, storage, management, display, and analysis of geographic and spatial data using any information that can be linked to a geographic location such as events, people, or environmental characteristics. A GIS stores data electronically in "layers" associated geographically. This geographic relationship is the key to mapping and spatial analysis. Overlaying the different layers of information and viewing them together can reveal patterns and relationships that might not otherwise be seen.

GIS is useful as an analytic and decision-making tool in every aspect of health care. Looking at spatial patterns of existing disease (prevalence) or new disease (incidence) is the basis for using GIS in health care. It allows for assessing the distribution and risk of disease in the community as a whole and in various geographic locations or population subgroups, as well as at different times.

Spatial statistics allow for testing of hypotheses about patterns and relationships seen in the maps and quantifies choices in decision making. These statistics consist of a set of statistical techniques that account for spatial relationship or spatial proximity. The advent of GISs allowed for the accurate computation of distance and direction between objects on a map, facilitating the analysis of spatial relationships. In health applications, analysis of point locations (such as health events, facilities, environmental sources) centers on identifying clustering, known as *spatial autocorrelation*. This is based on Tobler's first law of geography, which states that "everything is related to everything else, but near things are more related than distant things" (Tobler 1970). Additionally, distance between points calculated in the GIS can be used as one of the factors analyzed with spatial regression (Bailey and Gatrell 1995). It also forms the basis for spatial interaction analysis and the gravity model (Bailey and Gatrell 1995; Congdon 2000; Plane and Rogerson 1994). This is a test of the hypothesis that the volume of flow (e.g., people, goods, events) from one location to another is a function of proximity (distance), as well as size (land mass, population size, etc.) of the origin or the destination or both.

Like analysis of point locations, analysis of polygons or areas (for example, census tracts, neighborhoods, or regions) in health applications primarily centers on cluster detection, that is, spatial autocorrelation. An example of this is our study of late stage breast cancer rates described below. Polygons comprise the unit of analysis in spatial regression. In this type of regression, the spatial proximity of polygons and spatial autocorrelation is incorporated into the regression model, which distinguishes it from traditional regression techniques.

Data used in GIS applications described in this paper came from four main sources: the health care system itself, municipal and state departments, the US Census Bureau, and the GIS community. Individual patient and provider data on patient demographics, clinical characteristics, hospital events, and disease outcomes came from the Baystate Health patient medical record as well as selected hospital databases such as the operating room log and Human Resources employee database. The Massachusetts Department of Public Health (DPH) provided aggregate disease data (cases) from its cancer surveillance programs. The Springfield Police Department provided data on youth violent incidents. The US Census Bureau (US Census 2001) and the American Community Survey (US Census 2010) were the sources of population data on economic and demographic characteristics of the population by location, as well as counts for the population as a whole or for various demographic subgroups (e.g., by race, ethnicity, and gender). Using case counts from the Massachusetts DPH or Baystate Health hospitals or providers as numerators and census population counts as denominators, we calculated disease rates for the entire population of the hospital's service area or for different demographic subgroups according to geographic location. These types of data form the basis of much of the spatial statistical analysis carried out in GIS health care research beyond our own applications. Finally, the geographic spatial data we used were obtained from the US Census Bureau TIGER files (US Census 2000) for census boundaries, and shapefiles from MassGIS (MassGIS 2011).

APPLICATIONS

Patient Care

The focus of the health care system is the patient. Direct patient care includes treatment of disease when it occurs. GISs are applicable to the care of patients with both infectious and chronic disease. For the former, knowledge of the geographic origin of disease cases may provide answers as to the source of disease. This information may help in case diagnosis or may inform the choice of treatment, as will be illustrated by the following application.

One of the resident physicians at Baystate Medical Center, the largest hospital in the health care system, wanted to determine if geography was a risk factor for community-acquired, methicillin-resistant *Staphylococcus aureus* (MRSA) soft tissue infections in pediatric patients. He thought that mapping the home addresses of patients with resistant organisms could guide selection of an appropriate antibiotic before the culture results became available.

The resident obtained the addresses of patients with MRSA and methicillin-sensitive *S. aureus* (MSSA) from the medical record. Mapping these locations identified an obvious cluster in Springfield (Figure 2). The locations of MRSA and MSSA patients were then input into SatScan, cluster analysis software developed by the National Cancer Institute (Kulldorff 2010). SatScan verified that the cluster seen visually on the map was statistically significant, that is, it did not occur by chance. Because geography was identified as a significant risk factor for MRSA, it was concluded that MRSA colonization in the community was likely a predictor of methicillin-resistant infection. With this knowledge, new patients from high-risk areas (i.e., those with a preponderance of MRSA patients over MSSA patients) could be prescribed appropriate antibiotics for resistant organisms earlier in the course of treatment. Results of this study are published elsewhere (Tirabassi et al. 2005).

GISs also help identify disparities in treatment access and outcomes. Because geographic areas are often homogeneous by race, ethnicity, language, or economic status, looking at spatial patterns of disease or other health outcomes and relating them to demographic patterns may uncover health care disparities.

This is illustrated in a study on admissions at BMC for percutaneous coronary intervention (PCI), a widely used and potentially life-saving procedure for the treatment of coronary artery disease. PCI admission rates were calculated using census block groups[3] within a 10-mile radius of BMC. Figure 3 represents PCI admission rates for the period 1996–2001, by census block group, mapped separately by race and gender. Red block groups had admission rates of less than one per thousand. Block groups with other colors had admission rates from one to more than twenty per thousand. It is evident from the map that the majority of block groups had admission rates

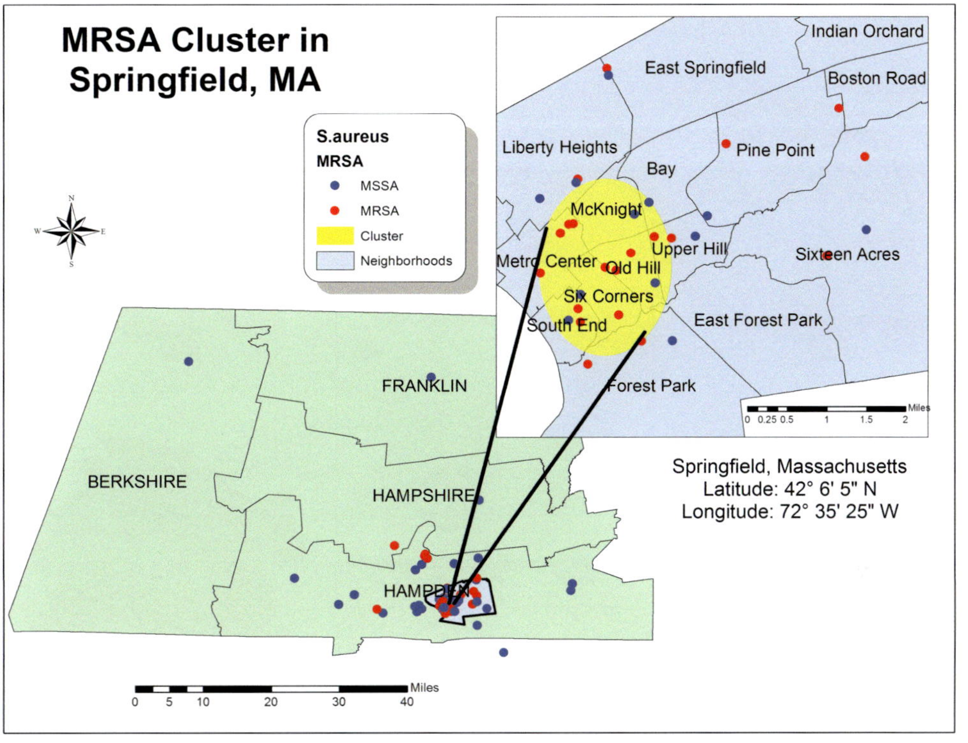

FIGURE 2 Cases of S. aureus in Springfield, MA, and Baystate Health service area, showing MRSA cluster in Springfield (adapted with permission from *Journal of Pediatric Surgery*, Elsevier Inc., © 2005).

greater than one per thousand for whites but less than one per thousand for blacks, for either gender.

The map highlights the disparity in PCI admissions for blacks compared with whites, despite known high rates of heart disease in the former. This information will be the starting point to investigate further whether real disparities exist and whether this can be attributed to referral bias, disparities in education or insurance, or other factors.

Epidemiological Research

GISs can be used to identify factors in disease etiology and treatment outcomes. As stated earlier, mapping disease patterns and overlaying various attributes of a geographic area allow visualization of the relationship of geography and disease, and they can generate hypotheses to be tested with spatial analysis.

This is exemplified by a study of late-stage breast cancer in Springfield, MA, contracted by the American Community Survey. We used visualization

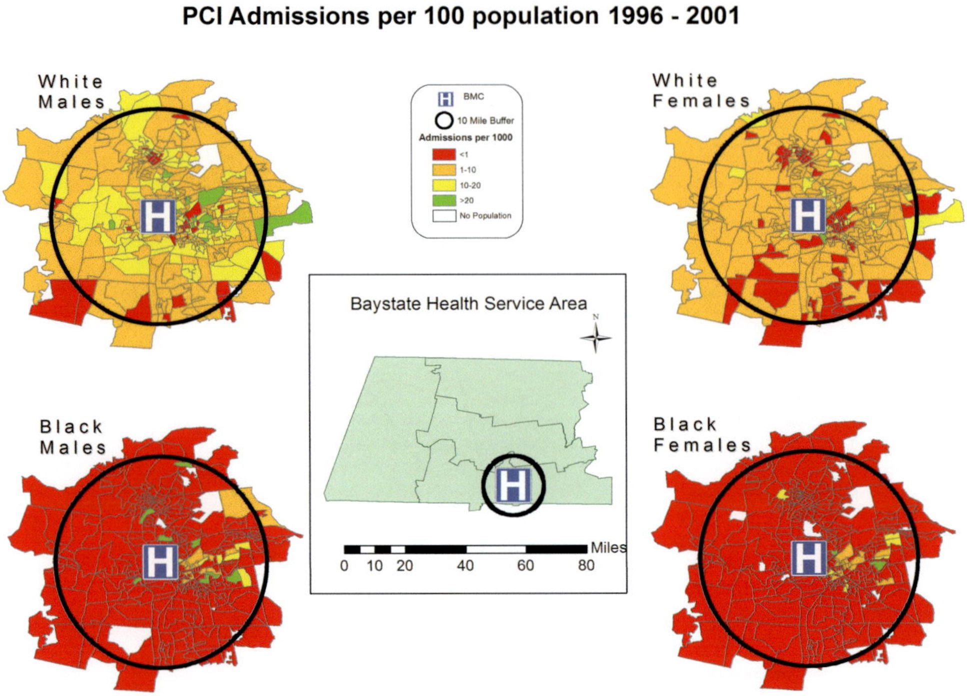

FIGURE 3 Admissions for percutaneous coronary intervention (PCI) within 10 miles of Baystate Medical Center (BMC).

and spatial analysis to identify geographically distributed demographic factors in advanced disease and to locate populations with high rates of these risk factors, implying an increased risk of advanced disease. To do this, we mapped the proportion of late-stage breast cancer cases out of all breast cancers by neighborhood (Figure 4). A high proportion in a neighborhood implies underutilization of screening mammography for female residents of that neighborhood. It can be seen in the figure that neighborhoods with a high proportion of late-stage cases also have high rates of poverty, minority populations, and linguistic isolation. This generated the hypothesis that socio-demographic factors play a role in late-stage disease. We tested this hypothesis and verified the relationship of these factors to late-stage disease by using spatial regression analysis. The risk of a woman's getting late-stage disease was greater in areas with higher rates of linguistic isolation and Hispanic ethnicity and lower median household income. These results support the design of "culturally appropriate" screening programs to target geographic areas of the city with high concentrations of these demographic subgroups so as to maximize breast cancer screening yield.

Baystate Health has applied a similar approach to explore geographic factors in disease at the scale of the human body. We employed clinical

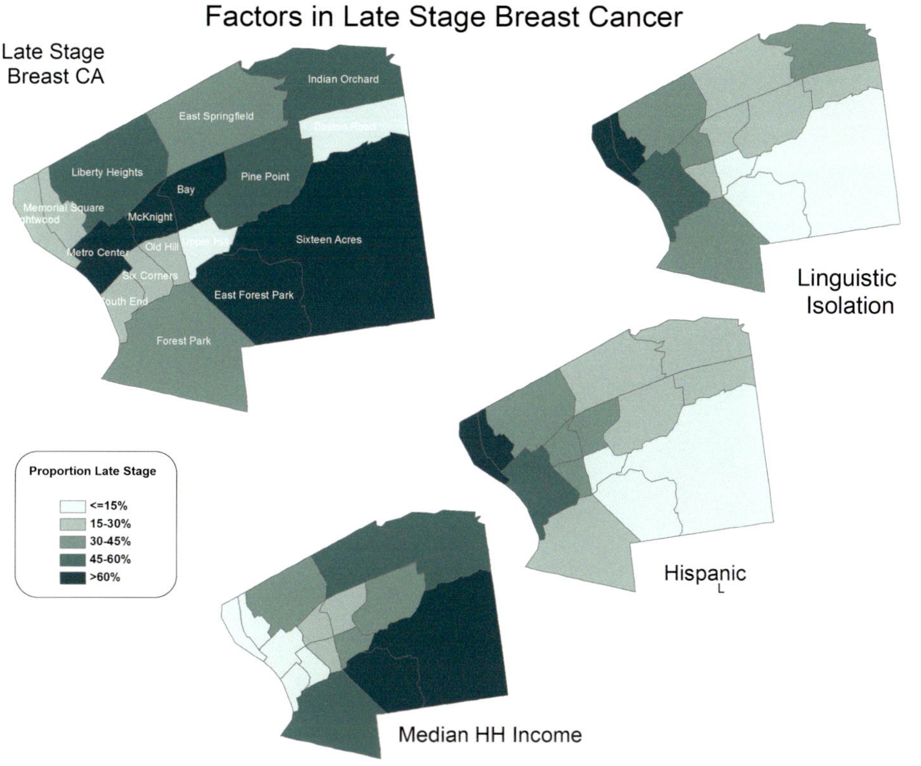

FIGURE 4 Proportion of late-stage breast cancer and demographic attributes by neighborhood in Springfield, MA.

data in a GIS to visualize and analyze the locations of anatomic features and their spatial relationship to one another. We used the results of transanal endoscopic microsurgery, a procedure to locate and remove benign polyps and cancerous lesions of the colon. Our purpose was to identify patient clinical and operative characteristics that might be related to outcomes such as difficulty of the procedure, operative complications, and patient prognosis.

The spatial relationship of anatomic features represented as polygons and lesions represented as points in the GIS formed the basis for visualization and spatial analysis in this study. We overlaid the precise location of lesions found on endoscopy (points) onto known anatomic regions (polygons). We used Moran's I statistic (Moran 1948) to detect significant clustering of lesions in different anatomic regions of the colon. The GIS was then used to visualize geographic patterns of clinical outcomes such as complications, development of cancer, or operative time (OT) needed to complete the procedure. Figure 5 is an example of a choropleth map of OT by anatomic region. The different color shades represent the mean OT for the lesions in each anatomic region. The map shows that for regions above the peritoneal reflection, mean OT was generally longer. Finally, we employed spatial regression analysis to identify

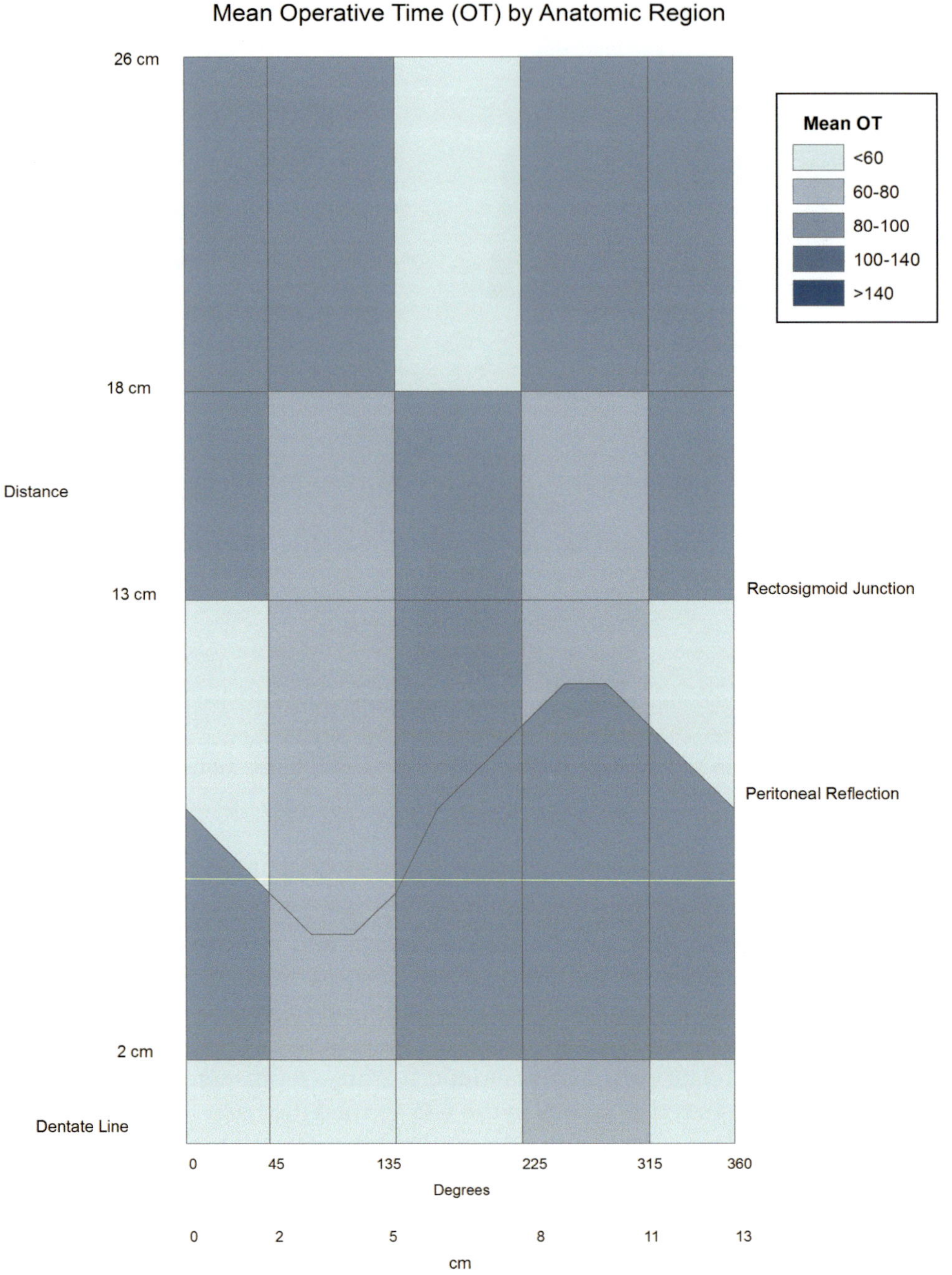

FIGURE 5 Mean operative time (OT) for anatomic regions of the colon (adapted with permission from *Journal of Gastrointestinal Surgery*, Elsevier Inc., © 2006).

clinical and spatial factors in OT. This showed that prolonged OT (greater than 90 minutes) was associated with lesions greater than 18 centimeters from the dentate line and with polyps greater than 4 centimeters in size (Ganai et al. 2006; Garb et al. 2007).

Prevention/Intervention

One aspect of patient care includes intervention to prevent the development or spread of disease or injury. We apply the results of our research to design prevention/intervention programs.

An example is provided by the previously mentioned project for the American Community Survey. Baystate Health's Injury Prevention Program worked with the Springfield Violence Prevention Task Force to examine violence in Springfield in an effort to reduce violent injuries. We looked at the geographic pattern of violent incidents involving youth in the after-school hours and overlaid the location of schools (Figure 6). The hypothesis was that violent incidents occurred in and around schools in this time period. If this proved to be true, school-based violence prevention programs might be effective.

We used GISs to visualize the pattern of flow of crime (at the police sector level) between an offender's home residence (origin) and incident location (destination) (Figure 7). This type of visualization was introduced

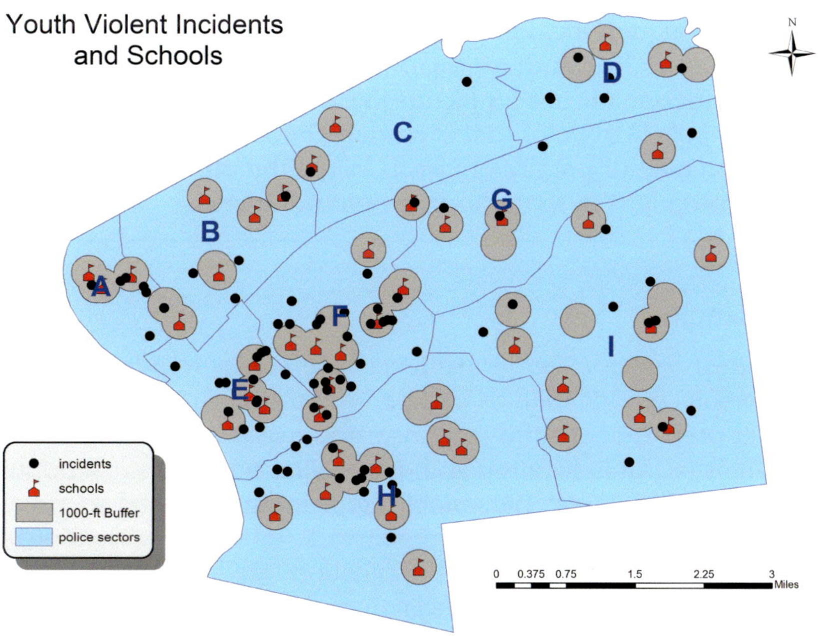

FIGURE 6 Youth violent incidents and schools in Springfield, MA.

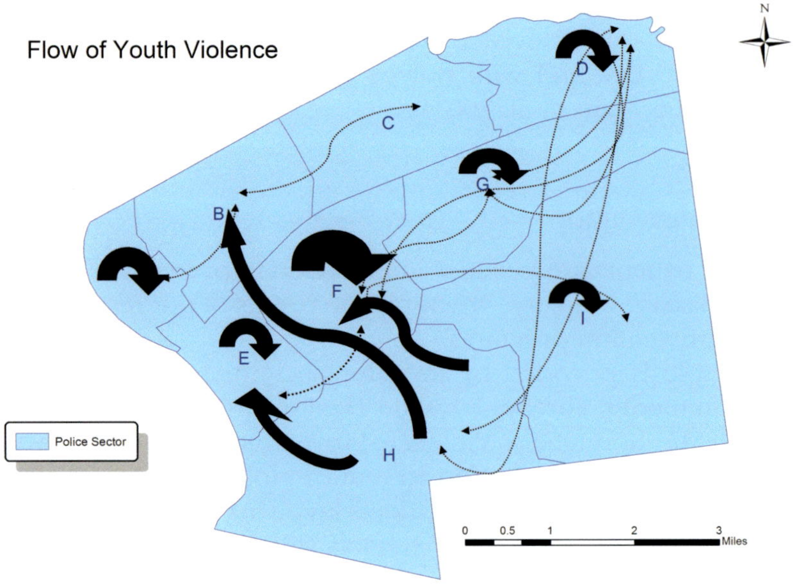

FIGURE 7 Flow of youth violence and police sectors in Springfield, MA.

by Tobler to map migration patterns (Tobler 1987). We can see from the flow map that the vast majority of incidents occurred in the same sector that the offender lived. This indicates that intervention/prevention programs in sectors with the highest incident rates would be beneficial, because potential offenders tended to live in these sectors. We applied the gravity model described above to formally test for factors that affected flow. We also added the number of schools in a sector to this model. The gravity model failed to confirm the importance of proximity to schools in this study, so we concluded that locating programs in the schools would not increase effectiveness.

Strategic Planning

GIS is an ideal tool for the global-level assessment required for strategic planning. Results of GIS analysis can be used to inform resource allocation, plan disaster preparedness and response, and marketing. In resource allocation, the GIS is useful in locating and quantifying both high-risk populations and resources (equipment, personnel, etc.). It can be used to predict the number of patients expected in a regionwide epidemic, assuming knowledge of disease incidence rates and population size for various segments of the population. It can be used in decision analysis for facilities planning and site location. And it can be used in marketing, to calculate patient share and locate patients who are not being reached.

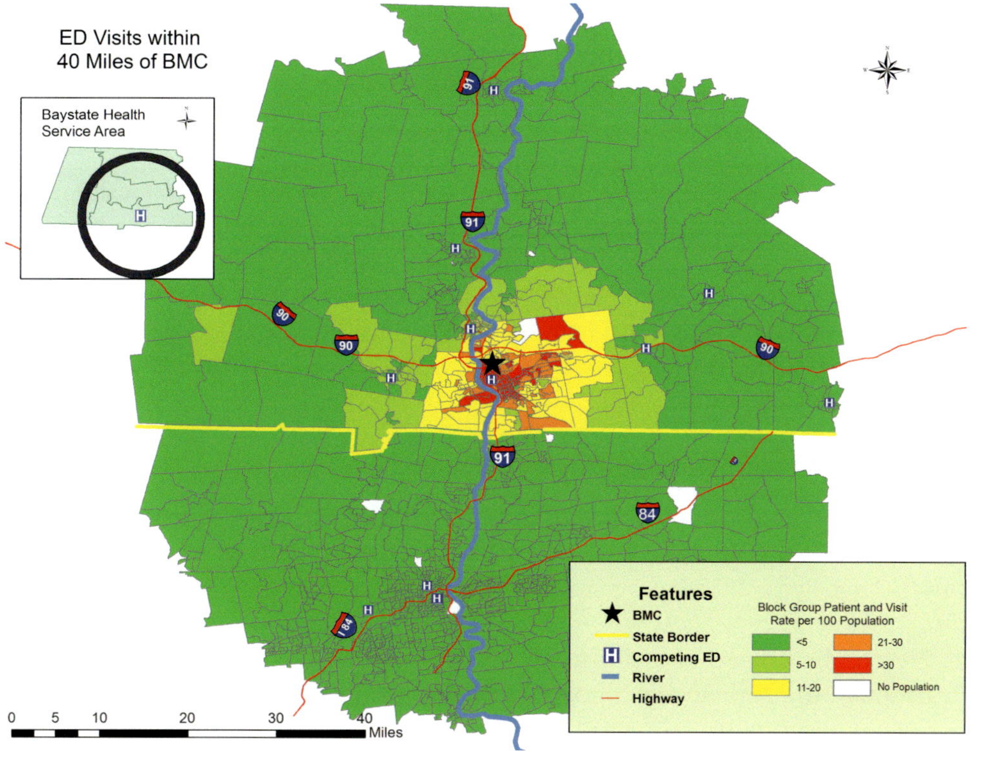

FIGURE 8 Flow of emergency room (ER) visits.

Resource Allocation

An example of how GISs and spatial analysis were used to optimize resource allocation is provided by a study of emergency room (ER) visits to BMC as part of an effort to reduce unnecessary visits to conserve resources. We again used flow analysis and the gravity model to identify factors that affect the flow of ER visits to the hospital from patients living within a 40-mile radius of BMC (Henneman et al. 2009). In this application, the measure of flow was the total number of ER visits to BMC from each census block group. The size of the origin was the block group population. Because there was only one destination (BMC), this was not included in the model. The measure of distance was the distance of each block group centroid to BMC. We also added other factors to the basic gravity model: a measure of attractiveness (which would increase the flow of visits) was block group proximity to major highways; and barriers (which would decrease the flow) were the Connecticut River and proximity to competing ERs.

The choropleth map in Figure 8 shows the visit rate per 100 persons for block groups within a 40-mile radius of BMC. Block groups with the highest rates appear in red and orange, those with intermediate rates are yellow, and those with the lowest rates are green. It is evident from the map that the block groups with the highest rates are closest to the hospital, with decreasing rates farther from the hospital. The Massachusetts-Connecticut state border (yellow line) is an obvious barrier, with a sharp drop in rates for block groups south of the border, in Connecticut.

The gravity model confirmed the visual impressions seen from the map. Total block group population was, as expected, a significant predictor of increased flow—the higher the block group population, the higher the volume of visits. Another significant factor that increased visit flow was location within the city of Springfield. Factors which significantly decreased visit flow were, as expected, driving distance from BMC and location west of the Connecticut River and south of the Connecticut border.

Disaster Planning, Preparedness, and Response

There are several ongoing activities associated with disaster planning, preparedness, and response, either in advance of a disaster or in the course of one:

1. Project the course of a disaster.
2. Estimate the size and location of affected populations.
3. Locate and quantify affected or special needs populations.
4. Assess surge capacity for area hospitals (beds and personnel).
5. Maintain a census of potential responders, equipment, and supplies and their locations in order to assess and allocate resources.

Because hospitals are first responders in a disaster, it is in the interest of effective response for hospitals to participate in the above-mentioned activities. GISs can help.

Estimating Affected Populations

Use of disaster modeling software in the GIS predicts what geographic areas are likely to be affected in an incident like the release of a hazardous plume. It is possible to combine incident information with population data to predict how many patients can be expected. With Baystate's human resources population database, we can also determine where our employees are located and how they could get to work if portions of the city were to become impassible in a disaster.

As part of Baystate Health's participation in a Springfield citywide disaster drill, we used the public domain modeling software ALOHA (Areal Locations of Hazardous Atmospheres) (NOAA 2004) to calculate the size and location of a toxic plume released, based on elevation, terrain, and current weather conditions (Figure 9). With a change in the wind or temperature,

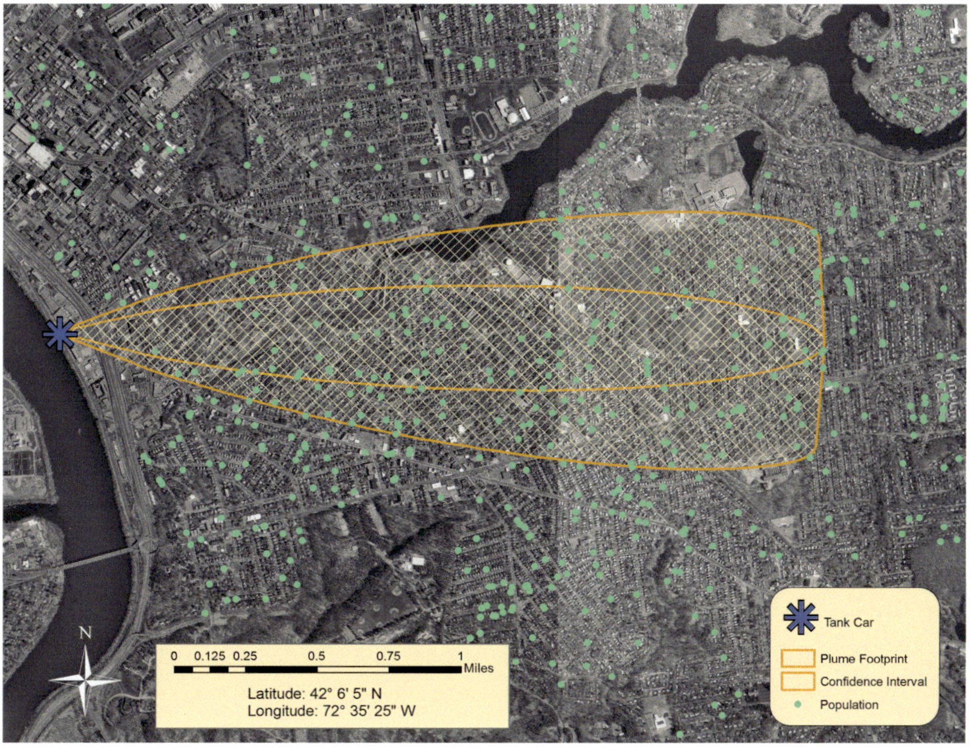

FIGURE 9 Modeling a disaster (adapted with permission from *Journal of Homeland Security and Emergency Management*, Berkeley Electronic Press, © 2007).

the location of the plume could shift and its footprint change. This modeling allowed us to predict what areas of the city were likely to be affected by the plume. By combining this footprint with population data for the area and utilizing GIS analytic techniques like areal interpolation (Lam 1980; Green 1990; Flowerdew and Green 1994; Flowerdew and Green 1991), our hospital was able to project the size of the affected population and how many patients could be expected. This method allowed us to use the population data we had for census block groups (source zones) to estimate the population under the plume (target zone). We used the GIS to calculate the intersection of these two layers through a polygon overlay operation. The result was a series of intersection zones. Population totals were calculated for the intersection zones using the areal weighting method—allocating population totals to each of the intersection zones based on the proportion of the source zone area represented.[3] The population totals for the intersection zones were then aggregated into the target zone (the plume) using the dissolve operation in the GIS, resulting in a total population count for the plume. Full details of the process can be found in Garb, Cromley, and Wait (2007).

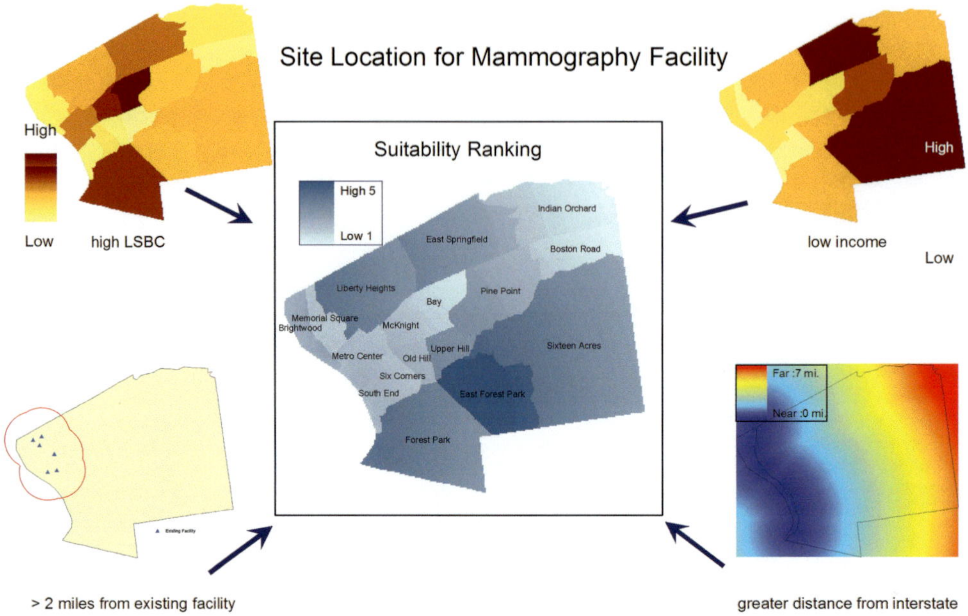

FIGURE 10 Decision analysis applied to choosing a mammography site.

From addresses in our human resources database we were also able to locate our employees (green dots), assess how many would themselves become patients (yellow dots), and plot alternate routes to work for the others using the ArcGIS Network Analyst routing software (Esri 2010).

Facilities Planning

Spatial decision analysis tools such as location/allocation, suitability modeling (Bailey and Gatrell 1995) and Multi-Criteria Evaluation (MCE) (Carver 1991) are methods of quantifying the decision-making process to make it more objective. It can be used by hospital administrators and clinical program designers to decide where to build new facilities, locate intervention programs, or allocate resources. Various criteria can be considered and combined using MCE. The result is a ranking of geographic areas according to their suitability for the desired usage. Different criteria can be weighted for their importance in the decision-making process. The selection and weighting of criteria can be varied to see the impact on the suitability ranking. This interactive process can test and model different scenarios and combinations of factors, using different weights for factors.[4]

Figure 10 is an example of how we used decision analysis to pick the best site for a mammography facility in Springfield. Administrators wanted to locate the facility in an area with high rates of late-stage breast cancer, low median income, far from existing mammography facilities, and close to a major interstate (peripheral figures). We used the raster calculator in ArcGIS (Esri 2010) to rank different neighborhoods in the city on the combined criteria. The middle figure shows the resulting suitability map based on these criteria. Neighborhoods with darker colors are more suitable, and ones with lighter colors are less suitable for a mammography facility.

Data Issues and Limitations

There are several issues in the use of data in a GIS. The first is varying quality of the data from different sources. Missing, erroneous or incomplete data, nonstandardized data formats, and lack of metadata (accompanying details about the source, quality, and usage of the data) may introduce varying degrees of error and bias when combining and utilizing this data. The kind of retrospective data on mortality and morbidity found in administrative datasets designed for purposes other than research will no doubt be less accurate and useful than prospective data designed for disease incidence registries.

Another issue pertaining to data quality and analysis of health data is the lag between environmental risk factors in disease and disease incidence. In GIS analysis of location as an etiologic factor in disease, it is highly probable that analyzing the characteristics of the current location of cases of disease is not related to etiologic factors which may have developed when the patients were living at different locations.

Another issue is the accuracy of geocoding,[5] which depends on correct addresses in standardized format. This may vary widely depending on the data source, and it can lead to errors in accurate placement of cases or events on a map, which are amplified when points are aggregated to calculate disease rates.

A further problem with using aggregate data such as disease rates or population counts from various sources is that they are not always in geographic units relevant to the problem under study. For example, Massachusetts state data on number of mammography screenings are collected and reported at the zip code level. Accurate base population data, which form the denominators for calculation of rates, are available only at the census block or block group level, which cannot be converted into zip codes. Even if it were possible to calculate accurate screening rates by postal zip code, these units would not be meaningful in locating neighborhoods in a city in need of enhanced mammography screening facilities, because zip code and neighborhood boundaries do not coincide. One solution to this is the application of areal interpolation techniques. We used this process to estimate the population total for the hazardous plume in our disaster preparedness example. Areal interpolation methods rely on the GIS primarily for calculating the area of the intersection zones and aggregating the population totals into target zones. As a result, census population counts or other data can be available for geographic units relevant to health care.

Another consequence of aggregating spatial data is known as the modifiable areal unit problem or MAUP (Openshaw 1983). It refers to the inconsistency of statistical results with different partitioning of the same geographic space, when partitioning occurs at different levels of aggregation (scale effect) or when different configurations of the same number of areal units at the same level of aggregation are used, forming areal units of different shapes and sizes (zoning effect).

Timely data are essential for applications in disaster preparedness and response, strategic planning, and resource allocation. They are less crucial in tracking disease prevalence over time. Population counts, widely used as denominators in calculating disease rates, are subject to this problem. The US Census, the major source of nationwide population data, is conducted only every 10 years. The American Community Survey (US Census 2010), which is also conducted by the US Census Bureau, although less comprehensive in scope, is conducted on an ongoing basis to give current estimates of the population. For disasters, estimates must be much more up-to-date, rather minute-to-minute, for data on affected populations or hospital census.

Sharing of health data also involves issues of confidentiality and ownership. Data sharing agreements between owners and users need to be put in place to assure proper use of data and acknowledgement of the source. Confidentiality of patient or case data needs to be assured as part of regulations on health-protected information according to the Health Insurance Portability and Accountability Act (HIPAA) (USDHHS 2011). Because of possible competition among hospitals for market share, they may be unwilling to share data on outcomes for research or require guarantees that their data will not be used to compete for patients.

Broader issues of confidentiality of GIS data exist. Maps of rare diseases at large geographic scales may allow identification of particular patients. Random re-assignment of point locations on large-scale maps, reducing the geographic scale at which data are displayed, and aggregating point data into polygons are three common solutions to this problem.

CONCLUSION

In this paper we have shown how GISs and spatial statistics have contributed to patient care, research, disease prevention and intervention, strategic planning, and the allocation of health care resources. Given the availability of accurate and timely spatial data and the proper application of the methodology, GISs and spatial statistics are extremely valuable tools in health care. Their use promotes a better understanding of the disease process, the population supported by the health care system, and the resources available in the service of better health. This leads to well-informed decisions by the health care system and its individual practitioners, effective allocation of its resources, and ultimately better service to its patients and the larger community.

NOTES

1. ESRI 22nd International User's Conference, San Diego, CA 2002.
2. ESRI International Health User's Conference, Washington, DC, 2004.
3. A census block group is a geographic unit used in census tabulations containing roughly 600–3,000 people, roughly demographically and economically homogeneous. Block groups are subdivisions of census tracts (US Census, "Summary File 1. 2000 Census of Population and Housing. Technical Documentation," in *Appendix B. Definitions of Subject Characteristics* (Washington, DC: US Government Printing Office, 2001; reprint, 4/1/01).
4. Other areal interpolation methods include the point-in-polygon, dasymetric and several regression methods. A discussion of these is beyond the scope of this paper, but it can be found in Flowerdew and Green as cited above.
5. Other areal interpolation methods include the point-in-polygon, dasymetric and several regression methods. A discussion of these is beyond the scope of this paper, but it can be found in Flowerdew and Green as cited above.
6. Geocoding is the process by which address data are converted to point locations on a map (i.e., assigned geographic coordinates such as latitude and longitude).

REFERENCES

Bailey, T., and A. C. Gatrell. 1995. *Interactive spatial data analysis.* Essex, England: Addison Wesley Longman, Ltd.

BaystateHealth. 2011. Baystate Health Mission. http://baystatehealth.com/Baystate/Main+Nav/About+Us. Last accessed August 8, 2011.

Carver, S. J. 1991.Integrating multi-criteria evaluation with geographical information systems. *International Journal Geographical Information Systems* 5: 321–339.

Congdon, P. 2000. A Bayesian approach to prediction using the gravity model, with an application to patient flow modeling. 2000. *Geographical Analysis* 32(3): 205–224.

Esri. 2010. *ArcGIS Version 10.0.* Redlands, CA.: Esri

Flowerdew, R., and M. Green. 1991. Data integration: Statistical methods for transferring data between several systems. In *Handling Geographical Information: Methodology and Potential Applications*, ed. I. Masser and M. J. Blakemore, 38–53. UK: Harlow Essex; New York: Longman Scientific & Technical; Wiley.

Flowerdew, R., and M. Green. 1994. Areal interpolation and types of data. In *Spatial Analysis and Gis*, ed. S. Fotheringham and P. Rogerson, 121–145. London: Taylor & Francis.

Ganai, S., J. L. Garb, P. Kanumuri, R. S. Rao, A. I. Alexander, and R. B. Wait. 2006. Mapping the rectum:Spatial analysis of transanal endoscopic microsurgical outcomes using GIS technology. 2006. *Journal of Gastrointestinal Surgery* 10(1): 22–31.

Garb, J. L., R. W. Cromley, and R. B. Wait. 2007. Estimating populations at risk for disaster preparedness and response. 2007. *Journal of Homeland Security and Emergency Management* 4(1): Article 3.

Garb, J. L., S. Ganai, R. Skinner, C. S. Boyd, and R. B. Wait. 2007. Using GIS for spatial analysis of rectal lesions in the human body. *International Journal of Health Geographics* 6 (11): 1–14.

Green, M. 1990. Statistical Models for Areal Interpolation. Paper presented at the EGIS '90: Proceedings, First European Conference on Geographical Information Systems, Utrecht, The Netherlands.

Henneman, P. L., J. L. Garb, G. A. Capraro, H. Li, H. A. Smithline, and R. B. Wait. 2009.Geography and travel distance impact emergency department visits. *J Emerg Med* 40 (3): 333–339.

Kulldorff, M. 2010. Software for the Spatial and Space-Time Scan Statistics Version 9.1. Information Management Services.

Lam, N. S.-N. 1980. *Methods and Problems of Areal Interpolation*. London, Ontario: University of Western Ontario.

MassGIS. 2011.Office of Geographic Information (Massgis). http://www.mass.gov/mgis/. Last accessed August 1, 2011.

Moran, P. A. P. 1948. The interpretation of statistical maps. *Journal of the Royal Statistical Society B* 19: 243–251.

NOAA. 2004. Aloha (Areal Locations of Hazardous Atmospheres) user's manual version. *Chemical Emergency Preparedness and Prevention Office. National Oceanic and Atmospheric Administration (NOAA) and the US Environmental Protection Agency (EPA)*, Washington, DC: US Government Printing Office.

Openshaw, S. 1983. *The Modifiable Areal Unit Problem. Concepts and Technologies in Modern Geography*. Vol. 38, Norwich, England: Geo Books.

Plane, D. A., and P. Rogerson. 1994. Modeling and forecasting migration: The gravity model. In *The Geographical Analysis of Population with Applications to Planning and Business*. New York: John Wiley.

Tirabassi, M. V., G. Wadie, K. P. Moriarty, J. L. Garb, S. H. Konefal, R. A. Courtney, B. F. Sachs, and R. B. Wait. 2005. Geographic information system localization of community-acquired mrsa soft tissue abscesses. *Journal of Pediatric Surgery* 40: 962–966.

Tobler, W. R. 1970. A computer movie simulating urban growth in the Detroit region. *Economic Geography* 46 (Suppl): 234–240.

Tobler, W. R. 1987. Experiments in migration mapping by computer. *The American Cartographer* 14 (2): 155–163.

US Census. 2000. *Tiger/Line Files, Redistricting Census*. Washington, DC: US Government Printing Office.

US Census. 2001.*US Census of Population and Housing: Summary Population and Housing Characteristics*. Washington, DC: US Government Printing Office.

US Census. 2010. *The American Community Survey*. Washington, DC: US Government Printing Office.

US DHHS. 2011. Health Information Privacy US Department of Health & Human Services, http://www.hhs.gov/ocr/privacy/. Last accessed August 1, 2011.

Applying GIS Methods to Public Health Research at Harvard University

JEFFREY C. BLOSSOM
Harvard University, Cambridge, MA, USA
JULIA L. FINKELSTEIN
Cornell University, Ithaca, NY, USA; Harvard University, Cambridge, MA, USA
WEIHE WENDY GUAN and BONNIE BURNS
Harvard University, Cambridge, MA, USA

The Center for Geographic Analysis (CGA) at Harvard University supports research and teaching that relies on geographic information. This includes supporting geographic analysis for public health research at Harvard. This article reviews geographic concepts that apply to public health, pertinent data available in geographic format, and GIS analytical techniques. The work-flow methodology the CGA has developed for conducting research with geographic data will be presented, highlighting successful practices to follow and pitfalls to avoid. Applications of this work flow are illustrated through an in-depth discussion of specific case studies in public health research at the university.

INTRODUCTION

The Center for Geographic Analysis (CGA) at Harvard University supports research and teaching that relies on geographic information. In this role, CGA provides support for geographic analysis in public health research and other disciplines across the university. Harvard University researchers relying on geographic information are abundant and cover dozens of different disciplines. Since its inception in 2006, the CGA has served members of the public health community at Harvard every month, with several months containing more than 50 active projects for public health or medical-related research or tasks. The majority of public health researchers aided by the CGA are from the Harvard School of Public Health and Harvard Medical School. On a less frequent basis, the CGA aids public health research for other Harvard entities including the Harvard Humanitarian Initiative and the Harvard Initiative for Global Health (Guan et al. 2011). The CGA's close collaboration with the Harvard Map Collection (HMC) and Harvard Geospatial Library (HGL) are essential in order to provide all researchers with the best possible service. The HMC holds 400,000 maps, more than 6,000 atlases, and thousands of reference books. HGL holds over 6,000 digital data layers ready for use in geographic information systems (GISs).

Discussed within the context of this existing infrastructure at Harvard, this article will draw on CGA's experience applying geographic analysis to public health research. Pertinent data available in geographic format will be reviewed, the full project workflow CGA employs to conduct projects will be articulated, and case studies in public health geography will be presented.

REVIEW OF GEOGRAPHIC DATA FOR USE IN SUPPORT OF PUBLIC HEALTH RESEARCH

Geographic data that support health research can be categorized as follows:

1. Data about health care capacities, such as health facilities, employment, and administration.
2. Data about the population and their health conditions and health care needs.
3. Data about the environment, both natural and social, that affect people's health.
4. Data about transportation and address location, which are essential in understanding accessibility for care, dissemination of medical supplies, transmission of infectious diseases, distribution of patients, and many other relationships among data of the above three categories.

We will examine each of these data categories, introduce the major data sources and popular data formats, and explain the most common usage of such data in health related research.

Data about Health Care Capacities

The US Department of Health and Human Services Health Resources and Services Administration (HRSA) maintains a Geospatial Data Warehouse and makes health care–related data available for download, including:

1. Health centers and look-alike sites.
2. Currently designated health professional shortage areas.
3. The National Sample Survey of Registered Nurses.
4. The Primary Care Service Areas project (a collaboration between HRSA and Dartmouth College).

Such data are in text or spreadsheet format, including postal addresses of the entities, which can be geocoded into spatial points data (see section below, "Data about Transportation and Address Location," for geocoding).

A summary of local health departments in the U.S. was published by Hua Lu and James Holt in 2009.[1] It was evident that local health services in the U.S. are fragmented, managed at different levels of local government agencies. It has been a challenge to develop a standard nationwide dataset to support effective collaboration.

Many states' GIS and health agencies maintain their own spatial health resource datasets for public use. Examples include Massachusetts[2] and New York.[3] In many states, such geospatial warehouses are often housed at state universities.

For data about health care providers, commercial data vendors are an alternative to public agencies. The ArcGIS Business Analyst is a licensed package of spatial data and analytical tools. It contains Infogroup Business Locations, which represents the locations of over 12 million private and public companies in the United States, among them health care facilities. It includes address information, estimated sales or assets, number of employees, franchise specialty information, and Standard Industrial Classification and North American Industry Classification System codes. These codes are four-digit numbers (standardized by the U.S. Government) that classify industries and are very useful in sifting out specific business types.

The availability of international health care data varies greatly from country to country, often depending on the national or provincial government agencies' data management practice. Health care provider information is harder to find in areas outside the United States The US National Geospatial-Intelligence Agency (NGA) maintains an international GeoNames service. It contains designations for medical centers, hospitals, and clinics.[4] The database is updated on a weekly basis, but locations are approximate and by no means complete for the globe.

Data about the Population and Health

Population data for health research can be further categorized into three categories. One is global population distribution and density data, which is aggregated and processed from nation-based census and other sources.[5] The second category is demographic health survey (DHS) data, which are surveys in many countries describing disease outbreak rates and other health indicators of the population, often published with map coordinates of survey clusters.[6] The third category is the more widely known national census data from many countries such as the U.S.,[7] Great Britan,[8] and Israel,[9] just to mention a few.

Population data are usually derived from interpolation and projection models, which provide continuous coverage for the globe and an estimated value for the times when no census was conducted. Data are often organized into tables, graphs, or grid formats, which require further processing to match administrative polygon units in a GIS. Five of these global population datasets are listed below.

1. Gridded Population of the World, v3[10]
2. United Nations Population Information Network[11]
3. Home HYDE—the Netherlands Environmental Assessment Agency[12]
4. LandScan[6]
5. International Database—US Census Bureau[13]

DHS data are plentiful. The World Health Organization (WHO) maintains a searchable database online,[14] which includes data on mortality and health status, diseases, coverage of services, risk factors, health systems, and world health statistics. The WHO Global InfoBase is a data warehouse that collects, stores, and displays information on chronic diseases and their risk factors for all WHO member states. Data is presented to download in graph, map, and data-table formats.

The DHS program[15] collects, analyzes, and disseminates data on population, health, HIV, and nutrition through more than 200 surveys in over 75 countries. Data are organized in administrative units that can be mapped to the administrative polygons.

UNICEF maintains a Web site that contains statistical information on the well-being of women and children around the globe.[16] It also supports the Multiple Indicator Cluster Surveys (MICS), which is a major source of global development data downloadable for users having a log-in.[17] The data are organized by country and year in SPSS format. It requires further processing to match with the country boundaries for global statistical analysis.

In the United States, national health survey data are available from many sources. The National Center for Health Statistics,[18] part of the Centers for Disease Control (CDC), provides downloadable tabular data. Some data are mappable by address geocoding or by matching table records to survey geographic units, such as administrative units or metropolitan and micropolitan statistical areas (MMSAs).

Behavioral Risk Factor Surveillance System (BRFSS), also sponsored by the CDC, provides downloadable GIS data.[19] These files contain data and documentation that are available in ZIP archive file format. The ZIP files contain BRFSS data that are mapped for both the states and MMSAs. These data files are a subset of the BRFSS data intended for use with a GIS package. Complete datasets and documentation for these data years are available in the BRFSS and SMART (self-monitoring, analysis, and reporting technology) sections of the site.[20]

CDC's WONDER, Wide-ranging Online Data for Epidemiologic Research, is a menu-driven system that provides access to a wide array of public health information by the CDC.[21] It allows for access to statistical research data published by the CDC, as well as reference materials, reports, and guidelines on health-related topics. Public-use data sets about mortality (deaths), cancer incidence, HIV and AIDS, tuberculosis, vaccinations, natality (births), census, and many other topics are available for query. The requested data are summarized and analyzed, with dynamically calculated statistics, charts, and maps. The data are ready for use in desktop applications such as word processors, spreadsheet programs, or statistical and geographic analysis packages. File formats available include plain text (ASCII), Web pages (HTML), and spreadsheet files (tab-separated values).

The Health and Medical Care Archive (HMCA)[22] is the data archive of the Robert Wood Johnson Foundation, the largest philanthropy devoted exclusively to health and health care in the United States. Operated by the Inter-university Consortium for Political and Social Research (ICPSR) at the University of Michigan, HMCA preserves and disseminates data collected by selected research projects funded by the foundation and facilitates secondary analyses of the data. The HMCA includes health care provider locations, household survey data, community disease information, and many more datasets used in numerous studies.

Local scale health surveys in the United States can be found at city or county government Web sites, such as the New York City Community Health Survey[23] and the Los Angeles County Health Assessment.[24] Some other countries publish their health survey results online as well. Examples are the China Health and Nutrition Survey[25] and the India National Family Health Survey.[26]

Census and demographic data are usually published by the respective countries' census organizations, as well as by commercial data vendors, who process the raw census data from the government and add value by applying statistical, geographic, or other analyses to produce derived demographic data that is more convenient for end users. In the United States, census data can be obtained from the US Census Bureau FactFinder[27] and a number of publicly accessible or subscription-based data providers, such as Geolytics,[28] Social Explorer,[29] ICPSR,[30] and Esri Community Analyst.[31]

Many other countries offer their census data through a fee-based service online or upon request. Examples include the China census data[32] and the India census data.[33] Most census data have their own geographic base units, either the same as local administration units (such as counties, districts, and townships in China), or a uniquely defined system (such as tracks, block groups, and blocks in the U.S.). The census data are usually organized in tabular format, which need to be matched to the geographic units for mapping or spatial analysis.

Data about the Environment

Many environmental conditions affect people's health. For example, the distribution of wetlands may affect the dispersion of malaria, while groundwater aquifer and the location of superfund sites may impact drinking water quality, which in turn affect residents' health. Because of the huge variety of data subjects that could belong to this category, we will not categorize data further by its content, but by the major source format instead, which includes remotely sensed image data, geo-referenced survey data, and statistical data.

The US Geological Survey (USGS) maintains a map-centric data discovery tool, Earth Explorer,[34] which provides public image data of different scales from global satellite images, national aerial photos, worldwide digital elevation models, land cover classifications, and weather monitoring images.

The commercial image data vendor, GeoEye, maintains an online image search tool GeoFUSE,[35] which allows users to find images they need and examine the cloud cover or other quality issues before submitting a purchase request. The Food and Agriculture Organization (FAO) of the United Nations maintains several statistical and spatial databases on agriculture, nutrition, fisheries, forestry, food aid, land use, and population.[36]

The US Environmental Protection Agency (EPA) maintains many public databases and tools for analyzing environmental data.[37] Its Geospatial Data Access Project provides downloadable files of environmental facilities or sites in various GIS formats, including extensible markup language (XML), keyhole markup language (KML), Esri Shapefile, and Esri Feature Class.[38] The EnviroMapper is an online mapping system for browsing environmental quality data interactively.[39]

The Esri Data and Maps and ArcGIS Business Analyst packages offer licensed users access to US parks and recreational land use data as well as food and beverage business locations and retail locations of tobacco and alcoholic beverages, and so on.

More specific local environmental data are often collected firsthand by researchers equipped with GPS receivers on the streets or in the field.

Data about Transportation and Address Location

Accurate and detailed transportation networks are critical for two purposes. One is for traffic routing, which provides information on the best route and travel time between any two points. The other is for address geocoding, which is the process of converting postal addresses into longitude and latitude coordinates. Datasets used for traffic routing and for address geocoding may look identical when displayed on a map—both appear to be linear networks. However, they require different preparation and contain different attributes on the street or road segments.

The most critical property of a traffic routing network dataset is connectivity among street or road segments. Other attributes in support of traffic routines include speed limits, one-way directions, turn restrictions, and vehicle height or weight limits. On the other hand, street networks in support of address geocoding require each street segment to contain street names and house number ranges, as well as other postal address components such as city and state names or zip codes. The geocoding software looks for matches between input and reference data, and when matches are found, the corresponding location is interpolated from the street segment whose value range contains the matching address number. Many of the commercial street network datasets are prepared for both traffic routing and address geocoding functions. The two combined allow for instant routing between a pair of user input addresses.

It is worth noting that both traffic routing and address geocoding datasets are readily available for North America and Europe, but not for many other parts of the world. Without a street level geocoder, addresses may be matched to zip code zones, town or city centers, or other geographic features. The locations obtained from such matching process is less precise than that from address geocoding, but nevertheless useful for some research purposes.

Information about foreign geographic feature names can be obtained from the GEOnet Names Server (GNS), developed and maintained by the NGA. The GNS database is the official repository of foreign place-name decisions approved by the U.S. Board on Geographic Names.[40]

The Geographic Names Information System (GNIS) is the U.S. federal and national standard for geographic nomenclature,[41] containing information about physical and cultural geographic features of all types in the United States, associated areas, and Antarctica. It includes current and historical place names, but not roads and highways. GNIS was developed by the USGS in support of the U.S. Board on Geographic Names as the official repository of domestic geographic names. Data were collected through a broad program of partnerships with federal, state, and local government agencies and other authorized contributors. "Hospital" is a category among the GNIS data types.[42]

Both address geocoding (using a street network) and location identification (matching place names with entries) in the GNIS or GNS achieve the purpose of mapping tabular records or descriptive data to a geographic location. Given that the vast majority of traditional health data reside in tabular files and other non-GIS file formats, many of which containing addresses—such as patient records, clinic records, and hospital records—geocoding is an essential feature. Once turned into locations, they can be studied through spatial analysis, revealing new patterns, relationships, trends, and meanings. The potential to identify address locations of patients raises a privacy issue that must be considered when using geocoded patient or other sensitive data. To preserve patient privacy, disassociating patient information such as names, Social Security numbers, health care system, or other individual identifiers from the geocoded address locations is necessary.

WORKFLOW FOR CONDUCTING PUBLIC HEALTH RESEARCH WITH GEOGRAPHIC DATA

Since its inception, the CGA has provided services in support of hundreds of Harvard research projects that have involved geographic information. To handle efficiently this large volume of services, a well-defined workflow has been developed, which is used by CGA personnel. This workflow involves several stages from initial consultation to final product creation, all of which are outlined below. When providing services for health researchers, there are specific considerations common to most clients that must be factored into the workflow cycle. This cycle involves the following general stages: initial consultation, project execution, and final delivery.

Initial Consultation

The initial consultation between a CGA staff member and a researcher interested in using geographic information usually originates from an e-mail or at the CGA help desk. The CGA general contact e-mail address (contact@help.cga.harvard.edu) is prominently displayed on the CGA Web site.[43] E-mails sent to this address are automatically forwarded to the in-boxes of several CGA staff members to ensure a response to all queries within one or two business days. In addition, e-mails sent to this address are automatically logged into a request-tracking ticketing system.[44] Each request ticket is assigned to the appropriate CGA member for resolution.

The CGA conducts a help desk every Tuesday afternoon both at the Harvard main campus in Cambridge and at the Harvard medical campus in the Longwood medical area in Boston. During this time, at least one CGA specialist is available at a computer lab at each location. These labs have high-powered desktop computers each with a variety of GIS software installed. This is an opportunity for any Harvard researcher to receive in-person consultation, hands-on troubleshooting assistance, or GIS data and software demonstrations from a CGA specialist. Appointments can be scheduled, or people can just drop in to receive help. Each help desk consultation or help session administered is logged into the CGA request-tracking ticketing system.

Whether initiated through the contact e-mail or help desk, the nature of requests varies, from a quick two-minute answer to a multiyear project involving multiple stages, deliverables, and personnel requirements. The requesting client's knowledge of using geographic information and GIS may also range from just having heard about GIS to an experienced GIS practitioner. This wide range of project complexity and client understanding requires a flexible, customized approach to handling each request.

During the initial consultation, the scope of work must be determined as soon as possible. This can be defined in the initial request, such as "How to convert a table of longitude, latitude coordinates into a shape file for use on a map?" or "Is there a GIS dataset available that contains hospital locations for Florida?" These clear procedural or information requests can usually be handled in a single reply; for example, sending the client a tutorial to resolve the former request, and extracting the requested data in the latter request. Typically, however, the scope of work determination is less straightforward.

To define the scope of work properly, the project objective must first be determined. The researcher usually has a very clear objective, for example, "I want a map that displays one mile buffers around hospitals in Chicago, fast food restaurants within these buffers, and a table listing the number of fast food restaurants within one mile of each hospital." Once the objective is established, then a scope of work required to achieve the objective can be developed. In defining the scope of work, the following must be taken into consideration: (1) datasets required to make the map or perform the analysis, (2) procedures and methodologies necessary to perform the work, (3) tools required to execute these procedures, and (4) deliverables needed and type of each deliverable (i.e., a Web map, statistical table, or geodatabase). The scope of work is documented in written form such that each component of the scope is clearly communicated.

Project Execution

Once the scope of work is determined, there are several ways to execute the project. The CGA's first approach is to equip the researcher to perform the work him- or herself. Harvard University has several proprietary GIS software programs licensed on a site-wide level, and it supports the use of many free and open-source software programs as well. Every semester the CGA conducts six different free, instructor-led training sessions at both the Cambridge and Boston campuses. These are intended for students or researchers who know little about GIS but want to learn the basics to apply to their coursework or research. More intensive, two-week "GIS institutes"

Center for Geographic Analysis
Harvard University

Center for Geographic Analysis
Project Specification

Template last updated: February 17, 2011

Project Identification	
Project ID **2011-XXX**	**Project Affiliation** School, Department
Project Title	
Contact Details	
Name	**Position**
Email	**Phone**
Project Specification	
Description	
Technical Overview	
Budget *(see CGA Financial Model Overview below)*	
Schedule	
Risk Risks and concerns	
Data Confidentiality Data for this project is (place an **x** next to all that apply): __ HRCI __ HCI __Non-confidential *(see Data Confidentiality overview below)*	
Phone	**Email** @cga.harvard.edu

Project Manager **Date**
Month/Day/Year

FIGURE 1 CGA Project Specification Document.

are held each summer and winter, geared at educating the graduate student-level researcher. The institute consists of lectures, lab exercises, discussions, and facility tours, culminating with each participant's presenting a GIS project featuring individual work. There are also many self-help tutorials and how-to documents available on the CGA Web site to help any Harvard personnel to use GIS.

Often it is not feasible for the researcher to perform the work. In these cases the CGA will schedule the work into their queue of service projects. For such projects, first-time clients receive 4 hours of CGA time for free, and then are charged $75 for each additional hour of work required. Using this consulting model has enabled the CGA to prioritize projects in order to meet project specific deadline schedules. A project specification document is filled out for these projects, wherein the scope of work, project methodology, budget, time line, and deliverables are documented and agreed upon by both parties (Figure 1).

The first stage of project execution involves gathering or creating the required datasets. As outlined above in the section Review of Geographic Data, etc., there are many datasets readily available for public health research, and various methods to geocode tabular data that may be necessary for use. The appropriate datasets are thus acquired as needed for the specific area of interest.

Once all datasets are acquired or created, the necessary methodology is applied to perform the GIS analysis. The methodology required to complete a project could use any number of GIS technologies and procedures. An overview of the general project methodology used in completing the major groupings of requests CGA receives will be discussed below. Detailed methodology for several specific projects will be presented further on in the article. The types of service projects CGA provides can usually be grouped into one of the following major categories: (1) geocoding and census variable extraction, (2) map creation for print publications, (3) dynamic Web map creation, and (4) GIS analysis and visualization.

Geocoding and Census Variable Extraction

Many researchers desire specific census demographic characteristics regarding their data for use in statistical regression modeling or analysis. If a researcher knows the level of geography and geographic area needed for census information (for example, all census tracts for the state of California), the CGA may provide an assisting role in pointing the researcher toward one of several methods to obtain demographic data for his or her area of interest or performing the data extraction itself. Care is taken in this process to ensure that the proper unique identifiers exist in attribute fields common to both datasets so that a table join can be performed. If a researcher needs to determine which census geographical unit their data are in, then CGA will first geocode the dataset using one of the methods listed in the section Review of Geographic Data, etc., above. Then a spatial join using ArcGIS software will be performed between the geocoded data and the desired level of census geography. An ArcGIS spatial join evaluates the geographic location of every feature in an input dataset (the geocoded data) against the join dataset (census GIS data) and appends the attributes of both datasets together into a new dataset. As a final step in this process, the data are often exported to comma separated value (.csv) format, for import into a statistical analysis software program.

Map Creation for Print Publications

Map creation for book, journal, dissertation, thesis, and other publications is performed on a nearl-daily basis at CGA. Both general reference and thematic maps are made, depending on a researcher's request. The application of best practice cartographic principles regarding the map layout, scale, projection, color, symbology, and type are used on these maps. Often explaining or demonstrating different variations of these principles with a researcher's data is necessary to produce the desired map. The audience for the map is taken into consideration, as is the final output media type. Printed maps are published in sizes ranging from 2 × 2 inches to 42 × 60 inches. The CGA has a 42-inch-wide plotter on which large format maps or posters can be plotted. In addition, maps are made in a wide variety of image formats and resolutions for use in presentations and publication on Web sites. Technology used to create the maps usually includes use of one or more GIS software programs (predominantly ArcGIS), and image-processing or graphic-design software.

Dynamic Web Map Creation

The ability to customize a variety of Web map application program interfaces (APIs) has created an increasing trend in dynamic Web map requests with various levels of functionality. The CGA publishes interactive Web maps using a variety of APIs including OpenLayers and Google Maps. Researchers readily recognize the utility of an interactive Web map embedded with their own data. This allows for entire research teams to view and interact with the same custom maps from anywhere in the world, fueling thought and collaboration. Technology used to create interactive Web maps is driven by user requests. The nature of the request (whether the researcher wants a handful of points with information window pop-up functionality or a Web map with complex symbolization capabilities and full database interaction) plays a large role in determining which software stacks are used to complete the request.

Enabling researchers to create their own Web maps is a major focus at the CGA. This has resulted in the CGA's building a series of Google Map mashup tutorials[45] and creating the WorldMap platform,[46] an open-source framework currently under development by the CGA designed for viewing and interpreting maps collaboratively. One can load data and maps from various sources in multiple formats and have flexibility in choosing how to create, share, and mix different datasets and maps together.

GIS Analysis and Visualization

The CGA aids public health researchers with many forms of GIS analysis. A critical first step in the workflow methodology of every GIS analysis project is recognizing what projected coordinate system is best to use for the type of analysis to be performed. Data layers are then projected onto the appropriate coordinate system. Some of the more common GIS analyses applied for public health researchers are the creation of straight-line and network buffers. Buffer creation enables proximity analysis, which, as described above, is a heavily applied spatial analysis method in public health research. Performing overlay and intersect between two map layers (for example, intersecting land cover and village regions to produce land-cover-type percentage values per village) is another common type of analysis desired by public health researchers at Harvard. Interpolation techniques such as inverse distance weighting, kriging, point density, and others are applied to datasets if needed. The CGA provides geostatistical analysis consulting as needed, and calls on a network of professors and researchers at Harvard for referral of specific questions. For many GIS analysis projects, the methodology is such that batch processing, macros, or software programming is required to best complete the job. Different programming languages such as Python, Java, .NET, and PHP are used when necessary. If specific programming skills required to complete the work do not exist within CGA, subcontactors are hired to write code. Animated PowerPoint slides, .gif images, and video files in all sorts of formats are produced when the temporal nature of a geographic dataset needs to be visualized.

Final Project Delivery

After the project execution stage concludes, final product delivery occurs. The end products to be delivered are always documented in the project specification document, which is updated and communicated to the client if the scope of work changes during the project execution stage. Project results might be tabular or GIS datasets, printed hard copy maps of various sizes, static map images for inclusion into print or Web publications, or interactive Web sites. For tabular or GIS dataset delivery, these data are sent to the researcher through e-mail or secure file transfer. A field key explaining what the data attributes or column names are is always included. Often a document listing the input data used and procedures employed to produce the data is also included. This usually completes the project workflow for tabular or GIS dataset delivery. For map, image, or Web site delivery, there is nearly always a revision process involved, and CGA factors this into the project specification. A draft map will be sent to the client for review and comment, then CGA will revise the map based on the comments and republish. This process is repeated until the researcher is satisfied with the map.

Once a dataset or map is deemed acceptable, the CGA specialist provides necessary metadata for the product and documents any processing procedures. This procedures document is saved into the project folder on CGA's file system and passed on to the researcher if requested. All project work is saved into individual project folders using a standard naming convention that includes the year the project was performed, project number, and client name. Subfolders within each project folder also have standardized names, so any CGA specialist is able to access and understand any project data if the need arises in the future. Project data are saved on a Netapp[47] file storage system. After two years of inactivity, project data are archived on flash memory storage media to free up space on the Netapp. In delivering Web maps hosted on the CGA Web map servers, Web sites are hosted for clients for one year. Subsequently, the researcher may opt to ensure permanence of a custom Web site for a yearly fee. Once the product, metadata, and documentation are delivered to the client's satisfaction, an invoice for the work is sent. Datasets produced that might be of use to others can be published into HGL with the client's permission.

CURRENT GIS RESEARCH IN PUBLIC HEALTH AT HARVARD UNIVERSITY

Many research projects are currently underway at Harvard that involve geographic analysis in the field of public health. Five of these projects will be highlighted in this section.

Nurses' Health Studies

The Nurses' Health Studies are among the most significant and longest-running epidemiological studies of women's health, established at the Department of Nutrition of the Harvard School of Public Health. Since 1976, investigators have followed over 238,000 registered nurses to examine risk factors for major noncommunicable diseases. This study brings together medical and public health researchers from the Harvard School of Public Health, Harvard Medical School, Brigham and Women's Hospital, Dana Farber Cancer Institute, Boston Children's Hospital, and Beth Israel Deaconess Medical Center. The Nurses' Health Study, established in 1976 by Dr. Frank Speizer, and the Nurses' Health Study II, established in 1989 by Dr. Walter Willett, are landmark epidemiological studies on women's health and noncommunicable diseases.

GIS regression approaches and geocoded residential addresses are being used to estimate different exposures and investigate associations between health outcomes and the environment. The following sections will highlight some of the major analyses being conducted in this study.

Spatio-Temporal Estimation of Particulate Matter Exposure

Public health researchers have been investigating the health effects of particulate matter (PM) air pollution as one of the components of the Nurses' Health Study. Yanosky et al. (2008) used GIS techniques to analyze data from the Nurses' Health Study; investigators used semiempirical models to predict spatially and temporally resolved long-term average outdoor concentrations of PM to successfully predict chronic fine and coarse particulate exposures for the northeastern and midwestern United States (Yanosky et al. 2009).

Researchers used a GIS-based spatial smoothing model to predict monthly outdoor PM10 concentrations (Yanosky, Paciorek, and Suh 2008), which included monthly smooth spatial terms and smooth regression terms of GIS-derived and meteorological predictors. Final model performance was strong (cross-validation $R^2 = 0.62$), with little bias ($-0.4\ \mu g\ m^{-3}$) and high precision ($6.4\ \mu g\ m^{-3}$). The final model performed better than a model with seasonal spatial terms (cross-validation $R^2 = 0.54$), and performed well in both urban and rural areas and across seasons and years. The addition of GIS-derived and meteorological predictors improved predictive performance over spatial smoothing (cross-validation $R^2 = 0.51$) or inverse distance weighted interpolation (cross-validation $R^2 = 0.29$) methods alone and increased the spatial resolution of predictions. The strong model performance demonstrated the suitability of these GIS-based spatial smoothing methods to estimate individual-specific chronic PM10 exposures for large populations.

Spatio-Temporal Estimation of PM Exposure and its Effects on Cardiovascular Disease

Researchers have applied GIS methods to investigate associations between environmental risk factors and health outcomes, using data from the Nurses' Health Study. In an analysis conducted by Puett et al. (2009), investigators examined the association of chronic particulate exposures with incident nonfatal myocardial infarction (MI), fatal coronary heart disease (CHD), and all-cause mortality in a prospective cohort of 66,250 women from the Nurses' Health Study in the northeastern United States (Puett et al. 2009). Researchers developed a spatio-temporal model to estimate monthly PM10 and $PM_{2.5}$ exposure between 1988 and 2002, using government monitoring data, geocoded residential addresses, and covariates calculated using GIS overlay analysis between address locations and census tract boundaries. Multivariate models included hypertension, family history of MI, hypercholesterolemia, body mass index (BMI, continuous), physical activity (<3, 3 to <9, 9 to <18, 18 to <27, or ≥ 27 metabolic equivalent hrs/week), smoking status (never, former, or current), diabetes, median house value, and household income for census tract of residence, season, and state of residence; these were stratified by age in months. GIS techniques were used to account for uncertainty and truncation in available data sources. In addition to the primary exposure, defined as the average exposure to $PM_{2.5}$ and $PM_{10-2.5}$ in the 12 months before the outcome of interest, other windows of exposure were considered, namely, 1, 3, 24, 36, and 48 months prior to exposure; $PM_{2.5}$ and

$PM_{10-2.5}$ were also assessed in separate single- and two-pollutant models. All multivariate models were also stratified by age in months and adjusted for state of residence (indicator variables), year (linear term), and season (indicator variables), to adjust for large-scale spatial mortality patterns that might be related to factors apart from pollution. Authors found increased risk of all-cause mortality (hazard ratio [HR], 1.26; 95% confidence interval [CI], 1.02–1.54) and fatal CHD (HR = 2.02; 95% CI, 1.07–3.78) associated with each 10-μg/m(3) increase in annual PM(2.5) exposure (Puett et al. 2008; Puett et al. 2009). Findings demonstrated that chronic PM(2.5) exposure was associated with risk of all-cause and cardiovascular mortality.

Association Between Residences in U.S. Northern Latitudes and Rheumatoid Arthritis

In order to examine the geographic variation in the occurrence of rheumatoid arthritis (RA), investigators analyzed geocoded addresses and incident case diagnosis of RA (or censoring of controls) in the Nurses' Health Study between 1988 and 2002. Generalized additive models were used to predict a continuous surface adjusted for known risk factors. Permutation tests were conducted to test for the importance of location and identify areas with statistically significant increased risk, compared with the entire study area. Spatial analyses demonstrated that women residing in high northern latitudes may be at greater risk for RA ($P < 0.05$). Findings also demonstrated the utility of applying GIS methods to traditional large-scale epidemiological studies to pose new research questions and generate hypotheses for future investigation.

The AfricaMap Project

AfricaMap is an open-source software project developed to support academic research and teaching and bring together resources from a variety of disciplines in a single geographic environment. This open-source system allows for the investigation, analysis, visualization, and communication of multidisciplinary, multisource and multiformat data, organized spatially and temporally.

This project was the first application of WorldMap, developed at the Center for Geographic Analysis (Lewis and Guan 2010). Since its Beta release in November of 2008, the AfricaMap framework has been implemented in several different locations including metro Boston, Chicago, East Asia, Vermont geological sites, Harvard Forest, and Paris. These Web mapping applications are used by individual researchers, and they have been incorporated into courses at Harvard University.

AfricaMap consists of a set of public digital base maps of the continent, viewable dynamically at a range of scales and composed of the best cartographic mapping publicly available. A gazetteer provides rapid navigation to specific locations across a vast landscape. As more detailed mapping becomes available, it is added to the system. Because of its decentralized architecture, there is (in theory) no hardware or software limitation to the amount of data that could be incorporated. Although currently focused on Africa, the Web-based mapping framework behind the project could be used to organize information for any region of the world. This model aggregates data using maps, rather than disciplines, authors, subjects, or indices.

AfricaMap serves the needs of researchers in multiple disciplines interested in Africa such as public health and medicine, including a common Web-accessible set of current and historical maps of Africa, a comprehensive gazetteer of African place names, and a repository for spatial and nonspatial datasets for research projects on Africa.

The AfricaMap project represents a framework for organizing African data from a variety of disciplines in a single environment. This allows researchers to explore public health research questions with the breadth and depth of data from other disciplines in a single environment. For example, researchers examining malarial transmission patterns in sub-Saharan Africa can explore environmental factors, vector sources, habitat reservoirs, soil type, land usage, urban planning, agriculture, socio-demographic data, and population health in a single environment and develop hypotheses for further analysis and investigation (Figure 2). Varied spatial information is also available to view and download for further study, including historical maps, topographic maps, historical trade routes, anthropological and ethnographic data, and epidemiological data.

AfricaMap supports collaborative public health research and teaching on Africa. This project brings together public health researchers from across Harvard University—including the Harvard School of Public Health, Harvard Medical School and affiliated hospitals, Harvard Humanitarian Initiative, Harvard Initiative for Global Health, and Faculty of Arts and Sciences—from a variety of disciplines including public health, medicine, infectious diseases, nutrition, epidemiology, biostatistics, demography, geography, sociology, and anthropology. Public health researchers can utilize the Projects layer in AfricaMap to search for ongoing or historic research projects, examine relevant publications and funding sources, and identify investigators and potential collaborators in a single environment. AfricaMap facilitates discovery and collaboration among researchers from across disciplines to examine health research questions and geographic analysis in Africa.

Child Physical Activity in the Built Environment

Childhood obesity is a public health issue that has risen to epidemic proportions in the past few decades (Koplan, Liverman, and Kraak 2005).

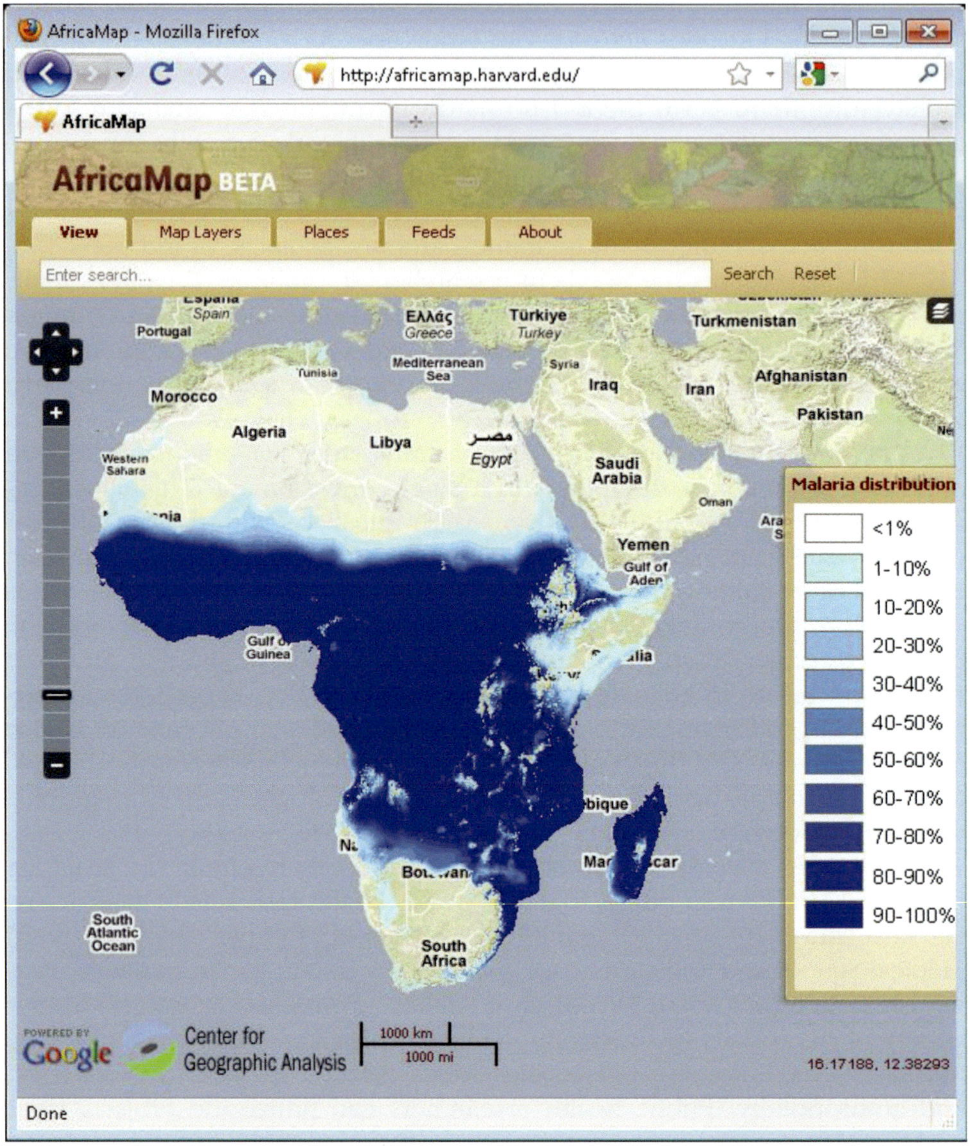

FIGURE 2 AfricaMap displaying malaria distribution.

Between 1970 and 2004 the prevalence of obesity almost tripled among U.S. preschoolers and adolescents and quadrupled among children aged 6 to 11 years (Ogden et al. 2006). Poor daily diet and lack of physical activity frequently lead to childhood obesity, and numerous factors figure into shaping these two behaviors, including personal and cultural beliefs, environmental conditions, societal influences, health care access, and individual physiology (National Institute of Health 2006).[48]

Recommendations by the American Academy of Pediatrics to prevent childhood obesity include getting at least 1 hour of physical activity per day, limiting sugary beverages and high-fat, fast food consumption, and switching dietary habits to include low-fat dairy products and high-fiber and calcium-rich foods.[49] It is common knowledge that physical activity can be increased through activities such as organized sports, but no intervention has yet sought to increase physical activity by increasing unstructured physical activities that include the use of one's built environment (Ogden et al. 2006). This includes sidewalks, open space, playgrounds, parks, and other areas freely accessible to children in which physical activity can occur. Assessing an individual's comprehensive use of the built environment throughout a given day in an attempt to find ways to enhance physical activity has had little previous study, and it is the focus of a current study[48] conducted by Harvard-affiliated medical professionals from Massachusetts General Hospital.

The study aims to collect objective information on adolescents' use of the built environment using GPS receivers and accelerometers (devices that measure one's movement or physical activity). By using GIS overlay analysis with the GPS and accelerometer data, the built environment elements most associated with physical activity in adolescents can be identified. Variations in use patterns of the built environment by age, gender, and socio-demographics can then be assessed. This objective analysis of where children are active or inactive throughout the course of an entire day may lead to discovery of methods for children to more effectively use the built environment for exercise.

The CGA is involved in this study by providing consultation regarding appropriate GPS devices with which to equip the children, writing a script that will automatically join GPS readings and accelerometer readings by date and time (using 30-second intervals), and performing overlay analysis using GIS. During December 2009, a preliminary study was conducted involving middle school children wearing a GPS and accelerometer for 7 consecutive days (Figure 3). The GPS and accelerometer data were joined by date and time. Locations were classified into categories in GIS using base-map data provided by MassGIS[50] (Figure 4).

Once classified, activity levels and locations were graphed for visual analysis and loaded into SAS for statistical analysis. This study is in the early stages, and it will collect activity and location information for the same group of children over several years.

The Surgical Safety Web Map

The Safe Surgery Saves Lives (SSSL) program has a mission of improving surgical care worldwide by ensuring adherence to proven standards of care in all countries.[51] Sponsored by WHO, the SSSL team is headquartered at the

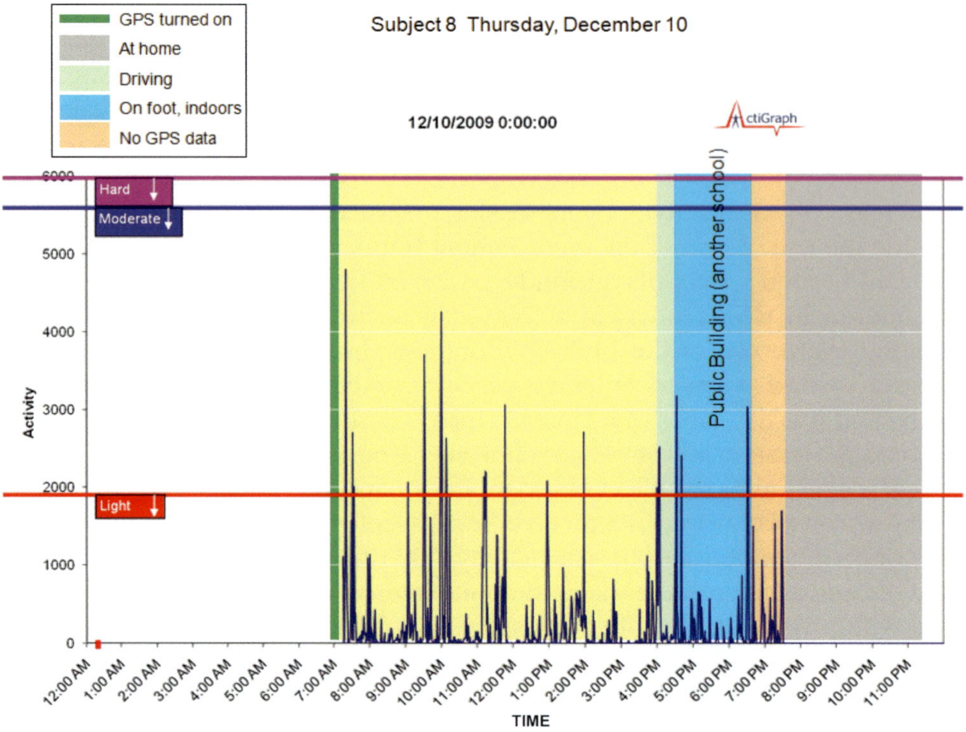

FIGURE 3 Graph of physical activity and locations.

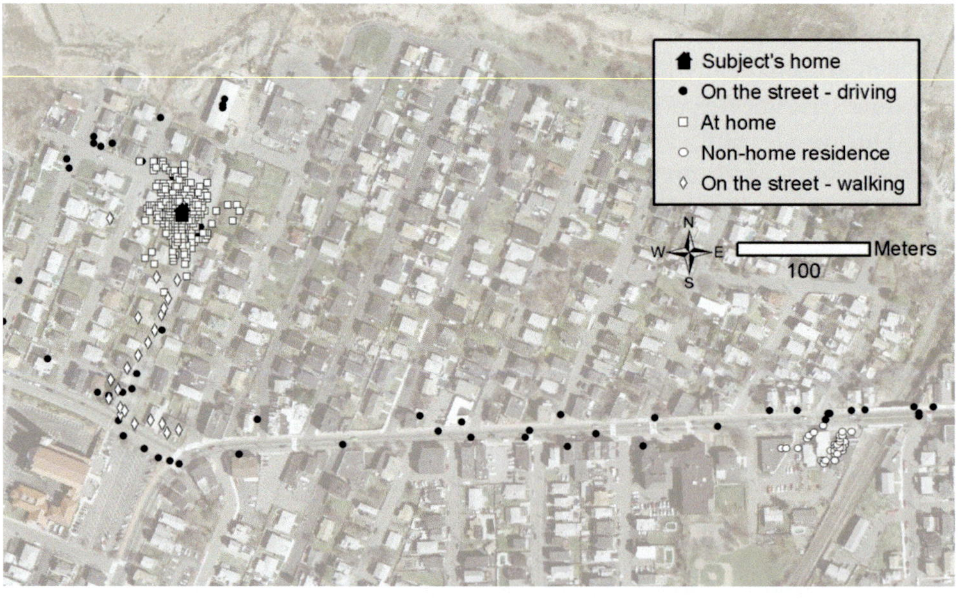

FIGURE 4 GPS location classifications on a MassGIS orthophoto.

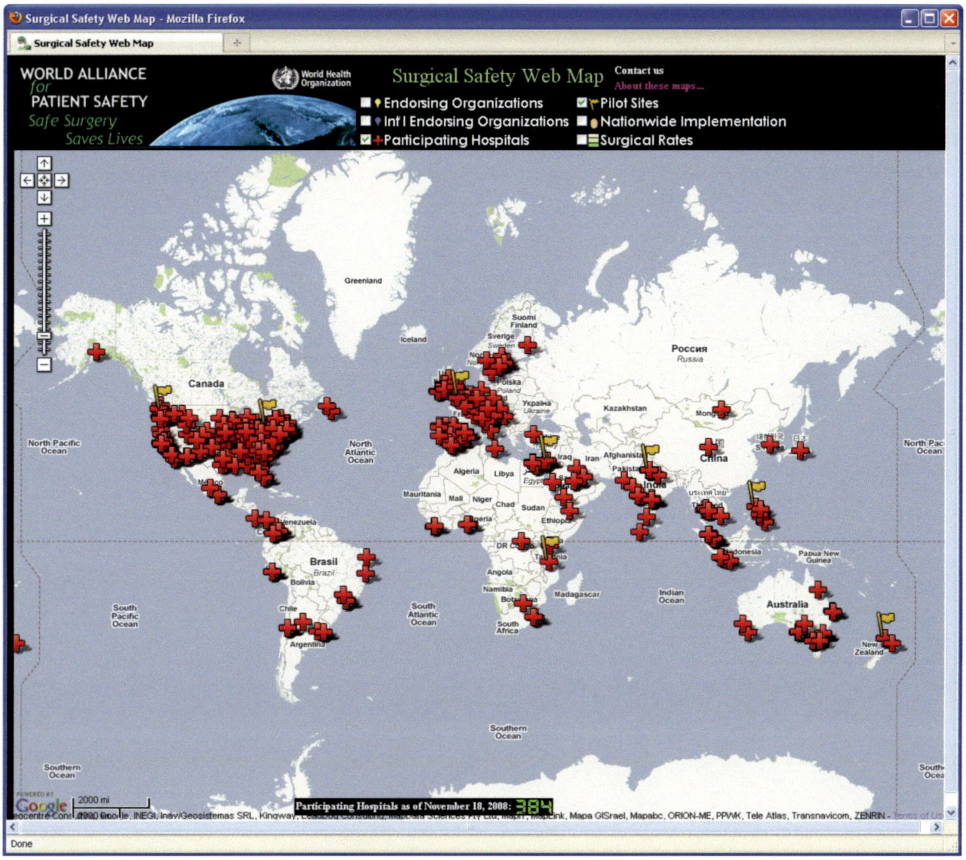

FIGURE 5 The Surgical Safety Web map from November, 2008, with 384 participating hospitals.

Harvard School of Public Health and led by Dr. Atul Gawande, an endocrine surgeon from Boston's Brigham and Women's Hospital. To improve surgical care worldwide, the team created a checklist (19 steps to be completed during any operation), tested the checklist in clinical settings in eight hospitals worldwide, and found that using the checklist reduced major complications from surgery by 36% and the rate of death resulting from surgery by 43% (Gawande 2009). These study results were sufficient justification to begin a worldwide dissemination effort to get as many hospitals as possible to use the checklist. In the summer of 2007, members from the SSSL team came to the CGA help desk to inquire about adding a mapping component to their project.

The team wanted a Web map displaying (1) distinct markers at the hospital locations that had registered to use the checklist and hospitals that were actively using the checklist and (2) a thematic map showing surgical rates per country, normalized by population (Figures 5 and 6). They wanted to

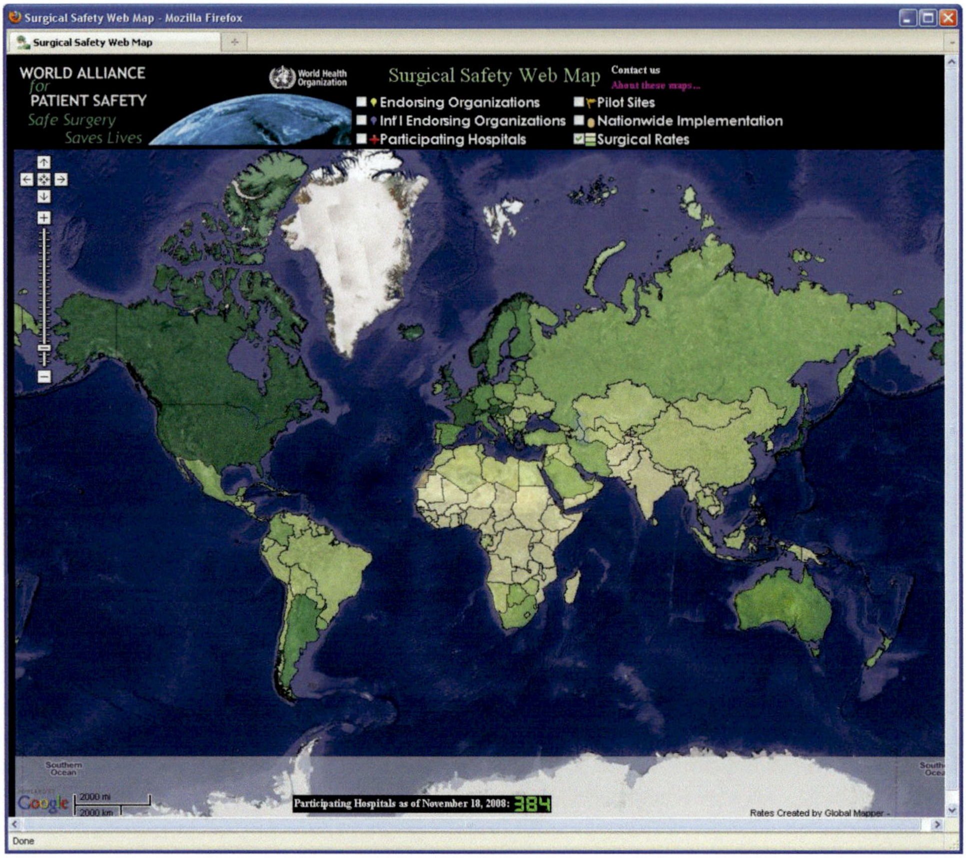

FIGURE 6 The Surgical Rates Thematic map overlay.

be able to update the map as new hospitals signed on, and wanted the map to have popup window functionality displaying the hospital name, city, and country upon a mouse click. The team wanted to use the map both internally to track progress of the checklist dissemination and for hospital information access and externally as a marketing tool to show hospital administrators, chief surgeons, and other decision makers the wide acceptance and proximity of hospitals using the checklist. The SSSL team liked the look, feel, and functionality of Google Maps, and wanted to use this as their basemap platform. In December 2007 the CGA published the Surgical Safety Web Map with the then 25 participating hospitals displayed as a KML file and the surgical rates map as a screen overlay.

The team quickly put the map to use, featuring it in presentations and referring potential checklist adaptors to it as their dissemination effort continued. New participating hospitals were sent to the CGA for inclusion on the map each month, and a new KML file was generated and published.

Team members also started using the map as a way to view the current status of the dissemination effort. Members could use the map to quickly get an idea of the participating hospitals in their area of interest, which are available worldwide to anyone with an Internet connection. This use of the map prompted a second phase in the Web map development. The team wanted to be able to update the map themselves as soon as hospitals signed up for the checklist. Also desired was an ability to access more information about the hospitals through the map such as the number of beds, number of physicians, contact person information, and whether devices such as pulse oximiters were available. The SSSL team wanted to be able to view and update this hospital information, yet restrict information access to the general public to the hospital name, city, and country. At this point the total hospital count was nearing 400, which exceeded the number of points that could be rendered on a Google Map mashup at once. Also, it was difficult to discern individual hospitals on the map in cities with many participating hospitals in close proximity. Because of this, the team wanted a list of hospitals in the viewable map area to be displayed interactively.

To accommodate the new Web map functionality requests, CGA transferred the hospital data layer into a PostgresSQL database, geospatially enabled with the PostGIS module. Mapserver was used to render the hospitals, and hospitals were symbolized according to whether they were registered or actively using the checklist. To enable the SSSL team to upload new hospitals, a data import program was written in Java, and the SSSL team was trained on how to geocode new hospitals using Batchgeocode.com to obtain longitude and latitude coordinates. The coordinates found for each new hospital were saved in columns in an MS Excel template that matched the PostGIS database schema. Once the template was populated with the hospital information and coordinates, it was saved into .csv format and uploaded to the database through the data import program. This upload program requires a login to access, ascertaining that the .csv file is in the right format. Once uploaded, the new hospitals immediately appear on the map, and each time the map is rendered it draws all the points in the database according to their coordinate locations. In addition, when a hospital is clicked on to identify it, a "For more hospital information" message appears in the information window that, when clicked on, prompts the user to enter a username and password. Upon authentication, a form appears listing all the hospital information in editable text forms. The longitude-latitude forms are editable as well, enabling position refinement of hospital locations. A new sidebar was added to the map, and programmed to display hospitals in the current view in a tabular fashion, enabling one to click on a hospital name in the list and see it identified on the map with its information displayed (Figure 7).

The final task was writing another Java program that allows for an export of the full database back to .csv format after logging in. This enabled

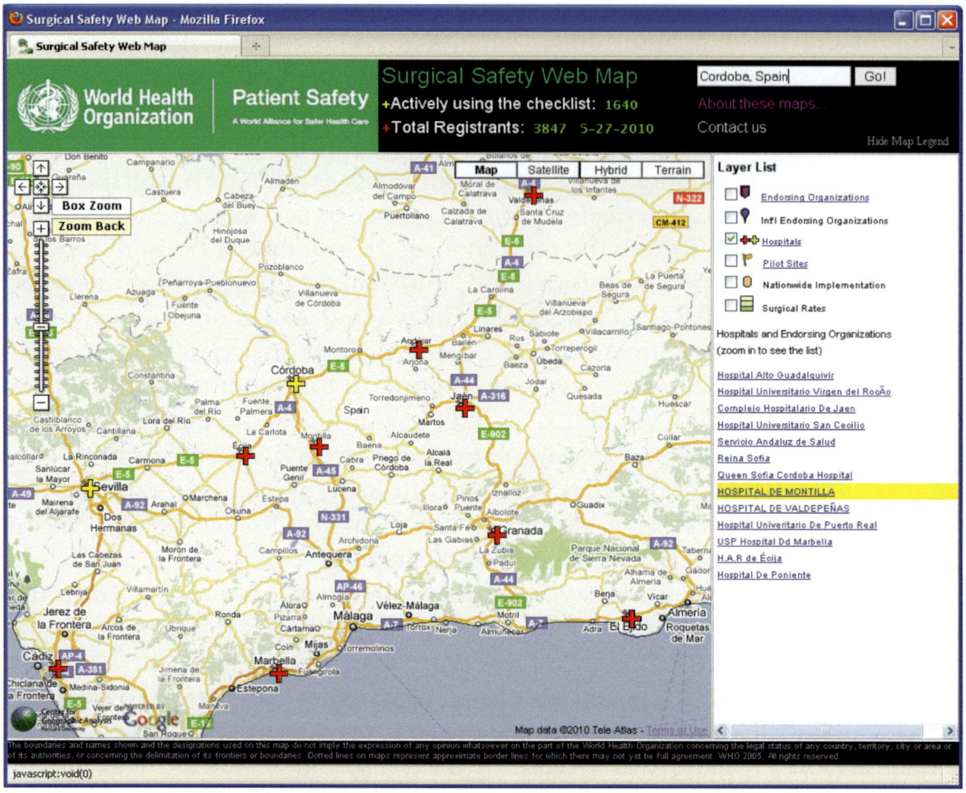

FIGURE 7 Updated Surgical Safety Web Map.

any member of the team to save out the latest version of the database, and interact with it in Excel, a database, or statistical program.

Once the new functionality was tested and rolled into the production Web map, the CGA's role of providing monthly update services was no longer needed. The SSSL team was now fully enabled to update the database and the map on their own. The database and map continue to be updated, and, as of this writing, they contain 3,924 hospitals that have signed up to use the checklist.

Enabling Health Researchers to Use GIS: The *Lancet* Publication

CGA's role of enabling public health researchers to use GIS technology is showcased in an article in the November 29, 2010, issue of *The Lancet*: "Health Professionals for a New Century: Transforming Education to Strengthen Health Systems in an Interdependent World" (Figure 8). The cover of this issue features global cartogram maps, as do several figures within the issue. The maps were produced by Dr. Ananda S. Bandyopadhyay, a

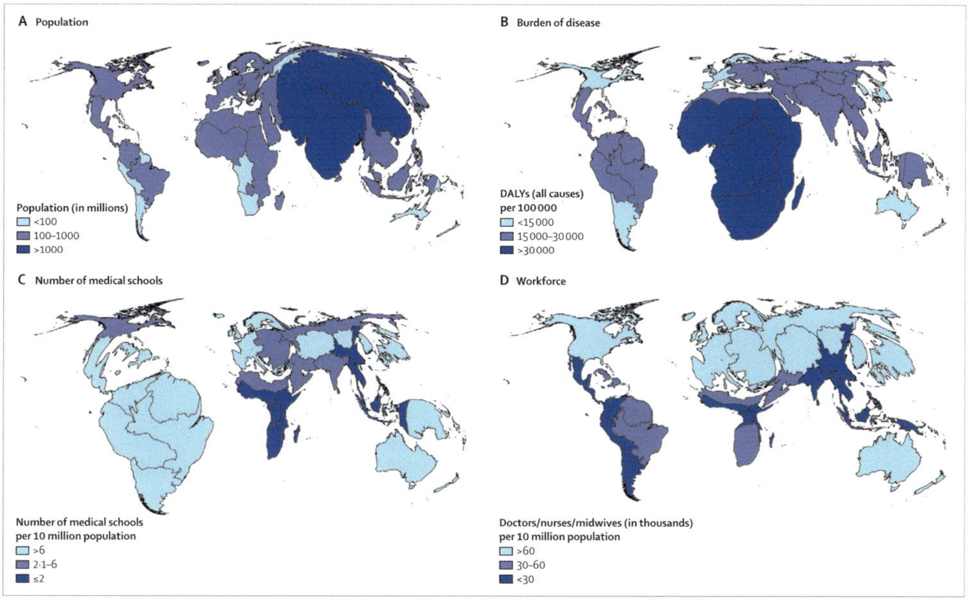

FIGURE 8 Map illustrations as published in *The Lancet*, 376 (9756), Julio Frenk, Lincoln Chen, Zulfiqar A. Bhutta, et al. Health professionals for a new century: Transforming education to strengthen health systems in an interdependent world. Pp. 1923–1957, © 2010, with permission from Elsevier.

graduate of the Harvard School of Public Health (HSPH) Master of Public Health Program. In performing his research at HSPH, Dr. Bandyopadhyay came to the CGA help desk to learn how to make maps and perform spatial analysis. Through CGA workshop training courses, the CGA GIS Institute, and several help desk sessions he became proficient in using many GIS analytical and cartographic tools. Dr. Bandyopadhyay was asked to join the *Lancet* research team, and his GIS skills enabled the production of these descriptive, informative maps, creating an unanticipated benefit to the publication that became one of its focal points.

CONCLUSION

The GIS infrastructure at Harvard, in addition to the services that the HGL, HMC, and CGA offer, provides a robust environment in which GIS can be applied to the realm of public health research. This article highlighted pertinent geographic data, the project workflow of the CGA, and case studies in public health research. These topics are prevalent in the Harvard research community today, and they are poised to grow and develop in the future.

NOTES

1. ESRI 2009 International Users Conference Proceedings Web site: http://proceedings.esri.com/library/userconf/health09/docs/monday/constructing_a_geospatial_database_of_united_states_local_health_departments.pdf
2. The Commonwealth of Massachusetts GIS Web site: http://www.mass.gov/mgis/
3. New York GIS Clearinghouse Web site: http://www.nysgis.state.ny.us/gisdata/
4. GeoNames Search Web site: http://geonames.nga.mil/ggmagaz
5. Oak Ridge National Laboratory Web site: http://www.ornl.gov/sci/landscan/
6. Demographic and Health Surveys Web site: http://www.measuredhs.com/
7. U.S. Census Bureau Web site: http://www.census.gov
8. United Kingdom Office for National Statistics Web site: http://www.ons.gov.uk/census/index.html
9. Israel Census of Population and Housing Web site: http://www.cbs.gov.il/mifkad/e-mifk.htm
10. Gridded Population of the World Web site: http://sedac.ciesin.columbia.edu/gpw/
11. United Nations Population Information Network Web site: http://www.un.org/popin/
12. PBL Netherlands Environmental Assessment Agency History Database of the Global Environment Web site: http://themasites.pbl.nl/en/themasites/hyde/index.html
13. U.S. Census Bureau International Data Base Web site: http://www.census.gov/ipc/www/idb/index.php
14. World Health Organization Data and Statistics Web site: http://www.who.int/research/en
15. Demographic and Health Surveys Web site: http://www.measuredhs.com/
16. UNICEF Childinfo Monitoring the Situation of Children and Women Web site: http://www.childinfo.org
17. UNICEF Childinfo MICS Web site: http://www.childinfo.org/mics.html
18. Centers for Disease Control and Prevention Web site: http://www.cdc.gov/nchs/
19. Centers for Disease Control Behavioral Risk Factor Surveillance System Web site: http://www.cdc.gov/brfss/maps/gis_data.htm
20. Centers for Disease Control Behavioral Risk Factor Surveillance System City and County Data Web site: http://apps.nccd.cdc.gov/BRFSS-SMART/index.asp
21. Centers for Disease Control WONDER Online Database Web site: http://wonder.cdc.gov
22. Health and Medical Care Archive of the Robert Wood Johnson Foundation Web site: http://www.icpsr.umich.edu/icpsrWeb/HMCA/index.jsp
23. New York City Department of Health and Mental Hygiene Web site: http://www.nyc.gov/html/doh/html/survey/survey.shtml
24. Los Angeles County Public Health Assessment Web site: http://www.publichealth.lacounty.gov/ha/HA_DATA.htm
25. The University of North Carolina Population Center China Health and Nutrition Web site: http://www.cpc.unc.edu/projects/china
26. National Family Health Survey of India Web site: http://www.nfhsindia.org/odata.html
27. U.S. Census Bureau American FactFinder Web site: http://factfinder.census.gov/home/saff/main.html?_lang=en
28. GeoLytics Web site: http://www.geolytics.com
29. Social Explorer Web Site: http://www.socialexplorer.com/pub/home/home.aspx
30. Inter-University Consortium for Political and Social Research Web site: http://www.icpsr.umich.edu/icpsrWeb/ICPSR/
31. ESRI Community Analyst Web site: http://communityanalyst.esri.com
32. All China Data Center: China Data Online Web site: http://chinadataonline.org/
33. Government of India Ministry of Home Affairs Census of India Web site: http://censusindia.gov.in
34. U.S.G.S. EarthExplorer Web site: http://edcsns17.cr.usgs.gov/NewEarthExplorer/
35. GeoEye GeoFUSE Online Maps Web site: http://geofuse.geoeye.com/maps/Map.aspx
36. Food and Agriculture Organization of the United Nations Web site: http://www.fao.org/corp/statistics/en/
37. United States Environmental Protection Agency Envirofacts Web site: http://www.epa.gov/enviro/index.html

38. U.S. Environmental Protection Agency Geospatial Data Download Service Web site: http://www.epa.gov/enviro/geo_data.html

39. U.S. EPA EnviroMapper Web site: http://www.epa.gov/emefdata/em4ef.home

40. U.S. Geological Survey Board on Geographic Names, Foreign Names Web site: http://geonames.usgs.gov/foreign/index.html

41. U.S. Geological Survey Board on Geographic Names, Domestic Names Web site: http://geonames.usgs.gov/domestic/index.html

42. GeoNames Forum Web site: http://forum.geonames.org/gforum/posts/list/5.page

43. Center for Geographic Analysis at Harvard University Web site: http://gis.harvard.edu

44. Best Practical RT: Request Tracker Web site: http://bestpractical.com/rt

45. Center for Geographic Analysis at Harvard University Google Maps Tutorial Web site: http://maps.cga.harvard.edu/gmaps_instruction/

46. WorldMap Alpha Web site: http://worldmap.harvard.edu

47. NetApp Web site: http://www.netapp.com/us

48. American Academy of Pediatrics Prevention and Treatment of Childhood Overweight and Obesity Web site: http://www.aap.org/obesity/families.html?technology=1

49. National Institute of Health Research Portfolio Online Reporting Tools Project Information Web site: http://projectreporter.nih.gov/project_info_description.cfm?aid=7962059&icde=7202284

50. The Commonwealth of Massachusetts GIS Web site: http://www.mass.gov/mgis/

51. World Health Organization Safe Surgery Saves Lives Web site: http://www.who.int/patientsafety/safesurgery/en

REFERENCES

Frenk, J., et al. 2010. Health professionals for a new century: Transforming education to strengthen health systems in an interdependent world. *Lancet* 376 (1): 1–3.

Gawande, A. 2009. *The Checklist Manifesto: How to Get Things Right*. New York: Henry Holt.

Guan, W. W., B. Burns, J. L. Finkelstein, and J. C. Blossom. 2011. Enabling geographic research across disciplines: Building an institutional infrastructure for geographic analysis at Harvard University. *Journal of Map & Geography Libraries* 7 (1): 36–60.

Higgs, G. 2004. A literature review of the use of GIS-based measures of access to health care services. *Health Services & Outcomes Research Methodology* 5 (1): 119–139.

Introduction to the "Working Group Report on Future Research Directions in Childhood Obesity Prevention and Treatment." 2007. *National Heart Lung and Blood Institute, National Institutes of Health*. http://www.nhlbi.nih.gov/meetings/workshops/child–obesity/index.htm

Jerrett, M., S. Gale, and C. Kontgis. 2010. Spatial modeling in environmental and public health research. *Int J Environ Res Public Health April* 7 (4): 1302–1329.

Koplan, J. P., C. T. Liverman, and V. I. Kraak (Eds.). 2005. Institute of Medicine of the National Academies. *Preventing Childhood Obesity*. Washington, DC: National Academy Press.

Lewis, B., and W. Guan. 2010. Jump-starting the next level of online geospatial collaboration: Lessons from AfricaMap. *Advances in Web-based GIS, Mapping Services and Applications*. Li, Dragicevic, and Veenendaal (Eds). Boca Raton, FL: CRC Press.

Martens, P., and L. Hall. 2000. Malaria on the move: Human population movement and malaria Transmission. *Emerg. Infect Dis. March/April* 6 (2): 103–109.

Ogden, C. L., M. D. Carroll, L. R. Curtin, M. A. McDowell, C. J. Tabak, and K. M. Flegal. 2006. Prevalence of overweight and obesity in the United States, 1999–2004. *Journal of the American Medical Association* 295 (13): 1549–1555.

Puett, R. C., J. E. Hart, J. D. Yanosky, C. Paciorek, J. Schwartz, H. Suh, F. E. Speizer, and F. Laden. 2009. Chronic fine and coarse particulate exposure, mortality, and coronary heart disease in the Nurses' Health Study. *Environmental Health Perspectives November* 117 (11): 1697–1701.

Puett, R. C., J. Schwartz, J. E. Hart, J. D. Yanosky, F. E. Speizer, H. Suh, C. J. Paciorek, L. M. Neas, and F. Laden. 2008. Chronic particulate exposure, mortality, and coronary heart disease in the Nurses' Health Study. *American Journal of Epidemiology* 168 (10): 1161–1168.

Yanosky, J., C. Paciorek, and H. Suh. 2009. Predicting chronic fine and coarse particulate exposures using spatio-temporal models for the Northeastern and Midwestern US. *Environ Health Perspect* 117 (1): 522–529.

Yanosky, J. D., C. J. Paciorek, J. Schwartz, F. Laden, R. C. Puett, and H. Suh. 2008. Spatio-temporal modeling of chronic PM10 exposure for the Nurses' Health Study. *Atmos. Environ.* 42 (18): 4047–4062.

From Snow to GIS Librarians: The Case for Health GIS and Informatics Within the Library

JAMES BOXALL
Dalhousie University, Halifax, Nova Scotia, Canada

The central question for map and geography librarians—or as we must add in this case, geospatial information managers—is What role is there for such managers in the process of health research? Health research includes, perhaps ironically, a greater emphasis on illness research and the "illness infrastructure" that we can consider as our hospitals, clinics, physicians, and other health care professionals such as pharmacists and nurse practitioners. Obviously, this may be considered a contentious view because we have always attempted to place emphasis on areas of preventive medicine that arise out of community health. So, What is our role in this system and its processes?

Perhaps the most well-known work on detecting and treating illness associated with geographically-based health research is that of Dr. John Snow in London in the mid-1800s. The famous series of Snow Maps, focusing on a wide variety of health topics such as income and housing standards and access to healthy resources (good food and water), has become the starting point for the field of epidemiology and community health. The Broad Street Pump Map has become a standard image in most texts and has been used in almost every presentation on the topic of geography and health. Even to this day, this work is celebrated yearly by the Broad Street Pump Society.

Now, 150 years later, we have gained many new insights about geographic information and health. The use of geographical analysis and of geographically referenced data to come to the conclusion that the water pump was central to the outbreak of cholera shows that place, space, and interaction were causal factors based upon geography, which could be understood only by focusing on the geographic information. Without the data and without the spatial context of the information, the outcome of the Broad Street cholera situation would have been much different.

The above, although an interesting story and clearly of great historical significance to the health research field, does not fully address the central question. Clearly, Snow was not in consultation with a map and geography librarian—or geospatial information manager. The situation today has much in common with Snow's time. One great difference is the plethora of studies, the total dollars of research investment, and the number of people within the fields of health care, health-related research, community health, and epidemiology. Today the underlying essentials of a reliance on geographic information and geospatial analysis is evident by the volume of research, policy, and practice—even though the rigor of practice and policy seems to sometimes differ from the outcomes of analysis and the recommendations of the research involved.

Without trying to describe the role of the information manager in any specific aspect of research, an interesting issue on its own, it is critical to state what the role of the manager is in the process of health research today. To do so, we have to accept one key feature of the research; nothing could be done if it were not for geographic technologies such as geographic information systems (GIS), remote sensing, and global positioning systems (GPS). Health research today relies upon a greater amount of data and a more sophisticated arsenal of geostatistics, data management, modeling, and even the presentation of results using cartography and online Web mapping. Any health research that includes "geographic reality" must, today, rely upon both the geographic technologies available and the geographic information resources at hand.

Herein is the essential role of the geospatial information manager and the issues for which that person is better suited to the collaborative process of health research (or illness studies). Librarians, archivists, and curators, as information managers, have always held to the principles of information organization and access, preservation and restoration, literacy, and use and promotion of the value of information to our research and public discourse. These building blocks are available to all disciplines, and yet even though they are available, they are also ignored or placed in a lower value proposition within the learning process. The obvious nature of the central role that information and data plays within research is actually not so obvious to everyone. If it were, many roles of the librarian would become nonessential.

Health research relies upon information that is timely, accurate, described, preserved (for longitudinal studies), and placed within a context that deals with copyright, privacy, and access. This is the domain of the geospatial information manager. If we could go back to the Snow period and place an information manager within that situation, we would find us as collaborators with Dr. Snow in managing all elements of information required for the study, and find additional sources that Dr. Snow may not have known about—and that is a very critical role. We have the ability, merely because we have designed the information access systems, to find those kernels of information and data not evident to the researcher, and for which the researcher may not have even thought about as having potential value. Therefore, an interesting idea might well be the role of the geospatial information manager becoming a collaborator—in the fullest sense—within the research process. For example, an ongoing issue in health research, and almost all forms or disciplines of research, is the loss of data. Data access, data description and data archiving are areas that do not have the full attention of researchers and research-granting councils. Those issues are central, or of great interest and professional concern, to our discipline.

We geospatial information managers are not health researchers per se. We are not epidemiologists or health care practitioners (although that may be true in some cases). We can, however, come to appreciate and understand the information needs of the health research field and assist that field in accessing and understanding the information required to conduct geographic research in those areas. We could also help the process of GIS education for the researchers by providing a starting point for GIS literacy efforts. Moreover, we can become part of the process by designing and delivering information services for both the provision of geospatial data, maps, historical spatial information, and research papers, and creation of robust services to deal with the preservation of health data and the overall management of the information and analytical processes.

Not every map and geography library—even those with a substantial capacity for GIS—will be able to participate fully in the process of health research. Some will be able to provide access to GIS hardware and software, some to access of basic geospatial data elements held within a collection, and some with the reference and research services associated with providing researchers access to the latest and best information for their projects. Some will be able to do more.

Two real-world examples illustrate the different paths this process could take. In the first, a doctoral student comes to a map/GIS library realizing that she needs some help with GIS and geospatial information access and use. This person needs to know what can be done and how to start doing it. The staff begins with a basic hour-long literacy "course" to introduce the value of GIS. From there, access to the software and data is provided, and the researcher is given multiple opportunities to return for help and guidance with the information and its structure, usefulness, and sources, as well as basic navigation through the software and related tools. The librarian teaches the student about what can be done and what is needed to do it. The student brings to the table a much greater understanding of geostatistics and epidemiology, but at the same time, a partnership forms between two people who know two sides of the process. The student ends up seeing the research as spatial and understands how spatial technologies and spatial information can play a key role in her research. The librarian does not do the research or direct the areas of emphasis or even determine the validity of the methods. He or she does, however, guide the process and provide access and input into the multitude of issues and potential pitfalls.

In our second case, a researcher in a pharmacy school approaches the manager of the geospatial information library to find out what resources the library has to add a spatial component to some emerging research areas within the pharmacy community. This had not been considered as an area of potential use or work that the library would ever support or even be asked to look into. The goal is to look at the distribution of prescriptions with drug addiction services and the use of such services with persons using fraudulent or multiple prescriptions among health care providers. The library does not provide the data in this case, but it does provide the experience to look at the information needs and how they should be used within a spatial context. This cannot be led by the library, but it can become a collaborative approach with the pharmacy school and other departments. At the outset, the library was asked to contribute with an overview of the technology and approach within the "spatial sciences." This could well be considered a form of information literacy. The library then ended up being listed as a collaborator on a research grant and was able to hire a student from a GIS program to add value to the work of the library, and this also meant a transfer of expertise from the student to the library, and vice versa.

The National Library of Medicine (NLM) and the National Institutes of Health (NIH) have helped and supported libraries' work with health-related information and data. The Digital Repository Report of 2007 (http://www.nlm.nih.gov/digitalrepository/NLM-DigRep-Report-rev 032007.pdf) outlines not only custodial responsibilities but makes note of the need for high level and focused attention (i.e., budgetary resources) on the infrastructure and technical architecture within such an effort. The NLM provided a blueprint that would instruct any needs assessment and planning process for any library looking at delivery of access services for spatial data, and in the more problematic aspects of preservation, archiving, and privacy. The key to this case is that the most essential issue needing attention is how to provide access to older datasets of longitudinal data banks—a very serious issue for health research! Spatial data permanence and lineage issues are true no matter what the subject matter of one's location.

There are, perhaps, many other cases that could be put forward that indicate the central role of map and geography librarians (or should one say "GIS Librarians" in these two cases?) toward providing data services and adding value to data access and preservation and, most of all, in generating metadata—an area that remains a weakness within the geospatial community. As the health GIS area continues to grow, these kinds of services and support should be reviewed by any library that has developed services with GIS or that has taken a more radical approach and actually become the hub of spatial data, software, hardware, and outreach services (teaching, research support, and internal research grants). There are also unique GIS and information needs to be considered, most of which fall under the heading of privacy, and the librarian should be forewarned that a solid understanding of both the issues and current research is essential before delving into an area where few have grasped the true potential of GIS—or have forgotten the lessons of Dr. Snow 150 years ago.

SUGGESTED SOURCES FOR FURTHER RESEARCH

Joyce, K. 2009. "To me it's just another tool to help understand the evidence": Public health decision-makers' perceptions of the value of geographical information systems (GIS). *Health & Place* 15: 831–840.

KamelBoulos, M. N. 2004. Towards evidence-based, GIS-driven national spatial health information infrastructure and surveillance services in the United Kingdom. *International Journal of Health Geographics* 3: 1.

Krieger, N. 2003. Place, space, and health: GIS and epidemiology. *Epidemiology* 14: 4.

LaRue, E. M. 2004. Using GIS to establish a public library consumer health collection. *Biomedical Digital Libraries* 1: 3.

MacEachren, A. M., et al., 2010. *International Journal of Health Geographics* 9: 23. http://www.ij-healthgeographics.com/content/9/1/23

Sui, D. Z. 2008. The wikification of GIS and its consequences: Or Angelina Jolie's new tattoo and the future of GIS. *Computers, Environment and Urban Systems* 32: 1–5.

Wilkinson, R. G., and K. E. Pickett. 2007. The problems of relative deprivation: Why some societies do better than others. *Social Science & Medicine* 65: 1965–1978.

Health-Related Geospatial Data and Social Media: Can You Harvest Geosocial Data?

JOHN A. OLSON
Syracuse University, Syracuse, New York, USA

Social media has been at the forefront of everyone's mind lately. Some of us are still wondering how to leverage and use social media to further our library's goals in reaching out to our patrons and users, let alone personal goals. But for some researchers, the question has been, "How can we mine these data and harvest the geospatial components to create meaningful datasets for mapping a specific topic or other need?" This has been on my mind as well. This column will begin to explore what is currently available to help mediate, sift, harvest, package, and display these geosocial data. I hope the sources and links shared here will encourage others to explore more deeply how social media data can be harvested and displayed from various outlets.

We will focus on searching for health-related data on the Web, determining their currency and assessing the correct level of geography to map it to. Just finding health-related data in this context can be quite a challenge! These health-related data sources will be for specific time periods and are finite in content and size. Conversely, with social media data the content is always growing and moving at a feverish rate, and it is difficult to tease out specific topics related to health. So, let us begin with some of the basic resources first.

BASIC RESOURCES: SITES WITH DOWNLOADABLE DATA

Following are a few of the in-depth statistical and geospatial data Web sites where health-related data can be discovered and downloaded. The data will either be as a stand-alone data file or it will be part of an interactive Web mapping tool. The sites Data.gov, http://www.data.gov/catalog, and Health Data.gov http://www.data.gov/health both contain raw and formatted geospatial datasets for health-related issues. Another of these is the Behavioral Risk Factor Surveillance System's interactive mapping portal found at the Centers for Disease Control (CDC) website, http://apps.nccd.cdc.gov/gisbrfss/default.aspx that has links to download data files separately or to display as part of their mapping portal. There are also sites that offer downloadable applications for use in mapping health-related data. The CDC has a list of pertinent geographic information system (GIS) Web applications as well, http://www.cdc.gov/gis/applications.htm.

The U.S. Department of Health and Human Services operates the Gateway to Data and Statistics data site that contains many links, http://www.hhs-stat.net/scripts/result.cfm?id=CWDR&lk=6. It also has its Health Resources and Services Administration Data Warehouse site, http://datawarehouse.hrsa.gov/pcsa2006.aspx that is filled with different types of health-related data.

For international data, the World Health Organizations (WHO's) Public Health Mapping and GIS Web page is a site where data can be viewed and downloaded, http://www.who.int/health_mapping/en/. The HealthMapper application is a WHO-specific software tool that must be downloaded to your computer before any of its data and maps can be used. The WHO also has an interactive Global Health Atlas http://apps.who.int/globalatlas/ where one can find and retrieve raw data, use an interactive mapping site, or download a number of prepared maps, statistics, and related resources for GIS purposes.

SOCIAL MEDIA SOURCES: SITES FOR COLLECTING AND DISSEMINATING GEOSOCIAL DATA

Now let's look at social media as an avenue to gather and share health-related data. There are some real challenges when searching for this type of data. Social media sites such as Twitter and Facebook are nebulous at best, and difficult to actually find data within them to harvest. Facebook offers a portal environment that provides access to sites like Healthmap to its friends that want to be kept up-to-date with health-related issues in a GIS framework. One can read the posts and click through on the links provided. In the case of Healthmap, its Facebook page URL sends you to their own site where a map displays the current feeds of disease outbreaks throughout the world. In this case, Facebook is more of a clearinghouse than an actual dataset provider.

Twitter, on the other hand, is a bit better for harvesting datasets. There are a variety of applications, tools and filters that can be used to display and harvest data from the raging torrent of Twitter feeds. Twitter displays the information on a constant, never-ending basis from people and from agencies like HealthGIS, CrisisMappers, or GeoCommons. The tweets from those sources can be harvested with some of the tools and apps listed below,

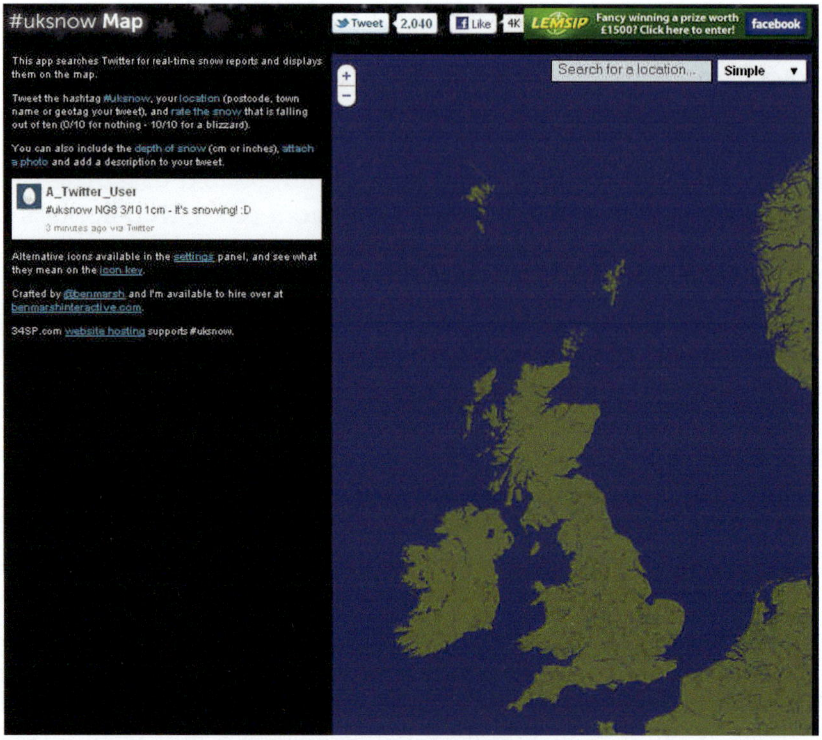

FIGURE 1 Screenshot of the #uksnow Map.

which can then be displayed or used to create your own map. One example of this capability is the #uksnow Map http:/ /uksnowmap.com/ (Figure 1).

Throughout the winter months this site displays different sized snowflakes that represent the number of twitters reporting snowfall by location within the United Kingdom. Check this site out next winter to see it in action.

So here are a few of the Twitter applications that can be used to harvest or display geospatial data twitter feeds. In all instances, the term, or *hashtag*, "#flu" was used.

1. Advanced Twitter search http://search.twitter.com/advanced allows you to search for terms within a designated distance from a particular place. The small map will display the location containing the search term. If only the map were bigger and actually displayed the source of the tweets!
2. TPS (Twitter Positioning System) http://tps.cumpleitup.com (Figure 2) allows searching by entering a term that can be a name, place, or topic, and then returns a map with proportional symbols from where those tweets are originating from. However, it allows for only a seven-day archive of tweets to search from.

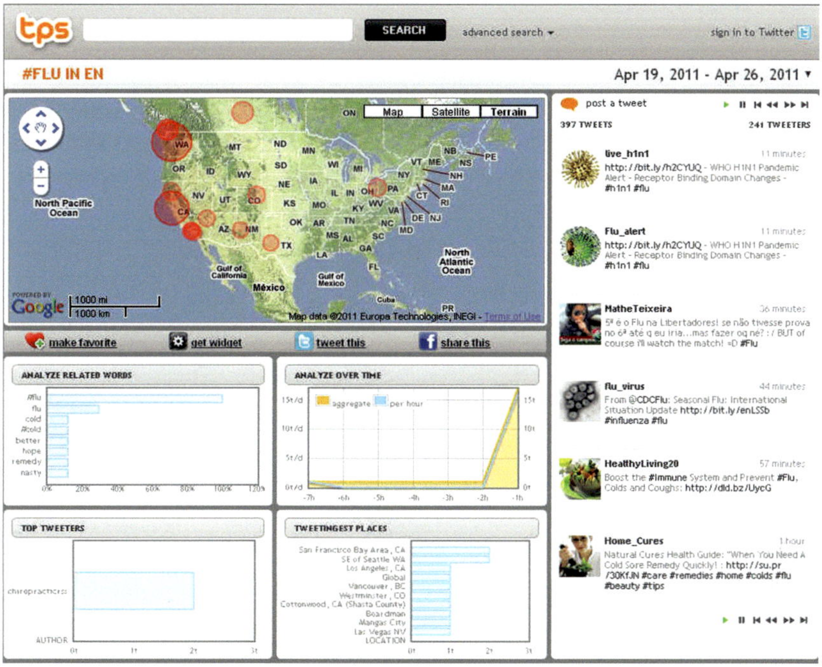

FIGURE 2 Twitter Positioning System (TPS) example.

3. Searchtastic.com http://www.searchtastic.com/index.php allows you to search for keywords and then export the data to an Excel file that has the location from which the twitter originated. Once again, searching using the #flu hashtag retrieved results that were downloaded to an Excel file. With some cleanup of the retrieved file, one could, in theory, then join the location field to a point layer file and map out concentrations of tweets in a GIS.

Esri is also getting into the Twitter game as well. Esri now has a Twitter Add-on app that you can download and use within ArcGIS Explorer (Figure 3). The add-on allows you to log into your Twitter account and then geo-locate twitter feeds that then display on a map either in a 2-D or in a 3-D environment. It also allows you to search for keywords worldwide and locates them as well on a map. Other layers can then be added, as well as other datasets, and one can use the twitter locations to reference or compare with other data and maps.

BEWARE OF SEARCH OUTCOMES!

What are the caveats to data harvesting? Be advised that the searches of almost any word will bring all manner of false results. Words that you use for

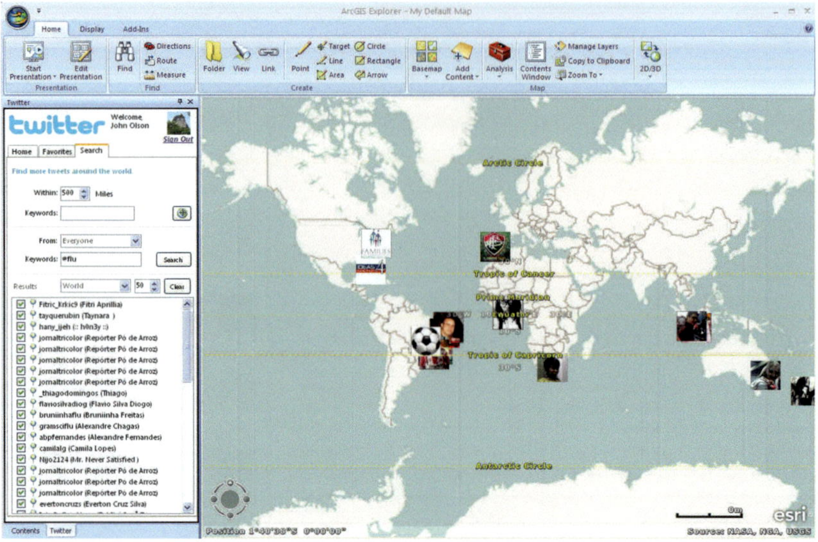

FIGURE 3 Twitter Add-In for ArcGIS Explorer (used with permission from Esri).

a search can also be used as slang, or can mean something totally different, or mean something else altogether in another language. One prime example is the word "cancer." Are you looking for tweets about the disease or the astrological sign? So, be on guard with how a given term is used, its specific terminology, how it is searched, the cleanliness of the data, and so forth. One will always need to be keeping these issues in mind when harvesting data from social networks to use in a GIS.

If you wish to delve deeper into twitter harvesting, look for tools and other applications at Twitdom.com, http://twitdom.com/ which has over 2,000 various tools and apps to use with Twitter, and the list is still growing.

CONCLUSIONS

As time, tools, and resources are applied to social media and GIS, the outcomes will be very interesting to watch, as well as be able to use. We will use these tools to mine for more than just health-related information, but also for other topics such as crime or disaster response. It appears that the sky's the limit with these technologies.

Social networking joined with mapping is, I believe, the next piece of technology fabric that will bring GIS to the next level of usability and access to the masses. It is poised to help users access, and assess, nonstatic datasets and continuous-feed data. It will also be easier to access geosocial data due to the varieties of mobile devices in the marketplace such as smartphones, tablets, and netbooks. In addition, mapping software will be easier to use and access from the cloud (i.e., ArcGIS Online). What will the future hold when we can leverage these types of data and GIS technology together?

Suggested Resources

KATHERINE H. WEIMER

Readers seeking to expand their GIS skills have numerous options. Books, websites, online courses, and other materials are readily available in most libraries. To get started, knowledge of basic GIS concepts is necessary. The fundamental concepts of GIS include the basics of geography and cartography, statistics and database design. Substantial knowledge is required to conduct the spatial analysis and creation of a visually accurate and meaningful map.

Next, one must understand the intricacies of available proprietary and open-source software packages. For those in a special subject area, such as health GIS, there are additional sources of information with which to enhance ones' skills. To that end, one must immerse oneself in the field. This study will not be quick or easy, but will provide the necessary depth to conduct the type of research included in this volume.

GENERAL GIS CONCEPTS

Albrecht, J. 2007. *Key concepts and techniques in GIS.* Thousand Oaks, Calif.: SAGE Publications.**

Bolstad, P. 2008. *GIS fundamentals: A first text on geographic information systems*, 3rd edition. White Bear Lake, Minn.: Eider Press.

Delaney, J. and K. Van Niel. 2007. *Geographical information systems: An introduction*, 2nd edition. New York: Oxford Press.**

DeMers, M. 2009. *Fundamentals of geographic information systems.* Hoboken, N.J.: John Wiley & Sons.

Harvey, F. 2008. A primer of GIS: Fundamental geographic and cartographic concepts. New York: Guilford Press.**

Hill, L. L. 2006. Georeferencing: The geographic associations of information. Cambridge, Mass.: MIT Press.**

Kemp, K. K., ed. 2008. *Encyclopedia of geographic information science.* Thousand Oaks, Calif.: SAGE Publications.**

Longley, P., M. Goodchild, D. Maguire, and D. Rhind. 2005. *Geographical information systems and science*, 2nd edition. Chichester, Sussex, UK: John Wiley & Sons.

Nyerges, T. L., H. Couclelis, and R. B. McMaster, eds. 2011. *The SAGE handbook of GIS and society.* Los Angeles: SAGE Publications.

Schuurman, N. 2004. *GIS: A short introduction.* Ames, Iowa: Blackwell Publishing.**

Shekhar, S. and H. Xiong, eds. 2008. *Encyclopedia of GIS.* New York: Springer.**

Wade, T. and S. Sommer, eds. 2006. A to Z GIS: An illustrated dictionary of geographic information systems. Redlands, Calif.: Esri Press.**

MAPMAKING AND DESIGN

These references provide guidance for those who create maps using GIS, but lack formal training in cartography.

Brewer, C. 2008. *Designed maps: A sourcebook for GIS users*. Redlands, Calif.: Esri Press.

Krygier, J. and D. Wood. 2005. *Making maps: A visual guide to map design for GIS*. New York: Guildford Press.**

Peterson, G. N. 2009. *GIS cartography: A guide to effective map design*. Boca Raton, FL.: CRC Press.

HANDS-ON SOFTWARE TRAINING

A number of books provide self-paced training to gain hands-on experience with GIS software. Some include a practice disk or a link to online resources.

Allen, D. W. 2009. *GIS tutorial 2: Spatial analysis workbook*. Redlands, Calif.: Esri Press.

Allen, D. W. and J. M. Coffey. 2011. *GIS tutorial 3: Advanced workbook*. Redlands, Calif.: Esri Press.

Clemmer, G. 2010. *The GIS 20: Essential skills*. Redlands, Calif.: Esri Press.

DeMers, M. N. 2009. *GIS for dummies*. Indianapolis, Ind.: John Wiley & Sons.

Gorr, W. L. and K. S. Kurland. 2011. *GIS tutorial 1: Basic workbook*. Redlands, Calif.: Esri Press. {NOTE: For ArcGIS 10, originally published as: GIS tutorial: workbook for ArcGIS 9 in 2005.}

Kropla, B. 2005. Beginning MapServer: Open source GIS development. Berkeley, Calif.: Apress.

Ormsby, T. 2010. *Getting to know ArcGIS Desktop*. Redlands, Calif.: Esri Press.

Price, M. H. 2010. *Mastering ArcGIS*, 4th edition. Dubuque, Iowa: McGraw Hill.

Sherman, G. E. 2008. *Desktop GIS: Mapping the planet with open source tools*. Raleigh, N.C.: Pragmatic Bookshelf.

MEDICAL AND PUBLIC HEALTH-RELATED GIS RESOURCES

Association of American Geographers. 2011. Establishing an NIH-wide geospatial infrastructure for medical research: Opportunities, challenges, and next steps: Report of the AAG-NIH workshop on geospatial infrastructure for medical research, 2011 http://www.aag.org/galleries/project-programs-files/NIH_GIS_Infras_Workshop_Report_Final_rev_title.pdf

Cromley, E. K. and S. McLafferty. 2011. *GIS and public health*, 2nd edition. New York: Guilford Press.

Curtis, A. and M. Leitner. 2006. Geographic information systems and public health: Eliminating perinatal disparity. Hershey, Pa.: IRM Press.

Dean, A. G., K. Sullivan and M. M. Soe. 2010. Epi Info™ and OpenEpi in epidemiology and clinical medicine: Health applications of free software. EpiInformatics.com.

Koch, T. 2011. *Disease maps: Epidemics on the ground*. Chicago, Ill.: University of Chicago Press.

Koch, T. 2005. Cartographies of disease: Maps, mapping, and medicine. Redlands, Calif.: Esri Press.

Kurland, K. S. and W. L. Gorr. 2006. *GIS tutorial for health*. Redlands, Calif.: Esri Press.

Lai, P. C., F. M. So, and K. W. Chan. 2009. S*patial epidemiological approaches in disease mapping and analysis*. Boca Raton, Fla.: CRC Press.

Skinner, R. 2010. GIS in hospital and healthcare emergency management. Boca Raton, Fla.: CRC Press.

WEB RESOURCES

Beyond published texts, many web pages include tutorials or descriptions of GIS concepts.

Esri. *Getting started with GIS.* http://www.esri.com/getting-started/index.html
Esri. *GIS.com, Geographic information systems.* http://www.gis.com/
Esri. *GIS dictionary.* http://support.esri.com/en/knowledgebase/Gisdictionary/browse
Federal Geographic Data Committee. *NSDI training (for metadata).* http://www.fgdc.gov/metadata/
GIS tutor. http://gistutor.com/ (includes tutorials for a variety of open source and proprietary software and web applications)
Harvard Map Collection. *GIS tutorials and exercises.* http://hcl.harvard.edu/libraries/maps/gis/tutorials.cfm
National Center for Geographic Information and Analysis. *NCGIA Core Curriculum in GIScience* http://www.ncgia.ucsb.edu/giscc/cc_outline.html (while no longer updated, many concepts still apply to current situations)
U.S. Geological Survey. *Geographic information systems* [poster] http://egsc.usgs.gov/isb/pubs/gis_poster/

(Titles reviewed in *CHOICE: Current Reviews for Academic Libraries* are denoted with ** at the end of the citation).

Index

Page numbers in *Italics* represent tables.
Page numbers in **Bold** represent figures.